Designing
Clinical Research

THIRD EDITION

STEPHEN B. HULLEY, M.D., M.P.H.
Professor and Chair, Department of Epidemiology & Biostatistics
Director, Clinical and Translational Sciences Training Program
University of California, San Francisco

STEVEN R. CUMMINGS, M.D.
Founding Director, San Francisco Coordinating Center
Senior Scientist, California Pacific Medical Center Research Institute
Professor Emeritus, University of California, San Francisco

WARREN S. BROWNER, M.D., M.P.H.
Scientific Director, Research Institute
Vice President, Academic Affairs
California Pacific Medical Center
Adjunct Professor, University of California, San Francisco

DEBORAH G. GRADY, M.D., M.P.H.
Professor of Epidemiology & Biostatistics, and of Medicine
Director, Women's Health Clinical Research Center
Associate Dean for Clinical & Translational Research
University of California, San Francisco

THOMAS B. NEWMAN, M.D., M.P.H.
Professor of Epidemiology & Biostatistics, and of Pediatrics
Chief, Division of Clinical Epidemiology
Attending Physician, Department of Pediatrics
University of California, San Francisco

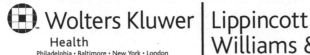

Wolters Kluwer | Lippincott
Health | Williams & Wilkins
Philadelphia · Baltimore · New York · London
Buenos Aires · Hong Kong · Sydney · Tokyo

Acquisitions Editor: Sonya Seigafuse
Managing Editor: Nancy Winter
Project Manager: Jennifer Harper
Manufacturing Coordinator: Kathleen Brown
Marketing Manager: Kimberly Schonberger
Designer: Stephen Druding
Production Services: Laserwords Private Limited, Chennai, India
Printer: Data Reproductions Corporation

© 2007 by LIPPINCOTT WILLIAMS & WILKINS, a Wolters Kluwer business
530 Walnut Street
Philadelphia, PA 19106 USA
LWW.com

Second edition, © 2001 Lippincott, Williams & Wilkins
First edition, © 1988 Williams & Wilkins

Library of Congress Cataloging-in-Publication Data
Designing clinical research / by Stephen B. Hulley ... [et al.].— 3rd ed.
    p. ; cm.
  Includes bibliographical references and index.
  ISBN-13: 978-0-7817-8210-4
  ISBN-10: 0-7817-8210-4
  1. Clinical trials. 2. Medicine—Research—Methodology.
3. Epidemiology—Research—Methodology. I. Hulley, Stephen B.
  [DNLM: 1. Epidemiologic Methods. 2. Research Design. WA 950 D457 2007]
  R853.C55D47 2007
  610.72—dc22   2006028271

Care has been taken to confirm the accuracy of the information presented and to describe generally accepted practices. However, the authors, editors, and publisher are not responsible for errors or omissions or for any consequences from application of the information in this book and make no warranty, expressed or implied, with respect to the currency, completeness, or accuracy of the contents of the publication. Application of this information in a particular situation remains the professional responsibility of the practitioner.

The authors, editors, and publisher have exerted every effort to ensure that drug selection and dosage set forth in this text are in accordance with current recommendations and practice at the time of publication. However, in view of ongoing research, changes in government regulations, and the constant flow of information relating to drug therapy and drug reactions, the reader is urged to check the package insert for each drug for any change in indications and dosage and for added warnings and precautions. This is particularly important when the recommended agent is a new or infrequently employed drug.

Some drugs and medical devices presented in this publication have Food and Drug Administration (FDA) clearance for limited use in restricted research settings. It is the responsibility of the health care provider to ascertain the FDA status of each drug or device planned for use in their clinical practice.

To purchase additional copies of this book, call our customer service department at (800) 638-3030 or fax orders to (301) 223-2320. International customers should call (301) 223-2300.

Visit Lippincott Williams & Wilkins on the Internet: at LWW.com. Lippincott Williams & Wilkins customer service representatives are available from 8:30 am to 6 pm, EST.

10 9 8 7 6

DRC0910

To our families and our students

CONTENTS

Section I: Basic Ingredients

Section II: Study Designs

Section III: Implementation

CONTRIBUTING AUTHORS

Norman Hearst M.D., M.P.H.
Professor of Family & Community Medicine, and of Epidemiology & Biostatistics
Attending Physician, Department of Family and Community Medicine
University of California, San Francisco

Michael A. Kohn M.D., M.P.P.
Associate Clinical Professor of Epidemiology & Biostatistics
Director, Data Management Consulting Services,
Clinical & Translational Sciences Institute
University of California, San Francisco

Bernard Lo, M.D.
Professor and Director, Program in Medical Ethics
Attending Physician, Department of Medicine, UCSF Medical Center
University of California, San Francisco

Jeffrey N. Martin, M.D., M.P.H.
Associate Professor of Epidemiology & Biostatistics, and of Medicine
Director, Training In Clinical Research Program
Attending Physician, Department of Medicine, San Francisco General Hospital
University of California, San Francisco

Thomas E. Novotny, M.D., M.P.H.
Professor in Residence, Epidemiology & Biostatistics
Director, International Programs, School of Medicine
University of California, San Francisco

INTRODUCTION

This book is about the science of doing clinical research in all its forms: translational research, clinical trials, patient-oriented research, epidemiologic studies, behavioral science and health services research. Codifying the nature of this broad-based science and how to do it is not straightforward, and there is no single approach that everyone agrees is best. Our first two editions drew on the terms and principles of epidemiology in a practical and reader-friendly way, emphasizing systematic and common sense approaches to the many judgments involved in designing a study.

The Third Edition of *Designing Clinical Research* (DCR) follows the same path, adding new developments along the way. New material on observational studies includes case-crossover designs, and the use of propensity scores, instrumental variables and Mendelian randomization to control confounding. Reorganized chapters on clinical trials introduce adaptive designs, and those on studying medical tests and on utilizing existing datasets present expanded options that will be attractive to beginning investigators. The chapter on research ethics is extensively updated, the one on data management entirely new (reflecting current approaches to information technology), and a rewritten chapter on study implementation and quality control introduces practicalities of study startup and regulatory issues ("Good Clinical Practices"). An updated chapter on getting funded brings help for the challenges facing young investigators.

The Third Edition is also fresh throughout, with updated examples and references in every chapter. And, perhaps most important, it reflects a continued maturation of our thinking, aided by feedback from nearly 1000 health professionals that we helped design their own studies in our Designing Clinical Research workshop in the past 6 years since DCR 2. The syllabus for that workshop, which can be used by others who wish to teach this material or desire a self-instruction guide, has been combined with useful tools like a sample size calculator on our new DCR Website at www.epibiostat.ucsf.edu/dcr/.

Many things have not changed in the Third Edition. It is still a simple book that leaves out unnecessary technicalities and invites the investigator to focus on the most important things: finding a good research question and planning an efficient, effective, ethical design. The two chapters on sample size estimation, which have received a larger number of favorable comments from readers than any other part of the book, continue to demystify the process and enable readers to make these calculations themselves without the need for formulas. We still use the feminine pronoun in the first half of the book, masculine in the second, reasoning that we are writing for clinical investigators of both genders. And we still do not address the important area of statistical analysis, nor how to go about disseminating the findings of clinical research—topics that many readers of this book will wish to pursue (1–5).

New investigators often find the choice of a research question to be the most difficult step in designing a project. Fortunately, studies tend to generate more questions than they answer, and an investigator's awareness of researchable questions will grow as she gains experience. In the meantime, she should seek out her own version of the most important companion to this book, a long-term relationship with an excellent mentor or two.

Other benefits come from experience. Clinical research becomes easier and more rewarding as investigators gain familiarity with the particulars of recruitment, measurement and design that pertain to their area of specialization. A higher percentage of their applications for funding are successful. They acquire staff and junior colleagues and develop lasting friendships with scientists working on the same topic in distant places. And because most increments in knowledge are small and uncertain—major scientific breakthroughs are rare—they begin to see substantial changes in the state of medicine as an aggregate result of their efforts.

It is gratifying to know many people who have used this book who have found they *like* doing research and have settled into a great career. For those with inquiring minds, the pursuit of truth can become a lifelong fascination. For perfectionists and craftsmen, there are endless challenges in creating an elegant study that produces conclusive answers to important questions at an affordable cost in time and money. And for those with the ambition to make a lasting contribution to society, there is the prospect that skill, tenacity and luck may lead to important advances in knowledge.

REFERENCES

1. Vittinghoff E, Glidden DV, Shiboski SC, et al. *Regression methods in biostatistics: linear, logistic, survival, and repeated measures models.* New York: Springer-Verlag, 2005.
2. Katz MH. *Multivariable analysis: a practical guide for clinicians,* 2nd ed. New York: Cambridge University Press, 2006.
3. Glantz SA. *Primer of biostatistics,* 5th ed. McGraw-Hill, 2005.
4. Browner WS. *Publishing and presenting clinical research,* 2nd ed. Philadelphia, PA: Lippincott Williams & Wilkins, 2006.
5. Fletcher RH, Fletcher SW. *Clinical epidemiology: the essentials,* 4th ed. Philadelphia, PA: Lippincott Williams & Wilkins, 2005.

ACKNOWLEDGMENTS

We are grateful to the Andrew P. Mellon Foundation for bringing us together more than two decades ago and stimulating the first edition; to our publisher for steadily inviting second and now third editions until resistance became futile; to our families for their patient support as we labored over this opus during family time; to many colleagues at UCSF and beyond, whose ideas and skills have influenced ours; to our students over the years, whose accomplishments have been fun to watch and stimulating to our thinking; and to our readers who have put this book to use.

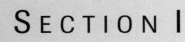

SECTION I

Basic Ingredients

1 Getting Started: The Anatomy and Physiology of Clinical Research

Stephen B. Hulley, Thomas B. Newman, and Steven R. Cummings

This chapter introduces clinical research from two viewpoints, setting up themes that run together through the book. One is the **anatomy** of research—what it's made of. This includes the tangible elements of the study plan: research question, design, subjects, measurements, sample size calculation, and so forth. An investigator's goal is to create these elements in a form that will make the project feasible, efficient, and cost-effective.

The other theme is the **physiology** of research—how it works. Studies are useful to the extent that they yield valid inferences, first about what happened in the study sample and then about how these study findings generalize to people outside the study. The goal is to minimize the errors, random and systematic, that threaten conclusions based on these inferences.

Separating the two themes is artificial in the same way that the anatomy of the human body doesn't make much sense without some understanding of its physiology. But the separation has the same advantage: it clarifies our thinking about a complex topic.

ANATOMY OF RESEARCH: WHAT IT'S MADE OF

The structure of a research project is set out in its **protocol**, the written plan of the study. Protocols are well known as devices for seeking grant funds, but they also have a vital scientific function: helping the investigator organize her research in a logical, focused, and efficient way. Table 1.1 outlines the components of a protocol. We introduce the whole set here, expand on each component in the ensuing chapters of the book, and return to put the completed pieces together in Chapter 19.

Research Question
The **research question** is the objective of the study, the uncertainty the investigator wants to resolve. Research questions often begin with a general concern that must be

3

TABLE 1.1	Outline of the Study Protocol
Element	**Purpose**
Research questions	What questions will the study address?
Background and significance	Why are these questions important?
Design	How is the study structured?
Time frame	
Epidemiologic approach	
Subjects	Who are the subjects and how will they be selected?
Selection criteria	
Sampling design	
Variables	What measurements will be made?
Predictor variables	
Confounding variables	
Outcome variables	
Statistical issues	How large is the study and how will it be analyzed?
Hypotheses	
Sample size	
Analytic approach	

narrowed down to a concrete, researchable issue. Consider, for example, the general question:

Should people eat more fish?

This is a good place to start, but the question must be focused before planning efforts can begin. Often this involves breaking the question into more specific components, and singling out one or two of these to build the protocol around. Here are some examples:

How often do Americans eat fish?

Does eating fish lower the risk of cardiovascular disease?

Is there a risk of mercury toxicity from increasing fish intake in older adults?

Do fish oil supplements have the same effects on cardiovascular disease as dietary fish?

Which fish oil supplements don't make people smell like fish?

A good research question should pass the "So what?" test. Getting the answer should contribute usefully to our state of knowledge. The acronym **FINER** denotes five essential characteristics of a good research question: it should be **feasible, interesting, novel, ethical,** and **relevant** (Chapter 2).

Background and Significance

The **background** and **significance** section of a protocol sets the proposed study in context and gives its rationale: What is known about the topic at hand? Why is the research question important? What kind of answers will the study provide? This section cites previous research that is relevant (including the investigator's own work) and indicates the problems with the prior research and what uncertainties remain. It specifies how the findings of the proposed study will help resolve these uncertainties and lead to new scientific knowledge and influence practice guidelines or public health policy. Often, work on the significance section will lead to modifications in the research question.

Design

The **design** of a study is a complex issue. A fundamental decision is whether to take a passive role in observing the events taking place in the study subjects in an **observational study** or to apply an intervention and examine its effects on these events in a **clinical trial** (Table 1.2). Among observational studies, two common designs are **cohort studies,** in which observations are made in a group of subjects that is followed over time, and **cross-sectional studies,** in which observations are made on a single occasion. Cohort studies can be further divided into **prospective** studies that begin in the present and follow subjects into the future, and **retrospective** studies that examine information and specimens that have been collected in the past. A third common option is the **case-control** design, in which the investigator compares a group of people who have a disease or condition with another group who do not. Among clinical trial options, the **randomized blinded trial** is usually the best design but nonrandomized or unblinded designs may be more suitable for some research questions.

No one approach is always better than the others, and each research question requires a judgment about which design is the most efficient way to get a satisfactory answer. The randomized blinded trial is often held up as the best design for establishing causality and the effectiveness of interventions, but there are many situations for which an observational study is a better choice or the only feasible option. The relatively low cost of case-control studies and their suitability for rare outcomes makes them attractive for some questions. Special considerations apply to choosing designs for studying diagnostic tests. These issues are discussed in Chapters 7 through 12, each dealing with a particular set of designs.

A typical sequence for studying a topic begins with observational studies of a type that is often called **descriptive**. These studies explore the lay of the land—for example, describing distributions of diseases and health-related characteristics in the population:

> *What is the average number of servings of fish per week in the diet of Americans with a history of coronary heart disease (CHD)?*

Descriptive studies are usually followed or accompanied by **analytic** studies that evaluate associations to permit inferences about cause-and-effect relationships:

> *Is there an association between fish intake and risk of recurrent myocardial infarction in people with a history of CHD?*

TABLE 1.2	Examples of Common Clinical Research Designs Used to Find Out Whether Fish Intake Reduces Coronary Heart Disease Risk

Study Design	Key Feature	Example
Observational Designs		
Cohort study	A group followed over time	The investigator measures fish intake at baseline and periodically examines subjects at follow-up visits to see if those who eat more fish have fewer coronary heart disease (CHD) events
Cross-sectional study	A group examined at one point in time	She interviews subjects about current and past history of fish intake and correlates results with history of CHD and current coronary calcium score
Case-control study	Two groups selected based on the presence or absence of an outcome	She examines a group of patients with CHD (the "cases") and compares them with a group who did not have CHD (the controls), asking about past fish intake
Clinical Trial Design		
Randomized blinded trial	Two groups created by a random process, and a blinded intervention	She randomly assigns subjects to receive fish oil supplements or placebo, then follows both treatment groups for several years to observe the incidence of CHD

The final step is often a **clinical trial** to establish the effects of an intervention:

Does treatment with fish oil capsules reduce total mortality in people with CHD?

Clinical trials usually occur relatively late in a series of research studies about a given question, because they tend to be more difficult and expensive, and to answer more definitively the narrowly focused questions that arise from the findings of observational studies.

It is useful to characterize a study in a single sentence that summarizes the design and research question. If the study has two major phases, the design for each should be mentioned.

This is a cross-sectional study of dietary habits in 50- to 69-year-old people with a history of CHD, followed by a prospective cohort study of whether fish intake is associated with low risk of subsequent coronary events.

This sentence is the research analog to the opening sentence of a medical resident's report on a new hospital admission: "*This 62-year-old white policewoman was well until 2 hours before admission, when she developed crushing chest pain radiating to the left shoulder.*" Some designs do not easily fit into the categories listed above, and classifying them with a single sentence can be surprisingly difficult. It is worth the effort—a precise description of design and research question clarifies the investigator's thoughts and is useful for orienting colleagues and consultants.

Study Subjects

Two major decisions must be made in choosing the study subjects (Chapter 3). The first is to specify **inclusion** and**exclusion criteria** that define the target population: the *kinds* of patients best suited to the research question. The second decision concerns how to **recruit** enough people from an accessible subset of this population to be the subjects of the study. For example, the study of fish intake in people with coronary heart disease (CHD) might identify subjects seen in the clinic with diagnosis codes for myocardial infarction, angioplasty, or coronary artery bypass grafting in their electronic medical record. Decisions about which patients to study represent trade-offs; studying a random sample of people with CHD from the entire country (or at least several different states and medical care settings) would enhance generalizability but be much more difficult and costly.

Variables

Another major set of decisions in designing any study concerns the choice of which variables to measure (Chapter 4). A study of fish intake in the diet, for example, might ask about different types of fish that contain different levels of Ω-3 fatty acids, and include questions about portion size, whether the fish was fried or baked, and whether the subject takes fish oil supplements.

In an analytic study the investigator studies the associations among variables to predict outcomes and to draw inferences about cause and effect. In considering the association between two variables, the one that occurs first or is more likely on biologic grounds to be causal is called the **predictor variable;** the other is called the **outcome variable.**[1] Most observational studies have many predictor variables (*age, race, sex, smoking history, fish and fish oil supplement intake*), and several outcome variables (*heart attacks, strokes, quality of life, unpleasant odor*).

Clinical trials examine the effects of an **intervention** (a special kind of predictor variable that the investigator manipulates), such as *treatment with fish oil capsules.* This design allows her to observe the effects on the outcome variable using **randomization** to control for the influence of **confounding variables**—other predictors of the outcome such as *intake of red meat* or *income level* that could be related to dietary fish and confuse the interpretation of the findings.

Statistical Issues

The investigator must develop plans for estimating sample size and for managing and analyzing the study data. This generally involves specifying a **hypothesis** (Chapter 5).

> *Hypothesis: 50- to 69-year-old women with CHD who take fish oil supplements will have a lower risk of myocardial infarction than those who do not.*

This is a version of the research question that provides the basis for testing the **statistical significance** of the findings. The hypothesis also allows the investigator to calculate the **sample size**—the number of subjects needed to observe the expected difference in outcome between study groups with reasonable probability or **power**

---

[1] Predictors are sometimes termed **independent variables** and outcomes **dependent variables,** but we find this usage confusing, particularly since independent means something quite different in the context of multivariate analyses.

(Chapter 6). Purely descriptive studies (*what proportion of people with CHD use fish oil supplements?*) do not involve tests of statistical significance, and thus do not require a hypothesis; instead, the number of subjects needed to produce acceptably narrow **confidence intervals** for means, proportions, or other descriptive statistics can be calculated.

PHYSIOLOGY OF RESEARCH: HOW IT WORKS

The goal of clinical research is to draw **inferences** from findings in the study about the nature of the universe around it (Fig 1.1). Two major sets of inferences are involved in interpreting a study (illustrated from right to left in Fig. 1.2). Inference #1 concerns **internal validity,** the degree to which the investigator draws the correct conclusions about what actually happened in the study. Inference #2 concerns **external validity** (also called **generalizability**), the degree to which these conclusions can be appropriately applied to people and events outside the study.

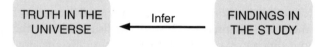

FIGURE 1.1. The findings of a study lead to inferences about the universe outside.

When an investigator plans a study, she reverses the process, working from left to right in the lower half of Fig. 1.2 with the goal of maximizing the validity of these inferences at the end of the study. She **designs a study plan** in which the choice of research question, subjects, and measurements enhances the external validity of the study and is conducive to **implementation** with a high degree of internal validity. In the next sections we address design and then implementation before turning to the errors that threaten the validity of these inferences.

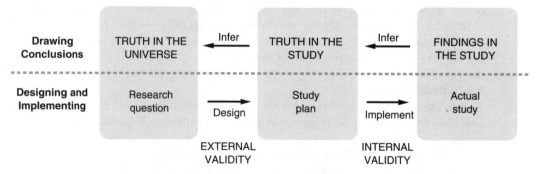

FIGURE 1.2. The process of designing and implementing a research project sets the stage for drawing conclusions from the findings.

Designing the Study
Consider the simple descriptive question:

> *What is the prevalence of regular use of fish oil supplements among people with CHD?*

This question cannot be answered with perfect accuracy because it would be impossible to study all patients with CHD and our approaches to discovering whether a person is taking fish oil are imperfect. So the investigator settles for a related question that *can* be answered by the study:

Among a sample of patients seen in the investigator's clinic who have a previous CHD diagnosis and respond to a mailed questionnaire, what proportion report taking fish oil supplements?

The transformation from research question to study plan is illustrated in Fig. 1.3. One major component of this transformation is the choice of a **sample** of subjects that will represent the **population.** The group of subjects specified in the protocol can only be a sample of the population of interest because there are practical barriers to studying the entire population. The decision to study patients in the investigator's clinic identified through the electronic medical record system is a compromise. This is a sample that is feasible to study but one that may produce a different prevalence of fish oil use than that found in all people with CHD.

The other major component of the transformation is the choice of **variables** that will represent the **phenomena of interest.** The variables specified in the study plan are usually proxies for these phenomena. The decision to use a self-report questionnaire to assess fish oil use is a fast and inexpensive way to collect information, but it will not be perfectly accurate. Some people may not accurately remember or record how much they take in a typical week, others may report how much they think they should be taking, and some may be taking products that they do not realize should be included.

In short, each of the differences in Fig. 1.3 between the research question and the study plan has the purpose of making the study more practical. The cost of this

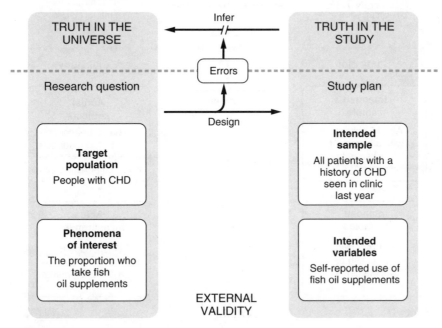

FIGURE 1.3. Design errors: if the intended sample and variables do not represent the target population and phenomena of interest, these errors may distort inferences about what actually happens in the population.

increase in practicality, however, is the risk that design changes may cause the study to produce a wrong or misleading conclusion because its design answers something different from the research question of interest.

Implementing the Study

Returning to Fig. 1.2, the right-hand side is concerned with implementation and the degree to which the actual study matches the study plan. At issue here is the problem of a wrong answer to the research question because the way the sample was actually drawn, and the measurements made, differed in important ways from the way they were designed (Fig. 1.4).

The actual sample of study subjects is almost always different from the intended sample. The plans to study all eligible patients with CHD, for example, could be disrupted by incomplete diagnoses in the electronic medical record, wrong addresses for the mailed questionnaire, and refusal to participate. Those subjects who are reached and agree to participate may have a different prevalence of fish oil use than those not reached or not interested. In addition to these problems with the subjects, the actual measurements can differ from the intended measurements. If the format of the questionnaire is unclear subjects may get confused and check the wrong box, or they may simply omit the question by mistake.

These differences between the study plan and the actual study can alter the answer to the research question. Figure 1.4 illustrates that errors in implementing the study join errors of design in leading to a misleading or wrong answer to the research question.

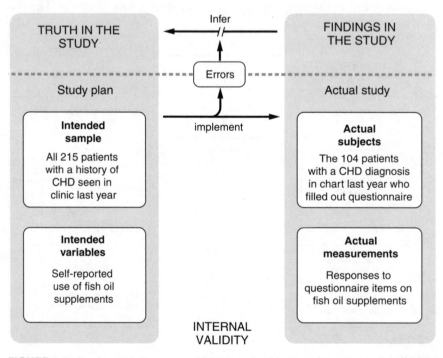

FIGURE 1.4. Implementation errors: if the actual subjects and measurements do not represent the intended sample and variables, these errors may distort inferences about what actually happened in the study.

Causal Inference

A special kind of validity problem arises in studies that examine the **association** between a predictor and an outcome variable in order to draw causal inference. If a cohort study finds an association between fish intake and CHD events, does this represent cause and effect, or is the fish just an innocent bystander in a web of causation that involves other variables? Reducing the likelihood of confounding and other rival explanations is one of the major challenges in designing an observational study (Chapter 9).

The Errors of Research

No study is free of errors, and the goal is to maximize the validity of inferences from what happened in the study sample to the nature of things in the population. Erroneous inferences can be addressed in the analysis phase of research, but a better strategy is to focus on design and implementation (Fig. 1.5), preventing errors from occurring in the first place to the extent that this is practical.

The two main kinds of error that interfere with research inferences are random error and systematic error. The distinction is important because the strategies for minimizing them are quite different.

Random error is a wrong result due to **chance**—sources of variation that are equally likely to distort estimates from the study in either direction. If the true prevalence of fish oil supplement use in 50- to 69-year-old patients with CHD is 20%, a well-designed sample of 100 patients from that population might contain exactly 20 patients who use these supplements. More likely, however, the sample would contain a nearby number such as 18, 19, 21, or 22. Occasionally, chance would produce a substantially different number, such as 12 or 28. Among several techniques for reducing the influence of random error (Chapter 4), the simplest is to increase

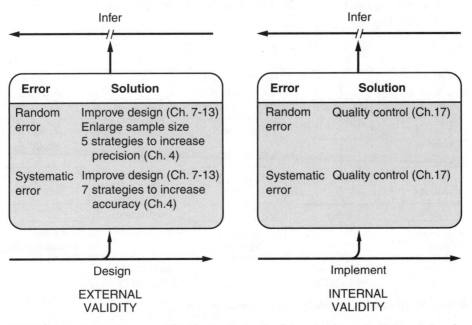

FIGURE 1.5. Research errors. This blown-up detail of the error boxes in Figures 1.3 and 1.4 reveals strategies for controlling random and systematic error in the design, implementation, and analysis phases of the study.

the sample size. The use of a larger sample diminishes the likelihood of a wrong result by increasing the **precision** of the estimate—the degree to which the observed prevalence approximates 20% each time a sample is drawn.

Systematic error is a wrong result due to **bias**—sources of variation that distort the study findings in one direction. An illustration is the decision in Fig. 1.3 to study patients in the investigator's clinic, where the local treatment patterns have responded to her interest in the topic and her fellow doctors are more likely than the US average to recommend fish oil. Increasing the sample size has no effect on systematic error. The only way to improve the **accuracy** of the estimate (the degree to which it approximates the true value) is to design the study in a way that either reduces the size of the various biases or gives some information about them. An example would be to compare results with those from a second sample of patients with CHD drawn from another setting, for example, examining whether the findings in patients seen in a cardiology clinic are different from those in patients in a gynecology clinic.

The examples of random and systematic error in the preceding two paragraphs are components of **sampling error,** which threatens inferences from the study subjects to the population. Both random and systematic errors can also contribute to **measurement error,** threatening the inferences from the study measurements to the phenomena of interest. An illustration of random measurement error is the variation in the response when the diet questionnaire is administered to the patient on several occasions. An example of systematic measurement error is the underestimation of the prevalence of fish oil use due to lack of clarity in how the question is phrased. Additional strategies for controlling all these sources of error are presented in Chapters 3 and 4.

The concepts presented in the last several pages are summarized in Fig. 1.6. Getting the right answer to the research question is a matter of designing and implementing the study in a fashion that keeps the extent of inferential errors at an acceptable level.

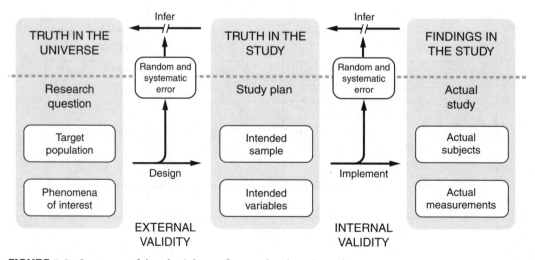

FIGURE 1.6. Summary of the physiology of research—how it works.

■ DESIGNING THE STUDY

Study Protocol

The process of developing the **study plan** begins with the one-sentence **research question** described earlier. Three versions of the study plan are then produced in sequence, each larger and more detailed than the preceding one.

- **Outline** of the elements of the study (Table 1.1 and Appendix 1.1). This one page beginning serves as a standardized checklist to remind the investigator to include all the components. As important, the sequence has an orderly logic that helps clarify the investigator's thinking on the topic.
- **Study protocol.** This expansion on the study outline can range from 5 to 25 or more pages, and is used to plan the study and to apply for grant support. The protocol parts are discussed throughout this book and put together in Chapter 19.
- **Operations manual.** This collection of specific procedural instructions, questionnaires, and other materials is designed to ensure a uniform and standardized approach to carrying out the study with good quality control (Chapters 4 and 17).

The research question and study outline should be written out at an early stage. Putting thoughts down on paper leads the way from vague ideas to specific plans and provides a concrete basis for getting advice from colleagues and consultants. It is a challenge to do it (ideas are easier to talk about than to write down), but the rewards are a faster start and a better project.

Appendix 1.1 provides an example of a study outline. These plans deal more with the anatomy of research (Table 1.1) than with its physiology (Fig. 1.6), so the investigator must remind herself to worry about the errors that may result when it is time to draw inferences about what happened in the study sample and how it applies to the population. A study's virtues and problems can be revealed by explicitly considering how the question the study is likely to answer differs from the research question, given the plans for acquiring subjects and making measurements, and given the likely problems of implementation.

With the study outline in hand and the intended inferences in mind, the investigator can proceed with the details of her protocol. This includes getting advice from colleagues, drafting specific recruitment and measurement methods, considering scientific and ethical appropriateness, changing the study question and outline, pretesting specific recruitment and measurement methods, making more changes, getting more advice, and so forth. This iterative process is the nature of research design and the topic of the rest of this book.

Trade-offs

Errors are an inherent part of all studies. The main issue is whether the errors will be large enough to change the conclusions in important ways. When designing a study, the investigator is in much the same position as a labor union official bargaining for a new contract. The union official begins with a wish list—shorter hours, more money, health care benefits and so forth. She must then make concessions, holding on to the things that are most important and relinquishing those that are not essential. At the end of the negotiations is a vital step: she looks at the best contract she could negotiate and decides if it has become so bad that it is no longer worth having.

The same sort of concessions must be made by an investigator when she transforms the research question to the study plan and considers potential problems in implementation. On one side are the issues of internal and external validity; on the other, feasibility. The vital last step of the union negotiator is sometimes omitted. Once the study plan has been formulated, the investigator must decide whether it adequately addresses the research question and whether it can be implemented with acceptable levels of error. Often the answer is no, and there is a need to begin the process anew. But take heart! Good scientists distinguish themselves not so much by their uniformly good research ideas as by their tenacity in turning over those that won't work and trying again.

SUMMARY

1. The **anatomy** of research is the set of tangible elements that make up the study plan: the **research question** and its **significance,** and the **design, study subjects,** and **measurement approaches.** The challenge is to design elements that are **fast, inexpensive,** and **easy** to implement.

2. The **physiology** of research is how the study works. The study findings are used to draw **inferences** about what happened in the study sample **(internal validity),** and about events in the world outside **(external validity).** The challenge here is to **design** and **implement** a study plan with adequate control over two major threats to these inferences: **random error** (chance) and **systematic error** (bias).

3. In designing a study the investigator may find it helpful to consider the relationships between the **research question** (what she wants to answer), the **study plan** (what the study is designed to answer), and the **actual study** (what the study will actually answer, given the errors of implementation that can be anticipated).

4. A good way to develop the **study plan** is to begin with a one-sentence version of the **research question** and expand this into an **outline** that sets out the study elements in a standardized sequence. Later on the study plan will be expanded into the **protocol** and the **operations manual.**

5. Good **judgment** by the investigator and advice from colleagues are needed for the many **trade-offs** involved, and for determining the overall viability of the project.

■ APPENDIX 1.1

Outline of a Study*

Element	Example
Title	Relationship between Level of Experience and Degree of Clinical Utility of Third Heart Sound Auscultation.
Research question	Do auscultatory assessments of third heart sound by more experienced physicians result in higher sensitivity and specificity for detecting left ventricular dysfunction than assessments by less experienced physicians?
Significance	1. Auscultation of third heart sounds is a standard physical examination indicator of heart failure that all medical students have learned for 100 years. 2. The degree to which this clinical assessment, which many physicians find difficult, actually detects abnormal left ventricular function has not been studied. 3. There are no studies of whether auscultatory measurements of third heart sounds by cardiology fellows and attendings are more accurate than those of residents and medical students.
Study design	Cross-sectional analytic study
Subjects	
• **Entry criteria**	Adults referred for left heart catheterization
• **Sampling design**	Consecutive sample of consenting patients
Variables	
• **Predictor**	Level of experience of physicians
• **Outcome**	1. Area under the receiver operating characteristic curve for third heart sound score (AUC) in relation to higher LV diastolic pressure by catheterization 2. AUC in relation to lower ejection fraction by cardiac echo 3. AUC in relation to B natriuretic protein
Statistical issues	Hypothesis: More experienced physicians will have more favorable AUCs
	Sample size (to be filled in after reading Chapter 6)

*Fortunately this study, designed and implemented by clinical investigators in training at our institution, found that more experienced physicians were better at detecting clinically significant third heart sounds (1).

■ REFERENCE

1. Marcus GM, Vessey J, Jordan MV, et al. Relationship between accurate auscultation of a clinically useful third heart sound and level of experience. *Arch Intern Med* 2006;166:1–7.

2 Conceiving The Research Question

Steven R. Cummings, Warren S. Browner,
and Stephen B. Hulley

The **research question** is the uncertainty about something in the population that the investigator wants to resolve by making measurements on her study subjects (Fig. 2.1). There is no shortage of good research questions, and even as we succeed in producing answers to some questions, we remain surrounded by others. Recent clinical trials, for example, have established that treatments that block the synthesis of estradiol (aromatase inhibitors) reduce the risk of breast cancer in women who have had early stage cancer (1). But now there are new questions: How long should treatment be continued, what is the best way to prevent the osteoporosis that is an adverse effect of these drugs, and does this treatment prevent breast cancer in patients with BRCA 1 and BRCA 2 mutations?

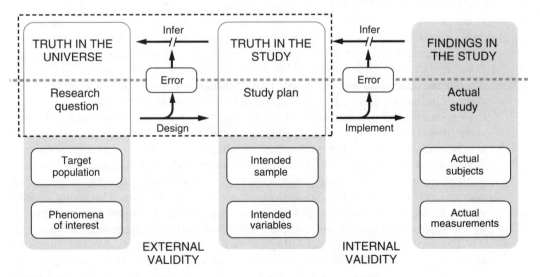

FIGURE 2.1. Choosing the research question and designing the study plan.

The challenge in searching for a research question is not a shortage of uncertainties; it is the difficulty of finding an important one that can be transformed into a feasible and valid **study plan**. This chapter presents strategies for accomplishing this in arenas that range from classical **clinical research** to the newly popular **translational research.**

ORIGINS OF A RESEARCH QUESTION

For an established investigator the best research questions usually emerge from the findings and problems she has observed in her own prior studies and in those of other workers in the field. A new investigator has not yet developed this base of experience. Although a fresh perspective can sometimes be useful by allowing a creative person to conceive new approaches to old problems, lack of experience is largely an impediment.

Mastering the Literature

It is important to master the published literature in an area of study; **scholarship** is a necessary ingredient to good research. A new investigator should conduct a thorough search of published literature in the area of study. Carrying out a systematic review is a great first step in developing and establishing expertise in a research area, and the underlying literature review can serve as background for grant proposals and research reports. Recent advances may be presented at research meetings or just be known to active investigators in a particular field long before they are published. Thus, mastery of a subject entails participating in meetings and building relationships with experts in the field.

Being Alert to New Ideas and Techniques

In addition to the medical literature as a source of ideas for research questions, all investigators find it helpful to **attend conferences** in which recent work is presented. As important as the presentations are the opportunities for informal conversations with other scientists during the breaks. A new investigator who overcomes her shyness and engages a speaker at the coffee break will often find the experience richly rewarding, and occasionally will find she has a new senior colleague. Even better, for a speaker known in advance to be especially relevant, it may be worthwhile to look up her recent publications and contact her in advance to arrange a meeting during the conference.

A **skeptical attitude** about prevailing beliefs can stimulate good research questions. For example, it has been widely believed that lacerations that extend through the dermis require sutures to assure rapid healing and a satisfactory cosmetic outcome. Alternative approaches that would not require local anesthetics and be faster, less expensive, and produce as good a cosmetic result were widely believed to be unachievable. However, Quinn et al. noted personal experience and case series evidence that wounds repair themselves regardless of whether wound edges are approximated. They carried out a randomized trial in which patients with hand lacerations less than 2 cm in length all received tap water irrigation and a 48-hour antibiotic dressing, but one group receive conventional sutures while the other did not. The group treated with sutures had a more painful and time-consuming treatment but subsequent blinded assessment revealed similar time to healing and cosmetic results (2).

The application of **new technologies** often generates new insights and questions about familiar clinical problems, which in turn can generate new paradigms (3).

Recent advances in imaging and in techniques for molecular and genetic analyses, for example, have spawned a large number of clinical research studies that have informed extraordinary advances in the use of these technologies in clinical medicine. Similarly, taking a new concept or finding from one field and applying it to a problem in a different field can lead to good research questions. Low bone density, for example, is widely recognized as a risk factor for fractures. Investigators applied this technology to other populations and found that women with low bone density have higher rates of cognitive decline (4), perhaps due to low levels of estrogen over a lifetime.

Keeping the Imagination Roaming

Careful **observation** of patients has led to many descriptive studies and is a fruitful source of research questions. **Teaching** is also an excellent source of inspiration; ideas for studies often occur while preparing presentations or during discussions with inquisitive students. Because there is usually not enough time to develop these ideas on the spot, it is useful to keep them in a computer file or notebook for future reference.

There is a major role for **creativity** in the process of conceiving research questions, imagining new methods to address old questions and having fun with ideas. There is also a need for **tenacity,** for returning to a troublesome problem repeatedly until a resolution is reached that feels comfortable. Some creative ideas come to mind during informal conversations with colleagues over lunch; others occur in brainstorming sessions. Many inspirations are solo affairs that strike while preparing a lecture, showering, perusing the Internet, or just sitting and thinking. Fear of criticism or seeming unusual can prematurely quash new ideas. The trick is to put an unresolved problem clearly in view and allow the mind to run freely toward it.

Choosing a Mentor

Nothing substitutes for experience in guiding the many judgments involved in conceiving and fleshing in a research question. Therefore an essential strategy for a new investigator is to apprentice herself to an experienced **mentor** who has the time and interest to work with her regularly. A good mentor will be available for regular meetings and informal discussions, encourage creative ideas, provide wisdom that comes from experience, help ensure protected time for research, open doors to networking and funding opportunities, encourage the development of independent work, and put the new investigator's name first on grants and publications whenever appropriate. Sometimes it is desirable to have more than one mentor, representing different disciplines. Good relationships of this sort can also provide tangible resources that are needed—office space, access to clinical populations, datasets and specimen banks, specialized laboratories, financial resources, and a research team. Choosing a mentor can be a difficult process, and is perhaps the single most important decision a new investigator makes.

CHARACTERISTICS OF A GOOD RESEARCH QUESTION

The characteristics of a good research question, assessed in the context of the intended study design, are that it be feasible, interesting, novel, ethical, and relevant (which form the mnemonic **FINER;** Table 2.1).

TABLE 2.1	FINER Criteria for a Good Research Question

Feasible

    Adequate number of subjects
    Adequate technical expertise
    Affordable in time and money
    Manageable in scope

Interesting

    Getting the answer intrigues the investigator and her friends

Novel

    Confirms, refutes or extends previous findings
    Provides new findings

Ethical

    Amenable to a study that institutional review board will approve

Relevant

    To scientific knowledge
    To clinical and health policy
    To future research

Feasible

It is best to know the practical limits and problems of studying a question early on, before wasting much time and effort along unworkable lines.

- *Number of subjects.* Many studies do not achieve their intended purposes because they cannot enroll enough subjects. A preliminary calculation of the sample size requirements of the study early on can be quite helpful (Chapter 6), together with an estimate of the number of subjects likely to be available for the study, the number who would be excluded or refuse to participate, and the number who would be lost to follow-up. Even careful planning often produces estimates that are overly optimistic, and the investigator should assure that there are enough eligible willing subjects. It is sometimes necessary to carry out a pilot survey or chart review to be sure. If the number of subjects appears insufficient, the investigator can consider several strategies: expanding the inclusion criteria, eliminating unnecessary exclusion criteria, lengthening the time frame for enrolling subjects, acquiring additional sources of subjects, developing more precise measurement approaches, inviting colleagues to join in a multicenter study, and using a different study design.
- *Technical expertise.* The investigators must have the skills, equipment, and experience needed for designing the study, recruiting the subjects, measuring the variables, and managing and analyzing the data. Consultants can help to shore up technical aspects that are unfamiliar to the investigators, but for major areas of the study it is better to have an experienced colleague steadily involved as a coinvestigator; for example, it is wise to include a statistician as a member of the research team from the beginning of the planning process. It is best to use familiar

and established approaches, because the process of developing new methods and skills is time-consuming and uncertain. When a new approach is needed, such as a questionnaire, expertise in how to accomplish the innovation should be sought.

- *Cost in time and money.* It is important to estimate the costs of each component of the project, bearing in mind that the time and money needed will generally exceed the amounts projected at the outset. If the projected costs exceed the available funds, the only options are to consider a less expensive design or to develop additional sources of funding. Early recognition of a study that is too expensive or time-consuming can lead to modification or abandonment of the plan before expending a great deal of effort.

- *Scope.* Problems often arise when an investigator attempts to accomplish too much, making many measurements at repeated contacts with a large group of subjects in an effort to answer too many research questions. The solution is to narrow the scope of the study and focus only on the most important goals. Many scientists find it difficult to give up the opportunity to answer interesting side questions, but the reward may be a better answer to the main question at hand.

Interesting

An investigator may have many motivations for pursuing a particular research question: because it will provide financial support, because it is a logical or important next step in building a career, or because getting at the truth of the matter is interesting. We like this last reason; it is one that grows as it is exercised and that provides the intensity of effort needed for overcoming the many hurdles and frustrations of the research process. However, it is wise to confirm that you are not the only one who finds a question interesting. Speak with mentors and outside experts before devoting substantial energy to develop a research plan or grant proposal that peers and funding agencies may consider dull.

Novel

Good clinical research contributes new information. A study that merely reiterates what is already established is not worth the effort and cost. The novelty of a proposed study can be determined by thoroughly reviewing the literature, consulting with experts who are familiar with ongoing research, and searching lists of projects that have been funded using the NIH Computer Retrieval of Information on Scientific Projects (CRISP). Although novelty is an important criterion, a research question need not be totally original—it can be worthwhile to ask whether a previous observation can be replicated, whether the findings in one population also apply to others, or whether improved measurement techniques can clarify the relationship between known risk factors and a disease. A confirmatory study is particularly useful if it avoids the weaknesses of previous studies.

Ethical

A good research question must be ethical. If the study poses unacceptable physical risks or invasion of privacy (Chapter 14), the investigator must seek other ways to answer the question. If there is uncertainty about whether the study is ethical, it is helpful to discuss it at an early stage with a representative of the institutional review board.

Relevant

Among the characteristics of a good research question, none is more important than its relevance. A good way to decide about relevance is to imagine the various outcomes that are likely to occur and consider how each possibility might advance scientific knowledge, influence practice guidelines and health policy, or guide further research. When relevance is uncertain, it is useful to discuss the idea with mentors, clinicians or experts in the field.

DEVELOPING THE RESEARCH QUESTION AND STUDY PLAN

It helps a great deal to write down the research question and a brief (one-page) outline of the **study plan** at an early stage (Appendix 1.1). This requires some self-discipline, but it forces the investigator to clarify her ideas about the plan and to discover specific problems that need attention. The outline also provides a basis for specific suggestions from colleagues.

Problems and Solutions

Two general solutions to the problems involved in developing a research question deserve special emphasis. The first is the importance of getting good advice. We recommend a research team that includes representatives of each of the major disciplines involved in the study, and that includes at least one senior scientist. In addition, it is a good idea to consult with specialists who can guide the discovery of previous research on the topic and the choice and design of measurement techniques. Sometimes a local expert will do, but it is often useful to contact individuals in other institutions who have published pertinent work on the subject. A new investigator may be intimidated by the prospect of writing or calling someone she knows only as an author in the *Journal of the American Medical Association,* but most scientists respond favorably to such requests for advice.

The second solution is to allow the study plan to gradually emerge from an iterative process of designing, reviewing, pretesting, and revising. Once the one-page study plan is specified, advice from colleagues will usually result in important changes. As the protocol gradually takes shape, a small pretest of the number and willingness of the potential subjects may lead to changes in the recruitment plan. The preferred imaging test may turn out to be prohibitively costly and a less expensive alternative sought. The qualities needed in the investigator for these planning stages of research are creativity, tenacity, and judgment.

Primary and Secondary Questions

Many studies have more than one research question. Experiments often address the effect of the intervention on more than one outcome; for example, the Women's Health Initiative was designed to determine whether reducing dietary fat intake would reduce the risk of breast cancer, but an important secondary hypothesis was to examine the effect on coronary events (5). Almost all cohort and case–control studies look at several risk factors for each outcome. The advantage of designing a study with several research questions is the efficiency that can result, with several answers emerging from a single study. The disadvantages are the increased complexity of designing and implementing the study and of drawing statistical inferences when there are multiple hypotheses (Chapter 5). A sensible strategy is to establish a single primary research question around which to focus the study plan and sample size estimate, adding secondary research questions about other predictors or outcomes that may also produce valuable conclusions.

TRANSLATIONAL RESEARCH

Translational research refers to studies of how to translate findings from the ivory tower into the "real world." Translational research (6) comes in two main flavors (Fig. 2.2):

- Applying basic science findings from laboratory research in clinical studies of patients (sometimes abbreviated as **T1** research), and
- Applying the findings of these clinical studies to alter health practices in the community (sometimes abbreviated as **T2** research).

Both forms of translational research require identifying a "translation" opportunity. Just as a literary translator first needs to find a novel or poem that merits translating, a translational research investigator must first identify a worthwhile scientific finding. Translational research projects are usually limited by the quality of the source material, so think "Tolstoy": the more valuable the result of a laboratory experiment or a clinical trial, the more likely a translational project will have merit. Pay attention to colleagues when they talk about their latest findings, to presentations at national meetings about novel methods, and to speculation about mechanisms in published reports.

Translating Research from the Laboratory to Clinical Practice (T1)

A host of **new tools** have become available for clinical investigations, including analysis of single nucleotide polymorphisms (SNPs), gene expression arrays, imaging and proteomics. From the viewpoint of a clinical investigator, there is nothing intrinsically different about any of these measurements or test results. The chapters on measurements will be useful in planning studies involving these types of measurements,

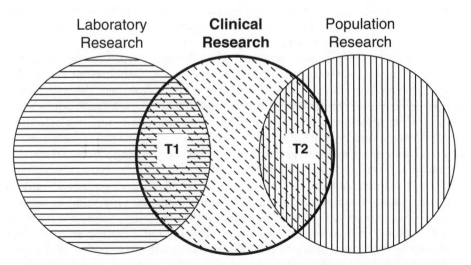

FIGURE 2.2. Transitional research is the component of clinical research that interacts with basic science research (hatched area T1) or with population research (hatched area T2).

as will the advice about study design, population samples, and sample size. Especially relevant will be the information about multiple hypothesis testing.

Compared with ordinary clinical research, being a successful T1 translational researcher requires having an additional skill set or identifying a collaborator with those skills. **Bench-to-bedside** research necessitates a thorough understanding of the underlying basic science. Although many clinical researchers believe that they can master this knowledge—just like many laboratory-based researchers believe doing clinical research requires no special training—in reality, the skills hardly overlap. For example, suppose a basic scientist has identified a gene that affects circadian rhythm in mice. A **clinical investigator** has access to a cohort study with data on sleep cycles in people and a bank of stored DNA, and wants to study whether there is an association between polymorphisms in the human homolog of that gene and sleep in people. In order to propose a T1 study looking at that association she needs collaborators who are familiar with that gene and with the advantages and limitations of the various methods of genotyping.

Similarly, imagine that a **laboratory-based investigator** has discovered a unique pattern of gene expression in tissue biopsy samples from patients with breast cancer. She should not propose a study of its use as a diagnostic test for breast cancer without collaborating with someone who understands the importance of test-retest reliability, receiver operating curves, sampling and blinding, and the effects of prior probability of disease on the applicability of her discovery. Good translational research requires expertise in more than one area. Thus a research team interested in testing a new drug needs scientists familiar with molecular biology, pharmacokinetics, pharmacodynamics, Phase I clinical trials, and the practice of medicine.

Translating Research from Clinical Studies to Populations (T2)

Studies that attempt to apply findings from clinical trials to larger and more diverse populations often require expertise in identifying high-risk or underserved groups, understanding the difference between screening and diagnosis, and knowledge of how to implement changes in health care delivery systems. On a practical level, this kind of research usually needs access to large groups of patients (or clinicians), such as those enrolled in health plans. Support and advice from the department chair, the chief of the medical staff at an affiliated hospital, or the leader of the local medical society, may be helpful when planning these studies.

Some investigators take a short cut when doing this type of translational research, studying patients in their colleagues' practices (e.g., a housestaff-run clinic in an academic medical center) rather than involving practitioners in the community. This is a bit like translating Aristophanes into modern Greek—it will still not be very useful for English-speaking readers. Chapter 18 emphasizes the importance of getting as far into the community as possible.

The sampling scheme is often a problem when studying whether research results can be applied in general populations. For example, in a study of whether a new office-based diet and exercise program will be effective in the community, it may not be possible to randomly assign individual patients. One solution would be to use physician practices as the unit of randomization; this will almost certainly require collaborating with an expert on cluster sampling and clustered analyses. Many T2 research projects use proxy "process" variables as their outcomes. For example, if clinical trials have established that a new treatment reduces mortality from sepsis, a translational research study might not need to have mortality as the outcome. Rather, it might examine different approaches to implementing the treatment protocol, and use the percentage of patients with sepsis who were placed on the protocol as the outcome of the study.

SUMMARY

1. All studies should start with a **research question** that addresses what the investigator would like to know. The goal is to find one that can be developed into a good study plan.

2. One key ingredient for developing a research question is **scholarship** that is acquired by a thorough and continuing review of the work of others, both published and unpublished. Another key ingredient is **experience,** and the single most important decision a new investigator makes is her choice of one or two senior scientists to serve as her **mentor(s).**

3. Good research questions arise from **medical articles** and **conferences,** from critical thinking about **clinical practices** and problems, from applying **new methods** to old issues, and from ideas that emerge from **teaching** and **daydreaming.**

4. Before committing much time and effort to writing a proposal or carrying out a study, the investigator should consider whether the research question and study plan are "FINER": **feasible, interesting, novel, ethical,** and **relevant.**

5. Early on, the research question should be developed into a one-page written **study plan** that specifically describes how many subjects will be needed, and how the subjects will be selected and the measurements made.

6. Developing the research question and study plan is an **iterative process** that includes consultations with advisors and friends, a growing familiarity with the literature, and pilot studies of the recruitment and measurement approaches. The qualities needed in the investigator are **creativity, tenacity,** and **judgment.**

7. Most studies have more than one question, but it is useful to focus on a **single primary question** in designing and implementing the study

8. **Translational research** is a type of clinical research that studies the application of basic science findings in clinical studies of patients **(T1)**, and how to apply these findings to improve health practices in the community **(T2)**; it requires collaborations from **laboratory** to **population-based investigators**, using the **clinical research methods** presented in this book.

REFERENCES

1. The ATAC Trialists Group. Anastrazole alone or in combination with tamoxifen versus tamoxifen alone for adjuvant treatment of postmenopausal women with early breast cancer: first results of the ATAC randomized trials. *Lancet* 2002;359:2131–2139.
2. Quinn J, Cummings S, Callaham M, et al. Suturing versus conservative management of lacerations of the hand: randomized controlled trial. *BMJ* 2002;325:299–301.

3. Kuhn TS. *The structure of scientific revolutions*. Chicago, IL: University of Chicago Press, 1962.
4. Yaffe K, Browner W, Cauley J, et al. Association between bone mineral density and cognitive decline in older women. *J Am Geriatr Soc* 1999;47:1176–1182.
5. Prentice RL, Caan B, Chlebowski RT, et al. Low-fat dietary pattern and risk of invasive breast cancer. *JAMA* 2006;295:629–642.
6. Zerhouni EA. US biomedical research: basic, translational and clinical sciences. *JAMA* 2005;294:1352–1358.

3 | Choosing the Study Subjects: Specification, Sampling, and Recruitment

Stephen B. Hulley, Thomas B. Newman,
and Steven R. Cummings

A good choice of study subjects serves the vital purpose of ensuring that the findings in the study accurately represent what is going on in the **population** of interest (Fig. 3.1). The protocol must specify a **sample** of subjects that can be studied at an acceptable cost in time and money, yet one that is large enough to control random error and representative enough to allow generalizing the study findings to populations of interest. An important precept here is that **generalizability** is rarely a simple yes-or-no matter; it is a complex qualitative judgment that is highly dependent on the investigator's choice of population and of sampling design.

We will come to the issue of choosing the appropriate *number* of study subjects in Chapter 6. In this chapter we address the process of **specifying** and **sampling** the *kinds* of subjects who will be representative and feasible. We also discuss strategies for **recruiting** these subjects to participate in the study.

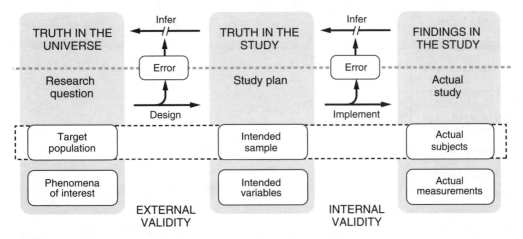

FIGURE 3.1. Choosing study subjects that represent the population.

BASIC TERMS AND CONCEPTS

Populations and Samples

A population is a complete set of people with a specified set of characteristics, and a sample is a subset of the population. In lay usage, the characteristics that define a population are geographic—*the population of Canada*. In research the defining characteristics are also clinical, demographic, and temporal:

- Clinical and demographic characteristics define the **target population,** the large set of people throughout the world to which the results will be generalized—*all teenagers with asthma,* for example.
- The **accessible population** is a geographically and temporally defined subset of the target population that is available for study—*teenagers with asthma living in the investigator's town this year.*
- The **study sample** is the subset of the accessible population that participates in the study.

Generalizing the Study Findings

The classic Framingham Study was an early approach to designing a study that would allow **inferences** from findings observed in a sample to be applied to a population (Fig. 3.2). The sampling design called for listing all the adult residents of the town and then asking every second person to participate. This "systematic" sampling design is not as tamperproof as a true random sample (as noted later in this chapter), but

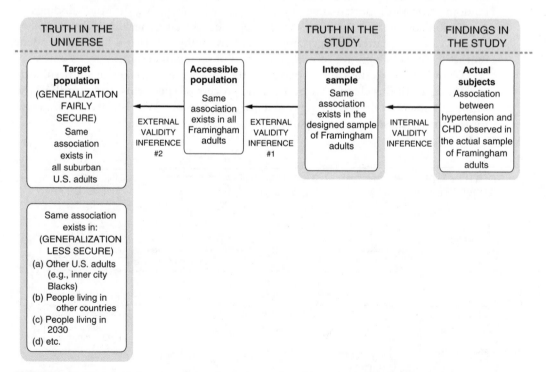

FIGURE 3.2. Inferences in generalizing from the study subjects to the target populations.

two more serious concerns were the facts that one-third of the Framingham residents selected for the study refused to participate, and that in their place the investigators accepted other residents who had heard about the study and volunteered (1). Because respondents are often healthier than nonrespondents, especially if they are volunteers, the characteristics of the actual sample undoubtedly differed from those of the intended sample. Every sample has some errors, however, and the issue is how much damage has been done. The Framingham Study sampling errors do not seem large enough to invalidate the conclusion that the findings of the study—that *hypertension is a risk factor for coronary heart disease (CHD)*—can be generalized to all the residents of Framingham.

The next concern is the validity of generalizing the finding that hypertension is a risk factor for CHD from the accessible population of Framingham residents to target populations elsewhere. This inference is more subjective. The town of Framingham was selected from the universe of towns in the world, not with a scientific sampling design, but because it seemed fairly typical of middle-class residential communities in the United States and was convenient to the investigators. The validity of generalizing the Framingham risk relationships to populations in other parts of the country involves the precept that, in general, analytic studies and clinical trials that address biologic relationships produce more widely generalizable results across diverse populations than descriptive studies that address distributions of characteristics. For example, the strength of hypertension as a risk factor for CHD is similar in Caucasian Framingham residents to that observed in inner city African Americans, but the prevalence of hypertension is much higher in the latter population.

Steps in Designing the Protocol for Acquiring Study Subjects

The inferences in Fig. 3.2 are presented from right to left, the sequence used for interpreting the findings of a completed study. An investigator who is planning a study reverses this sequence, beginning on the left (Fig. 3.3). She begins by specifying the clinical and demographic characteristics of the target population that will serve the research question well. She then uses **geographic** and **temporal criteria** to specify a study sample that is representative and practical.

SELECTION CRITERIA

An investigator wants to study the efficacy of *low dose testosterone versus placebo for enhancing libido in menopause*. She begins by creating selection criteria that define the population to be studied.

Establishing Inclusion Criteria

The inclusion criteria define the main characteristics of the target population that pertain to the research question (Table 3.1). Age is often a crucial factor. In this study the investigators might decide to focus on women in their fifties, reasoning that in this group the benefit-to-harm ratio of the drug might be optimal, but another study might include older decades. Incorporating African American, Hispanic, and Asian women in the study would appear to expand generalizability, but it's important to realize that the increase in generalizability is illusory unless there are enough women of each race to statistically test for the presence of an "interaction" (an effect in one

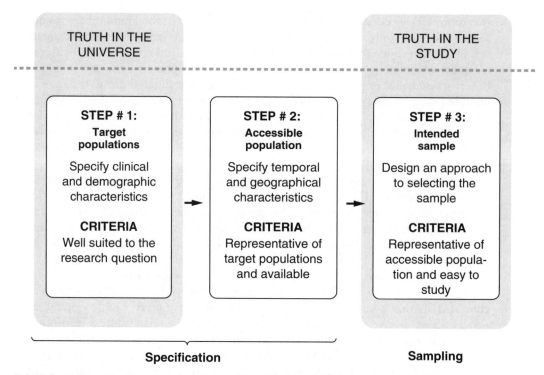

FIGURE 3.3. Steps in designing the protocol for choosing the study subjects.

race that is different from that in other races, Chapter 9); this is a large number, and most studies are not powered to discover such interactions.

Specifying clinical characteristics often involves difficult judgments, not only about which factors are important to the research question, but about how to define them. How, for example, would an investigator put into practice the criterion that the subjects be in "good general health"? She might decide not to include patients with diseases that might be worsened by the testosterone treatment (*atherosclerosis*) or interfere with follow-up (*metastatic cancer*).

The selection criteria that address the geographic and temporal characteristics of the accessible population may involve trade-offs between scientific and practical goals. The investigator may find that patients at her own hospital are an available and inexpensive source of subjects. But she must consider whether peculiarities of the local referral patterns might interfere with generalizing the results to other populations. On these and other decisions about inclusion criteria, there is no single course of action that is clearly right or wrong; the important thing is to make decisions that are sensible, that can be used consistently throughout the study, and that will provide a basis for knowing to whom the published conclusions apply.

Establishing Exclusion Criteria

Exclusion criteria indicate subsets of individuals who would be suitable for the research question were it not for characteristics that might interfere with the success of follow-up efforts, the quality of the data, or the acceptability of randomized treatment (Table 3.1). Clinical trials differ somewhat from observational studies in being more likely to have exclusions mandated by concern for the safety of the

TABLE 3.1	Designing Selection Criteria for a Clinical Trial of Low Dose Testosterone to Enhance Libido in Menopause	
	Design Feature	**Example**
Inclusion criteria (be specific)	Specifying populations relevant to the research question and efficient for study:	
	Demographic characteristics	White women 50 to 60 years old
	Clinical characteristics	Good general health Has a sexual partner
	Geographic (administrative) characteristics	Patients attending clinic at the investigator's hospital
	Temporal characteristics	Between January 1 and December 31 of specified year
Exclusion criteria (be parsimonious)	Specifying subsets of the population that will *not* be studied because of:	
	A high likelihood of being lost to follow-up	Alcoholic or plan to move out of state
	An inability to provide good data	Disoriented or have a language barrier*
	Being at high risk of possible adverse effects	History of myocardial infarction or stroke

* Alternatives to exclusion (when these subgroups are important to the research question) would be collecting nonverbal data or using bilingual staff and questionnaires.

participant (Chapter 10). A good general rule that keeps things simple and preserves the number of potential study subjects is to have as **few exclusion criteria** as possible.

Exclusion criteria can be a two-edged sword. Including alcoholics in the testosterone trial might provide subjects with low baseline libido, for example, but this potential advantage could be accompanied by greater problems with adherence to study treatment and with follow-up; the investigator may decide to exclude alcoholics if she believes that adherence to study protocol is the more important consideration. (She will then face the problem of developing specific criteria for classifying whether an individual is alcoholic.)

Clinical versus Community Populations

If the research question involves patients with a disease, hospitalized or clinic-based patients are easier to find, but selection factors that determine who comes to the hospital or clinic may have an important effect. For example, a specialty clinic at a tertiary care medical center tends to accumulate patients with serious forms of the disease that give a distorted impression of the commonplace features and prognosis. For research questions that pertain to diagnosis, treatment, and prognosis of patients in medical settings, sampling from primary care clinics can be a better choice.

Another common option in choosing the sample is to select subjects in the community who represent a healthy population. These samples are often recruited using mass mailings and advertising, and are not fully representative of a general population because they must (a) volunteer, (b) fit inclusion and exclusion criteria, and (c) agree to be included in the study. True "population-based" samples are difficult and expensive to recruit, but useful for guiding public health and clinical practice in the community. One of the largest and best examples is the National Health and Nutrition Examination Survey (NHANES), a probability sample of all US residents.

The size and diversity of a sample can be increased by collecting data by mail or telephone, by collaborating with colleagues in other cities, or by using preexisting data sets such as NHANES and Medicare. Electronically accessible datasets have come into widespread use in clinical research and may be more representative of national populations and less time-consuming than other possibilities (Chapter 13).

SAMPLING

Often the number of people who meet the selection criteria is too large, and there is a need to select a **sample** (subset) of the population for study.

Convenience Samples

In clinical research the study sample is often made up of people who meet the entry criteria and are easily accessible to the investigator. This is termed a **convenience sample.** It has obvious advantages in cost and logistics, and is a good choice for many research questions.

A convenience sample can minimize volunteerism and other selection biases by consecutively selecting every accessible person who meets the entry criteria. Such a **consecutive sample** is especially desirable when it amounts to taking the entire accessible population over a long enough period to include seasonal variations or other temporal changes that are important to the research question. The validity of using a sample is the premise that, for the purpose of answering the research question at hand, it sufficiently represents the target population. With convenience samples this requires a subjective judgment.

Probability Samples

Sometimes, particularly with descriptive research questions, there is a need for a scientific basis for generalizing the findings in the study sample to the population. Probability sampling, the gold standard for ensuring generalizability, uses a random process to guarantee that each unit of the population has a specified chance of being included in the sample. It is a scientific approach that provides a rigorous basis for estimating the fidelity with which phenomena observed in the sample represent those in the population, and for computing statistical significance and confidence intervals. There are several versions of this approach.

A **simple random sample** is drawn by enumerating the units of the population and selecting a subset at random. The most common use of this approach in clinical research is when the investigator wishes to select a representative subset from a population that is larger than she needs. To take a random sample of the cataract surgery patients at her hospital, for example, the investigator could list all such patients on the operating room schedules for the period of study, then use a table of random numbers to select individuals for study (Appendix 3.1).

A **systematic sample** resembles a simple random sample in first enumerating the population but differs in that the sample is selected by a preordained periodic process (e.g., the Framingham approach of taking every second person from a list of town residents). Systematic sampling is susceptible to errors caused by natural periodicities in the population, and it allows the investigator to predict and perhaps manipulate those who will be in the sample. It offers no logistic advantages over simple random sampling, and in clinical research it is rarely a better choice.

A **stratified random sample** involves dividing the population into subgroups according to characteristics such as sex or race and taking a random sample from each of these "strata." The subsamples in a stratified sample can be weighted to draw disproportionately from subgroups that are less common in the population but of special interest to the investigator. In studying the incidence of toxemia in pregnancy, for example, the investigator could stratify the population by race and then sample equal numbers from each stratum. This would yield incidence estimates of comparable precision from each racial group.

A **cluster sample** is a random sample of natural groupings (clusters) of individuals in the population. Cluster sampling is very useful when the population is widely dispersed and it is impractical to list and sample from all its elements. Consider, for example, the problem of reviewing the hospital records of patients with lung cancer selected randomly from a statewide list of discharge diagnoses; patients could be studied at lower cost by choosing a random sample of the hospitals and taking the cases from these. Community surveys often use a two-stage cluster sample: a random sample is drawn from city blocks enumerated on a map and a field team visits the blocks in the sample, lists all the addresses in each, and selects a subsample for study by a second random process. A disadvantage of cluster sampling is the fact that naturally occurring groups are often relatively homogeneous for the variables of interest; each city block, for example, tends to have people of uniform socioeconomic status. This means that the effective sample size will be somewhat smaller than the number of subjects, and that statistical analysis must take the clustering into account.

Summarizing the Sampling Design Options

The use of descriptive statistics and tests of statistical significance to draw inferences about the population from observations in the study sample is based on the assumption that a probability sample has been used. But in clinical research a random sample of the whole target population is almost never possible. Convenience sampling, preferably with a consecutive design, is a practical approach that is often suitable. The decision about whether the proposed sampling design is satisfactory requires that the investigator make a **judgment:** for the research question at hand, will the conclusions of the study be similar to those that would result from studying a true probability sample of the target population?

RECRUITMENT

The Goals of Recruitment

An important factor to consider in choosing the accessible population and sampling approach is the feasibility of recruiting study participants. There are two main goals:

(a) to recruit a sample that adequately **represents** the target population; and (b) to recruit **enough subjects** to meet the sample size requirements.

Achieving a Representative Sample

The approach to recruiting a representative sample begins in the design phase with choosing populations and sampling methods wisely. It ends with implementation, guarding against errors in applying the entry criteria to prospective study participants, and monitoring adherence to these criteria as the study progresses.

A particular concern, especially in observational studies, is the problem of **nonresponse.** The proportion of eligible subjects who agree to enter the study (the **response rate**) influences the validity of inferring that the sample represents the population. People who are difficult to reach and those who refuse to participate once they are contacted tend to be different from people who do enroll. The level of nonresponse that will compromise the generalizability of the study depends on the research question and on the reasons for not responding. A nonresponse rate of 25%, a good achievement in many settings, can seriously distort the observed prevalence of a disease when the disease itself is a cause of nonresponse. The degree to which this bias may influence the conclusions of a study can sometimes be estimated during the study with an intensive effort to acquire additional information on a sample of nonrespondents.

The best way to deal with nonresponse bias, however, is to minimize the number of nonrespondents. The problem of failure to make contact with individuals who have been chosen for the sample can be reduced by designing a systematic series of repeated contact attempts and by using various methods (mail, email, telephone, home visit). Among those contacted, refusal to participate can be minimized by improving the efficiency and attractiveness of the study (especially the initial encounter), by choosing a design that avoids invasive and uncomfortable tests, by using brochures and individual discussion to allay anxiety and discomfort, and by providing incentives such as reimbursing the costs of transportation and providing the results of tests. If language barriers are prevalent, they can be circumvented by using bilingual staff and translated questionnaires.

Recruiting Sufficient Numbers of Subjects

Falling short in the rate of recruitment is one of the commonest problems in clinical research. In planning a study it is safe to assume that the number of subjects who meet the entry criteria and agree to enter the study will be fewer, sometimes by several fold, than the number projected at the outset. The solutions to this problem are to estimate the magnitude of the recruitment problem empirically with a pretest, to plan the study with an accessible population that is larger than believed necessary, and to make contingency plans should the need arise for additional subjects. While the study is in progress it is important to closely monitor progress in meeting the recruitment goals and tabulate reasons for falling short of the goals; understanding the proportions of potential subjects lost to the study at various stages can lead to strategies for enhancing recruitment by reducing some of these losses.

Sometimes recruitment involves selecting patients who are already known to the members of the research team (e.g., in a study of a new treatment in patients attending the investigator's clinic). Here the chief concern is to present the opportunity for participation in the study fairly, making clear the advantages and disadvantages. In discussing the desirability of participation, the investigator must recognize the special ethical dilemmas that arise when her advice as the patient's physician might conflict with her interests as an investigator (Chapter 14).

Often recruitment involves contacting populations that are not known to the members of the research team. It is helpful if at least one member of the research team has previous experience with the approaches for contacting the prospective subjects. These include screening in work settings or public places such as shopping malls; sending out large numbers of mailings to listings such as driver's license holders; advertising on the Internet; inviting referrals from clinicians; carrying out retrospective record reviews; and examining lists of patients seen in clinic and hospital settings. Some of these approaches, particularly the latter two, involve concerns with privacy invasion that must be considered by the institutional review board.

It may be helpful to prepare for recruitment by getting the support of important organizations. For example, the investigator can meet with hospital administrators to discuss a clinic-based sample, and with the leadership of the medical society and county health department to plan a community screening operation or mailing to physicians. Written endorsements can be included as an appendix in applications for funding. For large studies it may be useful to create a favorable climate in the community by giving public lectures or by advertising through radio, TV, newspaper, fliers, websites, or mass mailings.

SUMMARY

1. All clinical research is based, philosophically and practically, on the use of a **sample** to represent a **population.**

2. The advantage of sampling is **efficiency;** it allows the investigator to draw inferences about a large population by examining a subset at relatively small cost in time and effort. The disadvantage is the source of **error** it introduces. If the sample is not sufficiently representative for the research question at hand, the findings may not **generalize** well to the population.

3. In designing a study the first step is to conceptualize the **target population** with a specific set of **inclusion criteria** that establish the demographic and clinical characteristics of subjects well suited to the research question, an appropriate **accessible population** that is geographically and temporally convenient, and a parsimonious set of **exclusion criteria** that eliminate subjects who are unethical or inappropriate to study.

4. The next step is to design an approach to **sampling** the population. A **convenience sample** is often a good choice in clinical research, especially if it is drawn **consecutively. Simple random sampling** can be used to reduce the size of a convenience sample if necessary, and **other probability sampling** strategies (stratified and cluster) are useful in certain situations.

5. Finally, the investigator must design and implement strategies for **recruiting** a sample of subjects that is large enough to meet the study needs, and that minimizes bias due to **nonresponse** and **loss to follow-up.**

APPENDIX 3.1

Selecting a Random Sample from a Table of Random Numbers

10480	15011	01536	81647	91646	02011
22368	46573	25595	85393	30995	89198
24130	48390	22527	97265	78393	64809
42167	93093	06243	61680	07856	16376
37570	33997	81837	16656	06121	91782
77921	06907	11008	42751	27756	53498
99562	72905	56420	69994	98872	31016
96301	91977	05463	07972	18876	20922
89572	14342	63661	10281	17453	18103
85475	36857	53342	53998	53060	59533
28918	79578	88231	33276	70997	79936
63553	40961	48235	03427	49626	69445
09429	93969	52636	92737	88974	33488
10365	61129	87529	85689	48237	52267
07119	97336	71048	08178	77233	13916
51085	12765	51821	51259	77452	16308
02368	21382	52404	60268	89368	19885
01011	54092	33362	94904	31273	04146
52162	53916	46369	58569	23216	14513
07056	97628	33787	09998	42698	06691
48663	91245	85828	14346	09172	30163
54164	58492	22421	74103	47070	25306
32639	32363	05597	24200	38005	13363
29334	27001	87637	87308	58731	00256
02488	33062	28834	07351	19731	92420
81525	72295	04839	96423	24878	82651
29676	20591	68086	26432	46901	20949
00742	57392	39064	66432	84673	40027
05366	04213	25669	26422	44407	44048
91921	26418	64117	94305	26766	25940

To select a 10% random sample, begin by enumerating (listing and numbering) every element of the population to be sampled. Then decide on a rule for obtaining an appropriate series of numbers; for example, if your list has 741 elements (which you have numbered 1 to 741), your rule might be to go vertically down each column using the first three digits of each number (beginning at the upper left, the numbers are 104, 223, etc.) and to select the first 74 different numbers that fall in the range of 1 to 741. Finally, pick a starting point by an arbitrary process. (Closing your eyes and putting your pencil on some number in the table is one way to do it.)

REFERENCE

1. Dawber TR. *The Framingham Study*. Cambridge, MA: Harvard University Press, 1980: 14–29.

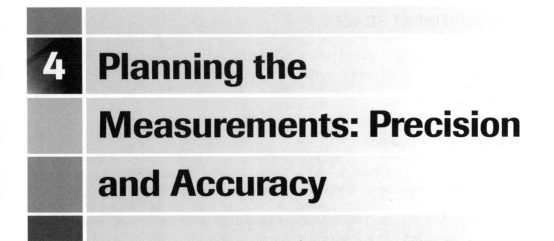

4 Planning the Measurements: Precision and Accuracy

Stephen B. Hulley, Jeffrey N. Martin and Steven R. Cummings

Measurements describe phenomena in terms that can be analyzed statistically. The validity of a study depends on how well the variables designed for the study represent the phenomena of interest (Fig. 4.1). How well does a prostate-specific antigen (PSA) level signal cancer in the prostate that will soon metastasize, for example, or an insomnia questionnaire detect amount and quality of sleep?

This chapter begins by considering how the choice of **measurement scale** influences the information content of the measurement. We then turn to the central goal of minimizing measurement error: how to design measurements that are relatively **precise** (free of random error) and **accurate** (free of systematic error), thereby enhancing the validity of drawing inferences from the study to the universe. We conclude with some considerations for clinical research, noting especially the advantages of storing specimens for later measurements.

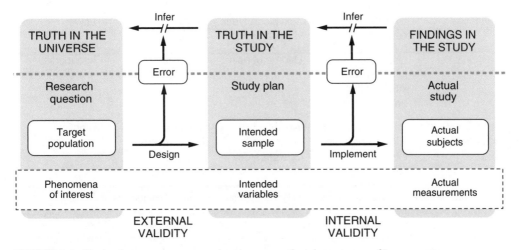

FIGURE 4.1. Designing measurements that represent the phenomena of interest.

MEASUREMENT SCALES

Table 4.1 presents a simplified classification of measurement scales and the information that results. The classification is important because some types of variables are **more informative** than others, adding power to the study and reducing sample size requirements.

Continuous Variables

Continuous variables are quantified on an infinite scale. The number of possible values of *body weight*, for example, is limited only by the sensitivity of the machine that is used to measure it. Continuous variables are rich in information.

A scale whose units are limited to integers (such as *the number of cigarettes smoked per day*) is termed **discrete.** Discrete variables that have a considerable number of possible values can resemble continuous variables in statistical analyses and be equivalent for the purpose of designing measurements.

Categorical Variables

Phenomena that are not suitable for quantification can often be measured by classifying them in categories. Categorical variables with two possible values (*dead or alive*) are termed **dichotomous.** Categorical variables with more than two categories (polychotomous) can be further characterized according to the type of information they contain.

Nominal variables have categories that are not ordered; *type O blood*, for example, is neither more nor less than *type B*; nominal variables tend to have a qualitative and absolute character that makes them straightforward to measure. **Ordinal** variables

TABLE 4.1	Measurement Scales			
Type of Measurement	**Characteristics of Variable**	**Example**	**Descriptive Statistics**	**Information Content**
Categorical*				
Nominal	Unordered categories	Sex; blood type; vital status	Counts, proportions	Lower
Ordinal	Ordered categories with intervals that are not quantifiable	Degree of pain	In addition to the above: medians	Intermediate
Continuous or ordered discrete[†]	Ranked spectrum with quantifiable intervals	Weight; number of cigarettes/day	In addition to the above: means, standard deviations	Higher

* Categorical measurements that contain only two classes (e.g., sex) are termed **dichotomous.**
[†] Continuous variables have an infinite number of values (e.g., weight), whereas discrete variables are limited to integers (e.g., number of cigarettes/day). Discrete variables that are ordered (e.g., arranged in sequence from few to many) and that have a large number of possible values resemble continuous variables for practical purposes of measurement and analysis.

have categories that do have an order, such as *severe, moderate, and mild pain.* The additional information is an advantage over nominal variables, but because ordinal variables do not specify a numerical or uniform difference between one category and the next, the information content is less than that of discrete variables.

Choosing a Measurement Scale

A good general rule is to prefer continuous variables, because the additional information they contain improves statistical efficiency. In a study comparing the antihypertensive effects of several treatments, for example, measuring *blood pressure in millimeters of mercury* allows the investigator to observe the magnitude of the change in every subject, whereas measuring it as *hypertensive versus normotensive* would limit the assessment. The continuous variable contains more information, and the result is a study with more power and/or a smaller sample size (Chapter 6).

The rule has some exceptions. If the research question involves the determinants of low birth weight, for example, the investigator would be more concerned with babies whose weight is so low that their health is compromised than with differences observed over the full spectrum of birth weights. In this case she is better off with a large enough sample to be able to analyze the results with a dichotomous outcome like the proportion of babies whose weight is below 2,500 g. Even when the categorical data are more meaningful, however, it is still best to collect the data as a continuous variable. This leaves the analytic options open: to change the cutoff point that defines low birth weight (she may later decide that 2,350 g is a better value for identifying babies at increased risk of developmental abnormalities), or to fall back on the more powerful analysis of the predictors of the full spectrum of weight.

Similarly, when there is the option of designing the number of response categories in an ordinal scale, as in a question about food preferences, it is often useful to provide a half-dozen categories that range from *strongly dislike* to *extremely fond of.* The results can later be collapsed into a dichotomy (*dislike and like*), but not vice versa.

Many characteristics, particularly symptoms (*pain*) or aspects of lifestyle, are difficult to describe with categories or numbers. But these phenomena often have important roles in diagnostic and treatment decisions, and the attempt to measure them is an essential part of the scientific approach to description and analysis. This is illustrated by the SF-36, a standardized questionnaire for assessing **quality of life** (1). The process of classification and measurement, if done well, can increase the objectivity of our knowledge, reduce bias, and provide a means of communication.

■ PRECISION

The **precision** of a variable is the degree to which it is reproducible, with nearly the same value each time it is measured. A beam scale can measure body weight with great precision, whereas an interview to measure quality of life is more likely to produce values that vary from one observer to the next. Precision has a very important influence on the power of a study. The more precise a measurement, the greater the statistical power at a given sample size to estimate mean values and to test hypotheses (Chapter 6).

Precision (also called reproducibility, reliability, and consistency) is a function of **random error** (chance variability); the greater the error, the less precise the measurement. There are three main sources of random error in making measurements.

- *Observer variability* refers to variability in measurement that is due to the observer, and includes such things as choice of words in an interview and skill in using a mechanical instrument.
- *Instrument variability* refers to variability in the measurement due to changing environmental factors such as temperature, aging mechanical components, different reagent lots, and so on.
- *Subject variability* refers to intrinsic biologic variability in the study subjects due to such things as fluctuations in mood and time since last medication.

Assessing Precision

Precision is assessed as the **reproducibility** of repeated measurements, either comparing measurements made by the same person (within-observer reproducibility) or different people (between-observer reproducibility). Similarly, it can be assessed within or between instruments.

The reproducibility of continuous variables is often expressed as the **within-subject standard deviation.** However, if a "Bland-Altman" plot (2) of the within-subject standard deviation versus that subject's mean demonstrates a linear association, then the preferred approach is the **coefficient of variation** (within-subject standard deviation divided by the mean). Correlation coefficients should be avoided (2). For categorical variables, **percent agreement** and the **kappa** statistic (3) are often used (Chapter 12).

Strategies for Enhancing Precision

There are five approaches to minimizing random error and increasing the precision of measurements (Table 4.2):

1. *Standardizing the measurement methods.* All study protocols should include operational definitions (specific instructions for making the measurements). This includes written directions on how to prepare the environment and the subject, how to carry out and record the interview, how to calibrate the instrument, and so forth (Appendix 4.1). This set of materials, part of the **operations manual,** is essential for large and complex studies and recommended for smaller ones. Even when there is only a single observer, specific written guidelines for making each measurement will help her performance to be uniform over the duration of the study and serve as the basis for describing the methods when the results are published.
2. *Training and certifying the observers.* Training will improve the consistency of measurement techniques, especially when several observers are involved. It is often desirable to design a formal test of the mastery of the techniques specified in the operations manual and to certify that observers have achieved the prescribed level of performance (Chapter 17).
3. *Refining the instruments.* Mechanical and electronic instruments can be engineered to reduce variability. Similarly, questionnaires and interviews can be written to increase clarity and avoid potential ambiguities (Chapter 15).
4. *Automating the instruments.* Variations in the way human observers make measurements can be eliminated with automatic mechanical devices and self-response questionnaires.
5. *Repetition.* The influence of random error from any source is reduced by repeating the measurement, and using the mean of the two or more readings. Precision will be substantially increased by this strategy, the primary limitation being the added cost and practical difficulties of repeating the measurements.

TABLE 4.2	Strategies for Reducing Random Error in Order to Increase Precision, with Illustrations from a Study of Antihypertensive Treatment		
Strategy to Reduce Random Error	**Source of Random Error**	**Example of Random Error**	**Example of Strategy to Prevent the Error**
1. Standardizing the measurement methods in an operations manual	Observer	Variation in blood pressure (BP) measurement due to variable rate of cuff deflation (sometimes faster than 2 mm Hg/second and sometimes slower)	Specify that the cuff be deflated at 2 mm Hg/second
	Subject	Variation in BP due to variable length of quiet sitting	Specify that subject sit in a quiet room for 5 minutes before BP measurement
2. Training and certifying the observer	Observer	Variation in BP due to variable observer technique	Train observer in standard techniques
3. Refining the instrument	Instrument and observer	Variation in BP due to digit preference (e.g., the tendency to round number to a multiple of 5)	Design instrument that conceals BP reading until after it has been recorded
4. Automating the instrument	Observer	Variation in BP due to variable observer technique	Use automatic BP measuring device
	Subject	Variation in BP due to emotional reaction to observer by subject	Use automatic BP measuring device
5. Repeating the measurement	Observer, subject, and instrument	All measurements and all sources of variation	Use mean of two or more BP measurements

For each measurement in the study, the investigator must decide how vigorously to pursue each of these strategies. This decision can be based on the importance of the variable, the magnitude of the potential problem with precision, and the feasibility and cost of the strategy. In general, the first two strategies (standardizing and training) should always be used, and the fifth (repetition) is an option that is guaranteed to improve precision whenever it is feasible and affordable.

ACCURACY

The **accuracy** of a variable is the degree to which it actually represents what it is intended to represent. This has an important influence on the **validity** of the

TABLE 4.3	The Precision and Accuracy of Measurements	
	Precision	**Accuracy**
Definition	The degree to which a variable has nearly the same value when measured several times	The degree to which a variable actually represents what it is supposed to represent
Best way to assess	Comparison among repeated measures	Comparison with a reference standard
Value to study	Increase power to detect effects	Increase validity of conclusions

Threatened by	Random error (chance) contributed by
	    The observer
	    The subject
	    The instrument
		Systematic error (bias) contributed by
		    The observer
		    The subject
		    The instrument

study—the degree to which the observed findings lead to the correct inferences about phenomena taking place in the study sample and in the universe.

Accuracy is different from precision in the ways shown in Table 4.3, and the two are not necessarily linked. If serum cholesterol were measured repeatedly using standards that had inadvertently been diluted twofold, for example, the result would be inaccurate but could still be precise (consistently off by a factor of 2). This concept is further illustrated in Figure. 4.2. Accuracy and precision do often go hand in hand however, in the sense that many of the strategies for increasing precision will also improve accuracy.

Accuracy is a function of **systematic error** (bias); the greater the error, the less accurate the variable. The three main classes of measurement error noted in the earlier section on precision each have counterparts here.

- *Observer bias* is a distortion, conscious or unconscious, in the perception or reporting of the measurement by the observer. It may represent systematic errors in the way an instrument is operated, such as a tendency to round down blood pressure measurements, or in the way an interview is carried out as in the use of leading questions.
- *Instrument bias* can result from faulty function of a mechanical instrument. A scale that has not been calibrated recently may have drifted downward, producing consistently low body weight readings.

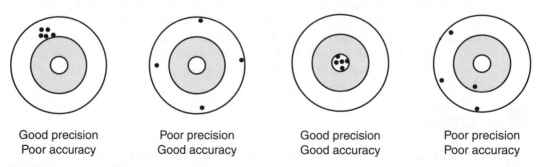

| Good precision | Poor precision | Good precision | Poor precision |
| Poor accuracy | Good accuracy | Good accuracy | Poor accuracy |

FIGURE 4.2. The difference between precision and accuracy.

- *Subject bias* is a distortion of the measurement by the study subject, for example, in reporting an event (respondent or recall bias). Patients with breast cancer who believe that alcohol is a cause of their cancer, for example, may exaggerate the amount they used to drink.

The accuracy of a measurement is best assessed by comparing it, when possible, to a **"gold standard"**—a reference technique that is considered accurate. For measurements on a continuous scale, the mean difference between the measurement under investigation and the gold standard across study subjects can be determined. For measurements on a dichotomous scale, accuracy in comparison to a gold standard can be described in terms of sensitivity and specificity (Chapter 12). For measurements on categorical scales with more than two response options, kappa can be used.

Validity

The degree to which a variable represents what is intended is difficult to assess when measuring subjective and abstract phenomena, such as pain or quality of life, for which there is no concrete gold standard. At issue is a particular type of accuracy termed **validity**—how well the measurement represents the phenomenon of interest. There are three ways to view and assess validity:

- *Content validity* examines how well the assessment represents all aspects of the phenomena under study—for example, including questions on social, physical, emotional, and intellectual functioning to assess quality of life—and often it uses subjective judgments (**face validity**) about whether the measurements seem reasonable.
- *Construct validity* refers to how well a measurement conforms to theoretical constructs; for example, if an attribute is theoretically believed to differ between two groups a measure of this attribute that has construct validity would show this difference.
- *Criterion-related* validity is the degree to which a new measurement correlates with well-accepted existing measures. A powerful version of this approach is **predictive validity,** the ability of the measurement to predict an outcome: the validity of a measure of depression would be strengthened if it was found to predict suicide.

The general approach to **validating** an abstract measure is to begin by searching the literature and consulting with experts in an effort to find a suitable instrument (questionnaire) that has already been validated. Using such an instrument has the advantage of making the results of the new study comparable to earlier work in the area, and may simplify and strengthen the process of applying for grants and publishing the results. Its disadvantage, however, is that an instrument taken off the shelf may be outmoded or not appropriate for the research question.

If existing instruments are not suitable for the needs of the study, then the investigator may decide to develop a new measurement approach and validate it herself. This can be an interesting challenge that leads to a worthwhile contribution to the literature, but it is fair to say that the process is often less scientific and conclusive than the word "validation" connotes (Chapter 15).

Strategies for Enhancing Accuracy

The major approaches to increasing accuracy include the first four of the strategies listed earlier for precision, and three additional ones (Table 4.4):

1. **Standardizing the measurement methods**
2. **Training and certifying the observers**

TABLE 4.4	Strategies for Reducing Systematic Error in Order to Increase Accuracy, with Illustrations from a Study of Antihypertensive Treatment		
Strategy to Reduce Systematic Error	**Source of Systematic Error**	**Example of Systematic Error**	**Example of Strategy to Prevent the Error**
1. Standardizing the measurement methods in an operations manual	Observer	Consistently high diastolic blood pressure (BP) readings due to using the point at which sounds become muffled	Specify the operational definition of diastolic BP as the point at which sounds cease to be heard
	Subject	Consistently high readings due to measuring BP right after walking upstairs to clinic	Specify that subject sit in quiet room for 5 minutes before measurement
2. Training and certifying the observer	Observer	Consistently high BP readings due to failure to follow procedures specified in operations manual	Trainer checks accuracy of observer's reading with a double-headed stethoscope
3. Refining the instrument	Instrument	Consistently high BP readings with standard cuff in subjects with very large arms	Use extra-wide BP cuff in obese patients
4. Automating the instrument	Observer	Conscious or unconscious tendency for observer to read BP lower in study group randomized to active drug	Use automatic BP measuring device
	Subject	BP increase due to proximity of attractive technician	Use automatic BP measuring device
5. Making unobtrusive measurements	Subject	Tendency of subject to overestimate compliance with study drug	Measure study drug level in urine
6. Calibrating the instrument	Instrument	Consistently high BP readings due to manometer being out of adjustment	Calibrate each month
7. Blinding	Observer	Conscious or unconscious tendency for observer to read BP lower in active treatment group	Use double-blind placebo to conceal study group assignment
	Subject	Tendency of subject to overreport side effects if she knew she was on active drug	Use double-blind placebo to conceal study group assignment

3. **Refining the instruments**
4. **Automating the instruments**
5. **Making Unobtrusive Measurements.** It is sometimes possible to design measurements that the subjects are not aware of, thereby eliminating the possibility that they will consciously bias the variable. A study of advice on healthy eating patterns for schoolchildren, for example, could measure the number of candy bar wrappers in the trash.
6. **Calibrating the Instrument.** The accuracy of many instruments, especially those that are mechanical or electrical, can be increased by periodic calibration using a gold standard.
7. **Blinding.** This classic strategy does not ensure the overall accuracy of the measurements, but it can eliminate **differential bias** that affects one study group more than another. In a double-blind clinical trial the subjects and observers do not know whether active medicine or placebo has been assigned, and any inaccuracy in measuring the outcome will be the same in the two groups.

The decision on how vigorously to pursue each of these seven strategies for each measurement rests, as noted earlier for precision, on the judgment of the investigator. The considerations are the magnitude of the potential impact that the anticipated degree of inaccuracy will have on the conclusions of the study and the feasibility and cost of the strategy. The first two strategies (standardizing and training) should always be used, calibration is needed for any instrument that has the potential to change over time, and blinding is essential whenever feasible.

■ OTHER FEATURES OF MEASUREMENT APPROACHES

Measurements should be **sensitive** enough to detect differences in a characteristic that are important to the investigator. Just how much sensitivity is needed depends on the research question. For example, a study of whether a new medication helps people to quit smoking could use an outcome measure that is relatively insensitive to the number of cigarettes smoked each day. On the other hand, if the question is the effect of reducing the nicotine content of cigarettes on the number of cigarettes smoked, the method should be sensitive to differences in daily habits of just a few cigarettes.

An ideal measurement is **specific,** representing only the characteristic of interest. The carbon monoxide level in expired air is a measure of smoking habits that is only moderately specific because it can also be affected by other exposures such as automobile exhaust. The overall specificity of assessing smoking habits can be increased by supplementing the carbon monoxide data with other measurements (such as self-report and serum cotinine level) that are not affected by air pollution.

Measurements should be **appropriate** to the objectives of the study. A study of stress as an antecedent to myocardial infarction, for example, would need to consider which kind of stress (psychological or physical, acute or chronic) was of interest before setting out the operational definitions for measuring it.

Measurements should provide an adequate **distribution of responses** in the study population. A measure of functional status is most useful if it produces values that range from high in some subjects to low in others. One of the main functions of pretesting is to ensure that the actual responses do not all cluster around one end of the possible range of response (Chapter 17).

Finally, there is the issue of **objectivity.** This is achieved by reducing the involvement of the observer and by increasing the structure of the instrument. The danger in these strategies, however, is the consequent tunnel vision that limits the scope of the observations and the ability to discover unanticipated phenomena. The best design is often a compromise, including an opportunity for acquiring subjective and qualitative data in addition to the main objective and quantitative measurements.

■ MEASUREMENTS ON STORED MATERIALS

Clinical research involves measurements on people that range across a broad array of domains (Table 4.5). Some of these measurements can only be made during a contact with the study subject, but many can be carried out later on biological **specimens** banked for chemical or genetic analysis, or on **images** from radiographic and other procedures filed electronically.

One advantage of such storage is the opportunity to reduce the cost of the study by making measurements only on individuals who turn out during follow-up to develop the condition of interest. A terrific approach to doing this is the nested case–control design (Chapter 7); paired blinded measurements can be made in a single analytic batch, eliminating the batch-to-batch component of random error. A second advantage is that scientific advances may lead to new ideas and measurement techniques that can be employed years after the study is completed.

The growing interest in **translational research** (Chapter 2) takes advantage of new measurements that have greatly expanded clinical research in the areas of **genetic and molecular epidemiology** (4,5). Measurements on specimens that contain DNA (e.g., saliva, blood) can provide information on genotypes that contribute to the

TABLE 4.5	Common Types of Measurements that Can Be Made on Stored Materials	
Type of Measurement	**Examples**	**Bank for Later Measurement**
Medical history	Diagnoses, medications, operations, symptoms, physical findings	Clinical charts
Psychosocial factors	Depression, family history	Voice recordings, videotapes
Anthropometric	Height, weight, body composition	Photographs
Biochemical measures	Serum cholesterol, plasma fibrinogen	Serum, plasma, urine, pathology specimens
Genetic/molecular tests	Single neucleotide polymorphisms, human leukocyte antigen type	DNA, immortal cell line
Imaging	Bone density, coronary calcium	X-rays, CT scans, MRI
Electromechanical	Arrhythmia, congenital heart disease	Electrocardiogram, echocardiogram

occurrence of disease or modify a patient's response to treatment. Measurements on serum can be used to study molecular causes or consequences of disease; for example, proteomic patterns may provide useful information for diagnosing certain diseases (6). It is important to consult with experts regarding the proper collection tubes and storage conditions in order to preserve the quality of the specimens and make them available for the widest spectrum of subsequent use.

IN CLOSING

Table 4.5 reviews the many kinds of measurements that can be included in a study. Some of these are the topic of later chapters in this book. In Chapter 9 we will address the issue of choosing measurements that will facilitate inferences about confounding and causality. And in Chapter 15 we will address the topic of questionnaires and other instruments for measuring information supplied by the study subject.

In designing measurements it is important to keep in mind the value of **efficiency** and **parsimony.** The full set of measurements should collect useful data at an affordable cost in time and money. Efficiency can be improved by increasing the quality of each item and by reducing the number of items measured. Collecting more data than are needed is a common error that can tire subjects, overwhelm the research team, and clutter data management and analysis. The result may be a more expensive study that paradoxically is less successful in answering the main research questions.

SUMMARY

1. Variables are either **continuous** (quantified on an infinite scale), **discrete** (quantified on a finite scale of integers), or **categorical** (classified in categories). Categorical variables are further classified as **nominal** (unordered) or **ordinal** (ordered); those that have only two categories are termed **dichotomous.**

2. Clinical investigators **prefer variables that contain more information** and thereby provide greater power and/or smaller sample sizes: continuous variables > discrete variables > ordered categorical variables > nominal and dichotomous variables.

3. The **precision** of a measurement (i.e., the reproducibility of replicate measures) is another major determinant of power and sample size. Precision is reduced by **random error** (chance) from three sources of variability: the observer, the subject, and the instrument.

4. Strategies for **increasing precision** that should be part of every study are to **operationally define** and **standardize methods** in an **operations manual,** and to **train** and **certify observers.** Other strategies that are often useful are **refining** the instruments, **automating** the instruments, and using the mean of **repeated measurements.**

5. The **accuracy** of a measurement (i.e., the degree to which it actually measures the characteristic it is supposed to measure) is a major key to inferring correct conclusions. **Validity** is a form of accuracy commonly used for abstract variables.

Accuracy is reduced by **systematic error** (i.e., bias) from the same three sources: the observer, the subject, and the instrument.

6. The **strategies for increasing accuracy** include all those listed for precision with the exception of repetition. In addition, accuracy is enhanced by **unobtrusive measures,** by **calibration,** and (in comparisons between groups) by **blinding.**

7. Individual measurements should be **sensitive, specific, appropriate,** and **objective,** and they should produce a **range of values.** In the aggregate, they should be broad but **parsimonious,** serving the research question at moderate cost in time and money.

8. Investigators should consider **storing banks of materials** for later measurements that can take advantage of new technologies and the efficiency of nested case–control designs.

APPENDIX 4.1

Operations Manual: Operational Definition of a Measurement of Grip Strength

The operations manual describes the method for conducting and recording the results of all the measurements made in the study. This example, from the operations manual of the Study of Osteoporotic Fractures, describes the use of a dynamometer to measure grip strength. To standardize instructions from examiner to examiner and from subject to subject, the protocol includes a script of instructions to be read to the participant verbatim.

Protocol for Measuring Grip Strength with the Dynamometer
Grip strength will be measured in both hands. The handle should be adjusted so that the participant holds the dynamometer comfortably. Place the dynamometer in the right hand with the dial facing the palm. The participant's arm should be flexed $90°$ at the elbow with the forearm parallel to the floor.

1. Demonstrate the test to the subject. While demonstrating, use the following description: "This device measures your arm and upper body strength. We will measure your grip strength in both arms. I will demonstrate how it is done. Bend your elbow at a $90°$ angle, with your forearm parallel to the floor. Don't let your arm touch the side of your body. Lower the device and squeeze as hard as you can while I count to three. Once your arm is fully extended, you can loosen your grip."
2. Allow one practice trial for each arm, starting with the right if she is right handed. On the second trial, record the kilograms of force from the dial to the nearest 0.5 kg.
3. Reset the dial. Repeat the procedure for the other arm.

   The arm should not contact the body. The gripping action should be a slow, sustained squeeze rather than an explosive jerk.

REFERENCES

1. Ware JE, Gandek B Jr. Overview of the SF-36 health survey and the International Quality of Life Assessment (IQOLA) Project. *Clin Epidemic* 1998;51:903–912.
2. Bland JM, Altman DG. Measurement error and correlation coefficients. *BMJ* 1996;313: 41–42; also, Measurement error proportional to the mean. *BMJ* 1996;313:106.
3. Cohen J. A coefficient of agreement for nominal scales. *Educ Psychol Meas* 1960;20:37–46.
4. Guttmacher AE, Collins FS. Genomic medicine: a primer. *NEJM* 2002;347:1512–1520.
5. Healy DG. Case-control studies in the genomic era: a clinician's guide. *http://neurology. thelancet.com.* 2006;5:701–707.
6. Liotta LA, Ferrari M, Petricoin E. Written in blood. *Nature* 2003;425:905.

5 Getting Ready to Estimate Sample Size: Hypotheses and Underlying Principles

Warren S. Browner, Thomas B. Newman, and Stephen B. Hulley

After an investigator has decided whom and what she is going to study and the design to be used, she must decide how many subjects to sample. Even the most rigorously executed study may fail to answer its research question if the sample size is too small. On the other hand, a study with too large a sample will be more difficult and costly than necessary. The goal of sample size planning is to estimate an **appropriate number** of subjects for a given study design.

Although a useful guide, sample size calculations give a deceptive impression of statistical objectivity. They are only as accurate as the data and estimates on which they are based, which are often just informed guesses. Sample size planning is a mathematical way of making a ballpark estimate. It often reveals that the research design is not feasible or that different predictor or outcome variables are needed. Therefore, sample size should be estimated early in the design phase of a study, when major changes are still possible.

Before setting out the specific approaches to calculating sample size for several common research designs in Chapter 6, we will spend some time considering the underlying principles. Readers who find some of these principles confusing will enjoy discovering that sample size planning does not require their total mastery. However, just as a recipe makes more sense if the cook is somewhat familiar with the ingredients, sample size calculations are easier if the investigator is acquainted with the basic concepts.

HYPOTHESES

The **research hypothesis** is a specific version of the research question that summarizes the main elements of the study—the sample, and the predictor and outcome variables—in a form that establishes the basis for tests of statistical significance. Hypotheses are not needed in descriptive studies, which describe how characteristics are distributed in a population, such as a study of the prevalence of a particular genotype among patients with hip fractures. (That does not mean, however, that you won't need to do a sample size estimate for a descriptive study, just that the methods for doing so, described in Chapter 6, are different). Hypotheses are needed for studies that will use tests of statistical significance to compare findings among groups, such as a study of whether that particular genotype is more common among patients with hip fractures than among controls. Because most observational studies and all experiments address research questions that involve making comparisons, most studies need to specify at least one hypothesis. If any of the following terms appear in the research question, then the study is not simply descriptive, and a hypothesis should be formulated: greater than, less than, causes, leads to, compared with, more likely than, associated with, related to, similar to, correlated with.

Characteristics of a Good Hypothesis
A good hypothesis must be based on a good research question. It should also be simple, specific, and stated in advance.

Simple versus Complex.   A simple hypothesis contains one predictor and one outcome variable:

> *A sedentary lifestyle is associated with an increased risk of proteinuria in patients with diabetes*

A complex hypothesis contains more than one predictor variable:

> *A sedentary lifestyle and alcohol consumption are associated with an increased risk of proteinuria in patients with diabetes*

Or more than one outcome variable:

> *Alcohol consumption is associated with an increased risk of proteinuria and of neuropathy in patients with diabetes*

Complex hypotheses like these are not readily tested with a single statistical test and are more easily approached as two or more simple hypotheses. Sometimes, however, a combined predictor or outcome variable can be used:

> *Alcohol consumption is associated with an increased risk of developing a microvascular complication of diabetes (i.e., proteinuria, neuropathy, or retinopathy) in patients with diabetes.*

In this example the investigator has decided that what matters is whether a participant has a complication, not what type of complication occurs.

Specific versus Vague.   A specific hypothesis leaves no ambiguity about the subjects and variables or about how the test of statistical significance will be applied. It uses concise operational definitions that summarize the nature and source of the subjects and how variables will be measured.

> *Use of tricyclic antidepressant medications, assessed with pharmacy records, is more common in patients hospitalized with an admission diagnosis of myocardial infarction at Longview Hospital in the past year than in controls hospitalized for pneumonia.*

This is a long sentence, but it communicates the nature of the study in a clear way that minimizes any opportunity for testing something a little different once the study findings have been examined. It would be incorrect to substitute, during the analysis phase of the study, a different measurement of the predictor, such as the self-reported use of pills for depression, without considering the issue of multiple hypothesis testing (a topic we discuss at the end of the chapter). Usually, to keep the research hypothesis concise, some of these details are made explicit in the study plan rather than being stated in the research hypothesis. But they should always be clear in the investigator's conception of the study, and spelled out in the protocol.

It is often obvious from the research hypothesis whether the predictor variable and the outcome variable are dichotomous, continuous, or categorical. If it is not clear, then the type of variables can be specified:

> *Alcohol consumption (in mg/day) is associated with an increased risk of proteinuria (>300 mg/day) in patients with diabetes.*

If the research hypothesis begins to get too cumbersome, the definitions can be left out, as long as they are clarified elsewhere in the protocol.

In-Advance versus After-the-Fact.   The hypothesis should be stated in writing at the outset of the study. Most important, this will keep the research effort focused on the primary objective. A single prestated hypothesis also creates a stronger basis for interpreting the study results than several hypotheses that emerge as a result of inspecting the data. Hypotheses that are formulated after examination of the data are a form of multiple hypothesis testing that can lead to overinterpreting the importance of the findings.

Types of Hypotheses

For the purpose of testing statistical significance, the research hypothesis must be restated in forms that categorize the expected difference between the study groups.

- *Null and alternative hypotheses.* The **null hypothesis** states that there is no association between the predictor and outcome variables in the population (*there is no difference in the frequency of drinking well water between subjects who develop peptic ulcer disease and those who do not*). The null hypothesis is the formal basis for testing statistical significance. Assuming that there really is no association in the population, statistical tests help to estimate the probability that an association observed in a study is due to chance.
- The proposition that there *is* an association (*the frequency of drinking well water is different in subjects who develop peptic ulcer disease than in those who do not*) is called the **alternative hypothesis.** The alternative hypothesis cannot be tested directly; it is accepted by default if the test of statistical significance rejects the null hypothesis (see later).
- *One- and two-sided alternative hypotheses.* A one-sided hypothesis specifies the direction of the association between the predictor and outcome variables. The hypothesis that drinking well water is more common among subjects who develop peptic ulcers is a one-sided hypothesis. A two-sided hypothesis states only that an association exists; it does not specify the direction. The hypothesis that subjects who develop peptic ulcer disease have a different frequency of drinking well water than those who do not is a two-sided hypothesis.

One-sided hypotheses may be appropriate in selected circumstances, such as when only one direction for an association is clinically important or biologically meaningful. An example is the one-sided hypothesis that a new drug for hypertension is more likely to cause rashes than a placebo; the possibility that the drug causes fewer rashes than the placebo is not usually worth testing (it might be if the drug had anti-inflammatory properties!). A one-sided hypothesis may also be appropriate when there is very strong evidence from prior studies that an association is unlikely to occur in one of the two directions, such as a study that tested whether cigarette smoking affects the risk of brain cancer. Because smoking has been associated with an increased risk of many different types of cancers, a one-sided alternative hypothesis (e.g., *that smoking increases the risk of brain cancer*) might suffice. However, investigators should be aware that many well-supported hypotheses (e.g., *that β-carotene therapy will reduce the risk of lung cancer, or that treatment with drugs that reduce the number of ventricular ectopic beats will reduce sudden death among patients with ventricular arrhythmias*) turn out to be wrong when tested in randomized trials. Indeed, in these two examples, the results of well-done trials revealed a statistically significant effect that was opposite in direction from the one supported by previous data (1–3). Overall, we believe that nearly all alternative hypotheses deserve to be two-sided.

It is important to keep in mind the difference between a **research hypothesis,** which is often one-sided, and the alternative hypothesis that is used when planning sample size, which is almost always two-sided. For example, suppose the research hypothesis is that recurrent use of antibiotics during childhood is associated with an increased risk of inflammatory bowel disease. That hypothesis specifies the direction of the anticipated effect, so it is one-sided. Why use a two-sided alternative hypothesis when planning the sample size? The answer is that most of the time, both sides of the alternative hypothesis (i.e., greater risk or lesser risk) are interesting, and the investigators would want to publish the results no matter which direction was observed. Statistical rigor requires the investigator choose between one- and two-sided hypotheses before analyzing the data; switching to a one-sided alternative hypothesis to reduce the *P* value (see below) is not correct. In addition (and this is probably the real reason that two-sided alternative hypotheses are much more common), most grant and manuscript reviewers expect two-sided hypotheses, and are critical of a one-sided approach.

UNDERLYING STATISTICAL PRINCIPLES

A hypothesis, such as that *15 minutes or more of exercise per day is associated with a lower mean fasting blood glucose level in middle-aged women with diabetes,* is either true or false in the real world. Because an investigator cannot study all middle-aged women with diabetes, she must test the hypothesis in a sample of that target population. As noted in Figure 1.6, there will always be a need to draw inferences about phenomena in the population from events observed in the sample.

In some ways, the investigator's problem is similar to that faced by a jury judging a defendant (Table 5.1). The absolute truth about whether the defendant committed the crime cannot usually be determined. Instead, the jury begins by presuming innocence: the defendant did not commit the crime. The jury must decide whether there is sufficient evidence to reject the presumed innocence of the defendant; the standard is known as **beyond a reasonable doubt.** A jury can err, however, by convicting an innocent defendant or by failing to convict a guilty one.

TABLE 5.1	The Analogy between Jury Decisions and Statistical Tests
Jury Decision	**Statistical Test**
Innocence: The defendant did not counterfeit money.	**Null hypothesis:** There is no association between dietary carotene and the incidence of colon cancer in the population.
Guilt: The defendant did counterfeit money.	**Alternative hypothesis:** There is an association between dietary carotene and the incidence of colon cancer.
Standard for rejecting innocence: Beyond a reasonable doubt.	**Standard for rejecting null hypothesis:** Level of statistical significance (α).
Correct judgment: Convict a counterfeiter.	**Correct inference:** Conclude that there is an association between dietary carotene and colon cancer when one does exist in the population.
Correct judgment: Acquit an innocent person.	**Correct inference:** Conclude that there is no association between carotene and colon cancer when one does not exist.
Incorrect judgment: Convict an innocent person.	**Incorrect inference (type I error):** Conclude that there is an association between dietary carotene and colon cancer when there actually is none.
Incorrect judgment: Acquit a counterfeiter.	**Incorrect inference (type II error):** Conclude that there is no association between dietary carotene and colon cancer when there actually is one.

In similar fashion, the investigator starts by presuming the null hypothesis of no association between the predictor and outcome variables in the population. Based on the data collected in her sample, the investigator uses statistical tests to determine whether there is sufficient evidence to reject the null hypothesis in favor of the alternative hypothesis that there is an association in the population. The standard for these tests is known as the **level of statistical significance.**

Type I and Type II Errors

Like a jury, an investigator may reach a wrong conclusion. Sometimes by chance alone a sample is not representative of the population and the results in the sample do not reflect reality in the population, leading to an erroneous inference. A **type I error** (false-positive) occurs if an investigator rejects a null hypothesis that is actually true in the population; a **type II error** (false-negative) occurs if the investigator fails to reject a null hypothesis that is actually not true in the population. Although type I and type II errors can never be avoided entirely, the investigator can reduce their likelihood by increasing the sample size (the larger the sample, the less likely that it will differ substantially from the population) or by manipulating the design or the measurements in other ways that we will discuss.

In this chapter and the next, we deal only with ways to reduce type I and type II errors due to **chance** variation, also known as random error. False-positive and false-negative results can also occur because of **bias,** but errors due to bias are not usually referred to as type I and II errors. Such errors are especially troublesome, because they may be difficult to detect and cannot usually be quantified using statistical methods or avoided by increasing the sample size. (See Chapters 1, 3, 4, and 7 through 12 for ways to reduce errors due to bias.)

Effect Size

The likelihood that a study will be able to detect an association between a predictor and an outcome variable in a sample depends on the actual magnitude of that association in the population. If it is large (*mean fasting blood glucose levels are 20 mg/dL lower in diabetic women who exercise than in those who do not*), it will be easy to detect in the sample. Conversely, if the size of the association is small (*a difference of 2 mg/dL*), it will be difficult to detect in the sample.

Unfortunately, the investigator does not usually know the exact size of the association; one of the purposes of the study is to estimate it! Instead, the investigator must choose the size of the association that she expects to be present in the sample. That quantity is known as the **effect size.** Selecting an appropriate effect size is the most difficult aspect of sample size planning (4). The investigator should first try to find data from prior studies in related areas to make an informed guess about a reasonable effect size. When data are not available, it may be necessary to do a small pilot study. Alternatively, she can choose the smallest effect size that in her opinion would be clinically meaningful (*a 10 mg/dL reduction in the fasting glucose level*).

Of course, from the public health point of view, even a reduction of 2 or 3 mg/dL in fasting glucose levels might be important, especially if it was easy to achieve. The choice of the effect size is always arbitrary, and considerations of feasibility are often paramount. Indeed, when the number of available or affordable subjects is limited, the investigator may have to work backward (Chapter 6) to determine the effect size that her study will be able to detect.

There are many different ways to measure the size of an association, especially when the outcome variable is dichotomous. For example, consider a study of whether middle-aged men are more likely to have impaired hearing than middle-aged women. Suppose an investigator finds that 20% of women and 30% of men 50 to 65 years of age are hard of hearing. These results could be interpreted as showing that men are 10% more likely to have impaired hearing than women (30% − 20%, the absolute difference), or 50% more likely ([30% − 20%] ÷ 20%, the relative difference). For sample size planning, both of the proportions matter; the sample size tables in this book use the smaller proportion (in this case, 20%) and the absolute difference (10%) between the groups being compared.

Many studies measure several effect sizes, because they measure several different predictor and outcome variables. For sample size planning, the sample size using the desired effect size for the most important hypothesis should be determined; the effect sizes for the other hypotheses can then be estimated. If there are several hypotheses of similar importance, then the sample size for the study should be based on whichever hypothesis needs the largest sample.

α, β, and Power

After a study is completed, the investigator uses statistical tests to try to reject the null hypothesis in favor of its alternative, in much the same way that a prosecuting attorney tries to convince a jury to reject innocence in favor of guilt. Depending on whether the null hypothesis is true or false in the target population, and assuming that the study is free of bias, four situations are possible (Table 5.2). In two of these, the findings in the sample and reality in the population are concordant, and the

TABLE 5.2	Truth in the Population versus the Results in the Study Sample: The Four Possibilities

	Truth in the Population	
Results in the Study Sample	**Association Between Predictor and Outcome**	**No Association Between Predictor and Outcome**
Reject null hypothesis	Correct	Type I error
Fail to reject null hypothesis	Type II error	Correct

investigator's inference will be correct. In the other two situations, either a type I or type II error has been made, and the inference will be incorrect.

The investigator establishes the maximum chance that she will tolerate of making type I and II errors in advance of the study. The probability of committing a type I error (rejecting the null hypothesis when it is actually true) is called α (**alpha**). Another name for α is the **level of statistical significance.**

If, for example, a study of the effects of exercise on fasting blood glucose levels is designed with an α of 0.05, then the investigator has set 5% as the maximum chance of incorrectly rejecting the null hypothesis if it is true (and inferring that exercise and fasting blood glucose levels are associated in the population when, in fact, they are not). This is the level of reasonable doubt that the investigator will be willing to accept when she uses statistical tests to analyze the data after the study is completed.

The probability of making a type II error (failing to reject the null hypothesis when it is actually false) is called β (**beta**). The quantity $[1 - \beta]$ is called **power,** the probability of correctly rejecting the null hypothesis in the sample if the actual effect in the population is equal to (or greater than) the effect size.

If β is set at 0.10, then the investigator has decided that she is willing to accept a 10% chance of missing an association of a given effect size if it exists. This represents a power of 0.90; that is, a 90% chance of finding an association of that size or greater. For example, suppose that exercise really would lead to an average reduction of 20 mg/dL in fasting glucose levels among diabetic women in the entire population. Suppose that the investigator drew a sample of women from the population on numerous occasions, each time carrying out the same study (with the same measurements and the same 90% power each time). Then in nine of every ten studies the investigator would correctly reject the null hypothesis and conclude that exercise is associated with fasting glucose level. This does not mean, however, that the investigator doing a single study will be unable to detect it if the effect actually present in the population was smaller, say, a 15 mg/dL reduction; it means simply that she will have less than a 90% likelihood of doing so.

Ideally, α and β would be set at zero, eliminating the possibility of false-positive and false-negative results. In practice they are made as small as possible. Reducing them, however, requires increasing the sample size; other strategies are discussed in Chapter 6. Sample size planning aims at choosing a sufficient number of subjects to keep α and β at an acceptably low level without making the study unnecessarily expensive or difficult.

Many studies set α at 0.05 and β at 0.20 (a power of 0.80). These are arbitrary values, and others are sometimes used: the conventional range for α is between 0.01 and 0.10, and that for β is between 0.05 and 0.20. In general, the investigator should use a low α when the research question makes it particularly important to avoid a type I (false-positive) error—for example, in testing the efficacy of a potentially dangerous medication. She should use a low β (and a small effect size) when it is especially important to avoid a type II (false-negative) error—for example, in reassuring the public that living near a toxic waste dump is safe.

P Value

The null hypothesis acts like a straw man: it is assumed to be true so that it can be knocked down as false with a statistical test. When the data are analyzed, such tests determine the **P value,** the probability of seeing an effect as big as or bigger than that in the study by chance if the null hypothesis actually were true. The null hypothesis is rejected in favor of its alternative if the P value is less than α, the predetermined level of statistical significance.

A "nonsignificant" result (i.e., one with a P value greater than α) does not mean that there is no association in the population; it only means that the result observed in the sample is small compared with what could have occurred by chance alone. For example, an investigator might find that men with hypertension were twice as likely to develop prostate cancer as those with normal blood pressure, but because the number of cancers in the study was modest this apparent effect had a P value of only 0.08. This means that even if hypertension and prostatic carcinoma were not associated in the population, there would be an 8% chance of finding such an association due to random error in the sample. If the investigator had set the significance level as a two-sided α of 0.05, she would have to conclude that the association in the sample was "not statistically significant." It might be tempting for the investigator to change her mind about the level of statistical significance, reset the two-sided α to 0.10, and report, "The results showed a statistically significant association ($P < 0.10$)," or switch to a one-sided P value and report it as "$P = 0.04$." A better choice would be to report that "The results, although suggestive of an association, did not achieve statistical significance ($P = 0.08$)."

This solution acknowledges that statistical significance is not an all-or-none situation. In part because of this problem, many statisticians and epidemiologists are moving away from hypothesis testing, with its emphasis on P values, to using confidence intervals to report the precision of the study results (5–7). However, for the purposes of sample size planning for analytic studies, hypothesis testing is still the standard.

Sides of the Alternative Hypothesis

Recall that an alternative hypothesis actually has two sides, either or both of which can be tested in the sample by using **one-** or **two-sided statistical tests.** When a two-sided statistical test is used, the P value includes the probabilities of committing a type I error in each of two directions, which is about twice as great as the probability in either direction alone. It is easy to convert from a one-sided P value to a two-sided P value, and vice versa. A one-sided P value of 0.05, for example, is usually the same as a two-sided P value of 0.10. (Some statistical tests are asymmetric, which is why we said "usually.")

In those rare situations in which an investigator is only interested in one of the sides and has so formulated the alternative hypothesis, sample size should be calculated accordingly. A one-sided hypothesis should never be used just to reduce the sample size.

Type of Statistical Test

The formulas used to calculate sample size are based on mathematical assumptions, which differ for each statistical test. Before the sample size can be calculated, the investigator must decide on the statistical approach to analyzing the data. That choice depends mainly on the type of predictor and outcome variables in the study. Table 6.1 lists some common statistics used in data analysis, and Chapter 6 provides simplified approaches to estimating sample size for studies that use these statistics.

ADDITIONAL POINTS

Variability

It is not simply the size of an effect that is important; its variability also matters. Statistical tests depend on being able to show a difference between the groups being compared. The greater the variability (or spread) in the outcome variable among the subjects, the more likely it is that the values in the groups will overlap, and the more difficult it will be to demonstrate an overall difference between them. Because measurement error contributes to the overall variability, less precise measurements require larger sample sizes (8).

Consider a study of the effects of two isocaloric diets (low fat and low carbohydrate) in achieving weight loss in 20 obese patients. If all those on the low-fat diet lost about 3 kg and all those on the low-carbohydrate diet failed to lose much weight (an effect size of 3 kg), it is likely that the low-fat diet really is better (Fig. 5.1A). On the other hand, suppose that although the average weight loss is 3 kg in the low-fat group and 0 kg in the low-carbohydrate group, there is a great deal of overlap between the two groups. (The changes in weight vary from a loss of 8 kg to a gain of 8 kg.) In this situation (Fig. 5.1B), although the effect size is still 3 kg, the greater variability will make it more difficult to detect a difference between the diets, and a larger sample size will be needed.

When one of the variables used in the sample size estimate is continuous (e.g., body weight in Figure 5.1), the investigator will need to estimate its variability. (See the section on the t test in Chapter 6 for details.) In the other situations, variability is already included in the other parameters entered into the sample size formulas and tables, and need not be specified.

Multiple and Post Hoc Hypotheses

When more than one hypothesis is tested in a study, especially if some of those hypotheses were formulated after the data were analyzed (*post hoc* hypotheses), the likelihood that at least one will achieve statistical significance on the basis of chance alone increases. For example, if 20 independent hypotheses are tested at an α of 0.05, the likelihood is substantial (64%; $[1 - 0.95^{20}]$) that at least one hypothesis will be statistically significant by chance alone. Some statisticians advocate adjusting the level of statistical significance when more than one hypothesis is tested in a study. This keeps the overall probability of accepting any one of the alternative hypotheses, when all the findings are due to chance, at the specified level. For example, genomic studies that look for an association between hundreds (or even thousands) of genotypes and a disease need to use a much smaller α than 0.05, or they risk identifying many false-positive associations.

One approach, named after the mathematician **Bonferroni,** is to divide the significance level (say, 0.05) by the number of hypotheses tested. If there were four

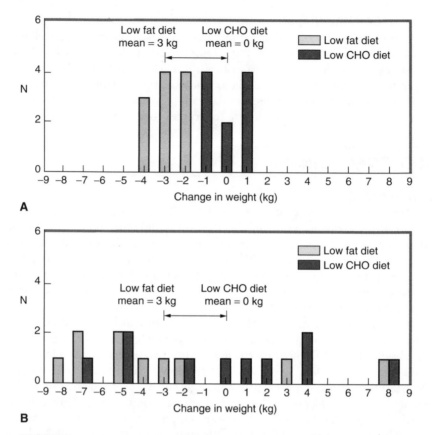

FIGURE 5.1. **A:** Weight loss achieved by two diets. All subjects on the low-fat diet lost from 2 to 4 kg, whereas weight change in those on the low-carbohydrate (CHO) diet varied from −1 to +1 kg. Because there is no overlap between the two groups, it is reasonable to infer that the low-fat diet is better at achieving weight loss than the low-carbohydrate diet (as would be confirmed with a t test, which has a P value < 0.0001). **B:** Weight loss achieved by two diets. There is substantial overlap in weight change in the two groups. Although the effect size is the same (3 kg) as in **A,** there is little evidence that one diet is better than the other (as would be confirmed with a t test, which has a P value of 0.19).

hypotheses, for example, each would be tested at an α of 0.0125 (i.e., 0.05 ÷ 4). This would require substantially increasing the sample size over that needed for testing each hypothesis at an α of 0.05.

We believe that a Bonferroni-type of approach to **multiple hypothesis** testing is usually too stringent. Investigators do not adjust the significance levels for hypotheses that are tested in separate studies. Why do so when several hypotheses are tested in the same study? In our view, adjusting α for multiple hypotheses is chiefly useful when the likelihood of making false-positive errors is high, because the number of tested hypotheses is substantial (say, more than ten) and the prior probability for each hypothesis is low (e.g., in screening a large number of genes for association with a phenotype). The first criterion is actually stricter than it may appear, because what matters is the number of hypotheses that are *tested*, not the number that are *reported*. Testing 50 hypotheses but only reporting or emphasizing the one or two P values that are less than 0.05 is misleading. Adjusting α for multiple hypotheses is especially important when the consequences of making a false-positive error are large, such as mistakenly concluding that an ineffective treatment is beneficial.

In general, the issue of what significance level to use depends more on the **prior probability** of each hypothesis than on the number of hypotheses tested. There is an analogy with the use of diagnostic tests that may be helpful (9). When interpreting the results of a diagnostic test, a clinician considers the likelihood that the patient being tested has the disease in question. For example, a modestly abnormal test result in a healthy person (a serum alkaline phosphatase level that is 15% greater than the upper limit of normal) is probably a false-positive test that is unlikely to have much clinical importance. Similarly, a P value of 0.05 for an unlikely hypothesis is probably also a false-positive result.

However, an alkaline phosphatase level that is 10 or 20 times greater than the upper limit of normal is unlikely to have occurred by chance (although it might be a laboratory error). So too a very small P value (say, <0.001) is unlikely to have occurred by chance (although it could be due to bias). It is hard to dismiss very abnormal test results as being false-positives or to dismiss very low P values as being due to chance, even if the prior probability of the disease or the hypothesis was low.

Moreover, the number of tests that were ordered, or hypotheses that were tested, is not always relevant. The interpretation of an elevated serum uric acid level in a patient with a painful and swollen joint should not depend on whether the physician ordered just a single test (the uric acid level) or obtained the result as part of a panel of 20 tests. Similarly, when interpreting the P value for testing a research hypothesis that makes good sense, it should not matter that the investigator also tested several unlikely hypotheses. What matters most is the reasonableness of the research hypothesis being tested: that it has a substantial prior probability of being correct. (Prior probability, in this **"Bayesian"** approach, is usually a subjective judgment based on evidence from other sources.) Hypotheses that are formulated during the design of a study usually meet this requirement; after all, why else would the investigator put the time and effort into planning and doing the study?

What about unanticipated associations that appear during the collection and analysis of a study's results? This process is sometimes called **hypothesis generation** or, less favorably, "data-mining" or a "fishing expedition." The many informal comparisons that are made during data analysis are a form of multiple hypothesis testing. A similar problem arises when variables are redefined during data analysis, or when results are presented for subgroups of the sample. Significant P values for data-generated hypotheses that were not considered during the design of the study are often due to chance. They should be viewed with interest but skepticism and considered a fertile source of potential research questions for future studies.

Sometimes, however, an investigator fails to specify a particular hypothesis in advance, although that hypothesis seems reasonable when it is time for the data to be analyzed. This might happen, for example, if others discover a new risk factor while the study is going on, or if the investigator just didn't happen to think of a particular hypothesis when the study was being designed. The important issue is not so much whether the hypothesis was formulated before the study began, but whether there is a reasonable prior probability based on evidence from other sources that the hypothesis is true (9).

There are some definite **advantages** to formulating more than one hypothesis when planning a study. The use of multiple unrelated hypotheses increases the efficiency of the study, making it possible to answer more questions with a single research effort and to discover more of the true associations that exist in the population. It may also be a good idea to formulate several **related hypotheses;** if the findings are consistent, the study conclusions are made stronger. Studies in patients with heart failure have found that the use of angiotensin-converting enzyme inhibitors is beneficial in reducing cardiac admissions, cardiovascular mortality, and total mortality. Had only one of these hypotheses been tested, the inferences from these studies would have been less definitive. Lunch may not be free, however, when multiple hypotheses are tested. Suppose that when these related and prestated hypotheses are tested, only one turns out to be statistically significant. Then the investigator must decide (and try to convince editors and readers) whether the significant results, the nonsignificant results, or both sets of results are true.

Primary and Secondary Hypotheses

Some studies, especially large randomized trials, specify some hypotheses as being "**secondary.**" This usually happens when there is one **primary hypothesis** around which the study has been designed, but the investigators are also interested in other research questions that are of lesser importance. For example, the primary outcome of a trial of zinc supplementation might be hospitalizations or emergency department visits for upper respiratory tract infections; a secondary outcome might be self-reported days missed from work or school. If the study is being done to obtain approval for a pharmaceutical agent, the primary outcome is what will matter most to the regulatory body. The sample size calculations are always focused on the primary hypothesis, and secondary hypotheses with insufficient power should be avoided. Stating a secondary hypothesis in advance does increase the credibility of the results. Stating a secondary hypothesis after the data have been collected and analyzed is another form of data dredging.

A good rule, particularly for clinical trials, is to establish in advance as many hypotheses as make sense, but specify just one as the **primary hypothesis,** which can be tested statistically without argument about whether to adjust for multiple hypothesis testing. More important, having a primary hypothesis helps to focus the study on its main objective and provides a clear basis for the main sample size calculation.

SUMMARY

1. **Sample size planning** is an important part of the design of both analytic and descriptive studies. The sample size should be estimated early in the process of developing the research design, so that appropriate modifications can be made.

2. Analytic studies and experiments need a **hypothesis** that specifies, for the purpose of subsequent **statistical tests,** the anticipated association between the main predictor and outcome variables. Purely descriptive studies, lacking the strategy of comparison, do not require a hypothesis.

3. Good hypotheses are **specific** about how the population will be sampled and the variables measured, **simple** (there is only one predictor and one outcome variable), and **formulated in advance.**

4. The **null hypothesis,** which proposes that the predictor and outcome variables are not associated, is the basis for tests of statistical significance. The **alternative**

hypothesis proposes that they are associated. Statistical tests attempt to reject the null hypothesis of no association in favor of the alternative hypothesis that there is an association.

5. An alternative hypothesis is either **one-sided** (only one direction of association will be tested) or **two-sided** (both directions will be tested). One-sided hypotheses should only be used in unusual circumstances, when only one direction of the association is clinically or biologically meaningful.

6. For analytic studies and experiments, the sample size is an estimate of the number of subjects required to detect an association of a given **effect size** and **variability** at a specified likelihood of making **type I** (false-positive) and **type II** (false-negative) **errors.** The maximum likelihood of making a type I error is called α; that of making a type II error, β. The quantity $(1 - \beta)$ is **power,** the chance of observing an association of a given effect size or greater in a sample if one is actually present in the population.

7. It is often desirable to establish more than one hypothesis in advance, but the investigator should specify a single **primary hypothesis** as a focus and for sample size estimation. Interpretation of findings from testing **multiple hypotheses** in the sample, including unanticipated findings that emerge from the data, is based on a judgment about the **prior probability** that they represent real phenomena in the population.

REFERENCES

1. The Alpha-Tocopherol, Beta Carotene Cancer Prevention Study Group. The effect of vitamin E and beta carotene on the incidence of lung cancer and other cancers in male smokers. *N Engl J Med* 1994;330:1029–1035.
2. Echt DS, Liebson PR, Mitchell LB, et al. Mortality and morbidity in patients receiving encainide, flecainide, or placebo. The Cardiac Arrhythmia Suppression Trial. *N Engl J Med* 1991;324:781–788.
3. The Cardiac Arrhythmia Suppression Trial II Investigators. Effect of the antiarrhythmic agent moricizine on survival after myocardial infarction. *N Engl J Med* 1992;327:227–233.
4. Van Walraven C, Mahon JL, Moher D, et al. Surveying physicians to determine the minimal important difference: implications for sample-size calculation. *J Clin Epidemiol* 1999;52: 717–723.
5. Daly LE. Confidence limits made easy: interval estimation using a substitution method. *Am J Epidemiol* 1998;147:783–790.
6. Goodman SN. Toward evidence-based medical statistics. 1: The *P* value fallacy. *Ann Intern Med* 1999;130:995–1004.
7. Goodman SN. Toward evidence-based medical statistics. 2: The Bayes factor. *Ann Intern Med* 1999;130:1005–1013.
8. McKeown-Eyssen GE, Tibshirani R. Implications of measurement error in exposure for the sample sizes of case-control studies. *Am J Epidemiol* 1994;139:415–421.
9. Browner WS, Newman TB. Are all significant *P* values created equal? The analogy between diagnostic tests and clinical research. *JAMA* 1987;257:2459–2463.

Estimating Sample Size and Power: Applications and Examples

Warren S. Browner, Thomas B. Newman, and Stephen B. Hulley

Chapter 5 introduced the basic principles underlying sample size calculations. This chapter presents several cookbook techniques for using those principles to estimate the sample size needed for a research project. The first section deals with sample size estimates for an analytic study or experiment, including some special issues that apply to these studies such as multivariate analysis. The second section considers studies that are primarily descriptive. Subsequent sections deal with studies that have a fixed sample size, strategies for maximizing the power of a study, and how to estimate the sample size when there appears to be insufficient information from which to work. The chapter concludes with common errors to avoid.

At the end of the chapter, there are tables and formulas in the appendixes for several basic methods of estimating sample size. In addition, there is a calculator on our website (www.epibiostat.ucsf.edu/dcr/), and there are many sites on the Web that can provide instant interactive sample size calculations; try searching for "sample size" *and* "power" *and* "interactive". Most statistical packages can also estimate sample size for common study designs.

SAMPLE SIZE TECHNIQUES FOR ANALYTIC STUDIES AND EXPERIMENTS

There are several variations on the recipe for estimating sample size in an analytic study or experiment, but they all have certain steps in common:

1. State the **null hypothesis** and either a **one-** or **two-sided alternative hypothesis.**
2. Select the appropriate **statistical test** from Table 6.1 based on the type of predictor variable and outcome variable in those hypotheses.
3. Choose a reasonable **effect size** (and **variability,** if necessary).

TABLE 6.1	Simple Statistical Tests for Use in Estimating Sample Size*	

| | Outcome Variable | |
Predictor Variable	**Dichotomous**	**Continuous**
Dichotomous	Chi-squared test[†]	t test
Continuous	t test	Correlation coefficient

* See text for what to do about ordinal variables, or if planning to analyze the data with another type of statistical test.
[†] The chi-squared test is always two-sided; a one-sided equivalent is the Z statistic.

4. Set α and β. (Specify a two-sided α unless the alternative hypothesis is clearly one-sided.)
5. Use the appropriate table or formula in the appendix to estimate the sample size.

Even if the exact value for one or more of the ingredients is uncertain, it is important to estimate the sample size early in the design phase. Waiting until the last minute to prepare the sample size can be a rude awakening: it may be necessary to start over with new ingredients, which may mean redesigning the entire study. This is why this subject is covered early in this book.

Not all analytic studies fit neatly into one of the three main categories that follow; a few of the more common exceptions are discussed in the section called "Other Considerations and Special Issues."

The t Test

The **t test** (sometimes called "Student's t test," after the pseudonym of its developer) is commonly used to determine whether the mean value of a continuous outcome variable in one group differs significantly from that in another group. For example, the t test would be appropriate to use when comparing the mean depression scores in patients treated with two different antidepressants, or the mean change in weight among two groups of participants in a placebo-controlled trial of a new drug for weight loss. The t test assumes that the distribution (spread) of the variable in each of the two groups approximates a normal (bell-shaped) curve. However, the t test is remarkably robust, so it can be used for almost any distribution unless the number of subjects is small (fewer than 30 to 40) or there are extreme outliers.

To estimate the sample size for a study that will be analyzed with a t test (see Example 6.1), the investigator must

1. State the null hypothesis and whether the alternative hypothesis is one- or two-sided.
2. Estimate the effect size (E) as the difference in the mean value of the outcome variable between the study groups.
3. Estimate the variability of the outcome variable as its standard deviation (S).
4. Calculate the standardized effect size (E/S), defined as the effect size divided by the standard deviation of the outcome variable.
5. Set α and β.

The **effect size** and **variability** can often be estimated from previous studies in the literature and consultation with experts. Occasionally, a small pilot study will be necessary to estimate the standard deviation of the outcome variable (also see the Section "How to estimate sample size when there is insufficient information," later in this chapter). When the outcome variable is the change in a continuous measurement (e.g., change in weight during a study), the investigator should use the standard deviation of the change in that variable (not the standard deviation of the variable itself) in the sample size estimates. The standard deviation of the change in a variable is usually smaller than the standard deviation of the variable; therefore the sample size will also be smaller.

The **standardized effect size** is a unitless quantity that makes it possible to estimate a sample size when an investigator cannot obtain information about the variability of the outcome variable; it also simplifies comparisons between the effect sizes of different variables. (The standardized effect size equals the effect size divided by the standard deviation of the outcome variable. For example, a 10 mg/dL difference in serum cholesterol level, which has a standard deviation in the population of about 40 mg/dL, would equal a standardized effect size of 0.25.) The larger the standardized effect size, the smaller the required sample size. For most studies, the standardized effect size will be >0.1. Effect sizes smaller than that are difficult to detect (they require very large sample sizes) and usually not very important clinically.

Appendix 6A gives the sample size requirements for various combinations of α and β for several standardized effect sizes. To use Table 6A, look down its leftmost column for the standardized effect size. Next, read across the table to the chosen values for α and β for the sample size required per group. (The numbers in Table 6A assume that the two groups being compared are of the same size; use the formula below the table or an interactive Web-based program if that assumption is not true.)

Example 6.1 Calculating Sample Size When Using the *t* Test

Problem: The research question is whether there is a difference in the efficacy of salbutamol and ipratropium bromide for the treatment of asthma. The investigator plans a randomized trial of the effect of these drugs on FEV$_1$ (forced expiratory volume in 1 second) after 2 weeks of treatment. A previous study has reported that the mean FEV$_1$ in persons with treated asthma was 2.0 liters, with a standard deviation of 1.0 liter. The investigator would like to be able to detect a difference of 10% or more in mean FEV$_1$ between the two treatment groups. How many patients are required in each group (salbutamol and ipratropium) at α (two-sided) = 0.05 and power = 0.80?

Solution: The ingredients for the sample size calculation are as follows:

1. **Null Hypothesis:** *Mean FEV$_1$ after 2 weeks of treatment is the same in asthmatic patients treated with salbutamol as in those treated with ipratropium.*
   Alternative Hypothesis *(two-sided): Mean FEV$_1$ after 2 weeks of treatment is different in asthmatic patients treated with salbutamol from what it is in those treated with ipratropium.*
2. *Effect Size = 0.2 liters (10% × 2.0 liters).*
3. *Standard Deviation of FEV$_1$ = 1.0 liter.*

> 4. *Standardized Effect Size = effect size ÷ standard deviation = 0.2 liters ÷ 1.0 liter = 0.2.*
> 5. *α (two-sided) = 0.05; β = 1 - 0.80 = 0.20. (Recall that β = 1 − power.)*
>
> *Looking across from a standardized effect size of 0.20 in the leftmost column of Table 6A and down from α (two-sided) = 0.05 and β = 0.20, 394 patients are required **per group**. This is the number of patients in each group who need to complete the study; even more will need to be enrolled to account for dropouts. This sample size may not be feasible, and the investigator might reconsider the study design, or perhaps settle for only being able to detect a larger effect size. See the section on the t test for paired samples ("Example 6.8") for a great solution.*

The t test is usually used for comparing continuous outcomes, but it can also be used to estimate the sample size for a dichotomous outcome (e.g., in a case–control study) if the study has a continuous predictor variable. In this situation, the t test compares the mean value of the predictor variable in the cases with that in the controls.

There is a convenient **shortcut** for approximating sample size using the t test, when more than about 30 subjects will be studied and the power is set at 0.80 ($\beta = 0.2$) and α (two-sided) is set at 0.05 (1). The formula is

Sample size (per equal-sized group) = $16 \div$ (standardized effect size)^2.

For Example 6.1, the shortcut estimate of the sample size would be $16 \div 0.2^2 = 400$ per group.

The Chi-Squared Test

The **chi-squared test** (χ^2) can be used to compare the proportion of subjects in each of two groups who have a dichotomous outcome. For example, the proportion of men who develop coronary heart disease (CHD) while being treated with folate can be compared with the proportion who develop CHD while taking a placebo. The chi-squared test is always two-sided; an equivalent test for one-sided hypotheses is the **one-sided Z test.**

In an experiment or cohort study, effect size is specified by the difference between P_1, the proportion of subjects expected to have the outcome in one group, and P_2, the proportion expected in the other group. In a case–control study, P_1 represents the proportion of cases expected to have a particular risk factor, and P_2 represents the proportion of controls expected to have the risk factor. Variability is a function of P_1 and P_2, so it need not be specified.

To estimate the sample size for a study that will be analyzed with the chi-squared test or Z test to compare two proportions, the investigator must

1. State the null hypothesis and decide whether the alternative hypothesis should be one- or two-sided.
2. Estimate the effect size and variability in terms of P_1, the proportion with the outcome in one group, and P_2, the proportion with the outcome in the other group.
3. Set α and β.

Appendix 6B gives the sample size requirements for several combinations of α and β, and a range of values of P_1 and P_2. To estimate the sample size, look down the leftmost column of Tables 6B.1 or 6B.2 for the smaller of P_1 and P_2 (if necessary rounded to the nearest 0.05). Next, read across for the difference between P_1 and P_2. Based on the chosen values for α and β, the table gives the sample size required per group.

Example 6.2 Calculating Sample Size When Using the Chi-Squared Test

Problem: The research question is whether elderly smokers have a greater incidence of skin cancer than nonsmokers. A review of previous literature suggests that the 5-year incidence of skin cancer is about 0.20 in elderly nonsmokers. At α (two-sided) = 0.05 and power = 0.80, how many smokers and nonsmokers will need to be studied to determine whether the 5-year skin cancer incidence is at least 0.30 in smokers?

Solution: The ingredients for the sample size calculation are as follows:

1. **Null Hypothesis:** *The incidence of skin cancer is the same in elderly smokers and nonsmokers.*
   Alternative Hypothesis *(two-sided): The incidence of skin cancer is different in elderly smokers and nonsmokers.*
2. *P_2 (incidence in nonsmokers) = 0.20; P_1 (incidence in smokers) = 0.30. The smaller of these values is 0.20, and the difference between them ($P_1 - P_2$) is 0.10.*
3. *α (two-sided) = 0.05; β = 1 - 0.80 = 0.20.*

Looking across from 0.20 in the leftmost column in Table 6B.1 and down from an expected difference of 0.10, the middle number for α (two-sided) = 0.05 and β = 0.20 is the required sample size of 313 smokers and 313 nonsmokers. If the investigator had chosen to use a one-sided alternative hypothesis, given that there is a great deal of evidence suggesting that smoking is a carcinogen and none suggesting that it prevents cancer, the sample size would be 251 smokers and 251 nonsmokers.

Often the investigator specifies the effect size in terms of the **relative risk** (risk ratio) of the outcome in two groups of subjects. For example, an investigator might study whether women who use oral contraceptives are at least twice as likely as nonusers to have a myocardial infarction. In a cohort study (or experiment), it is straightforward to convert back and forth between relative risk and the two proportions (P_1 and P_2), since the relative risk is just P_1 divided by P_2 (or vice versa).

For a case–control study, however, the situation is a little more complex because the relative risk must be approximated by the **odds ratio,** which equals $[P_1 \times (1 - P_2)] \div [P_2 \times (1 - P_1)]$. The investigator must specify the odds ratio (OR) and P_2 (the proportion of controls exposed to the predictor variable). Then P_1 (the proportion of cases exposed to the predictor variable) is

$$P_1 = \frac{OR \times P_2}{(1 - P_2) + (OR \times P_2)}$$

For example, if the investigator expects that 10% of controls will be exposed to the oral contraceptives ($P_2 = 0.1$) and wishes to detect an odds ratio of 3 associated with the exposure, then

$$P_1 = \frac{(3 \times 0.1)}{(1 - 0.1) + (3 \times 0.1)} = \frac{0.3}{1.2} = 0.25$$

The Correlation Coefficient

Although the **correlation coefficient** (r) is not used frequently in sample size calculations, it can be useful when the predictor and outcome variables are both continuous. The correlation coefficient is a measure of the strength of the linear association between the two variables. It varies between -1 and $+1$. Negative values indicate that as one variable increases, the other decreases (like blood lead level and IQ in children). The closer the absolute value of r is to 1, the stronger the association; the closer to 0, the weaker the association. Height and weight in adults, for example, are highly correlated in some populations, with $r \approx 0.9$. Such high values, however, are uncommon; many biologic associations have much smaller correlation coefficients.

Correlation coefficients are common in some fields of clinical research, such as behavioral medicine, but using them to estimate the sample size has a disadvantage: correlation coefficients have little intuitive meaning. When squared (r^2) a correlation coefficient represents the proportion of the spread (variance) in an outcome variable that results from its linear association with a predictor variable, and vice versa. That's why small values of r, such as those ≤ 0.3, may be statistically significant if the sample is large enough without being very meaningful clinically or scientifically, since they "explain" at most 9% of the variance.

An alternative—and often preferred—way to estimate the sample size for a study in which the predictor and outcome variables are both continuous is to dichotomize one of the two variables (say, at its median) and use the t test calculations instead. This has the advantage of expressing the effect size as a "difference" between two groups.

To estimate sample size for a study that will be analyzed with a correlation coefficient, the investigator must

1. State the null hypothesis, and decide whether the alternative hypothesis is one or two-sided.
2. Estimate the effect size as the absolute value of the smallest correlation coefficient (r) that the investigator would like to be able to detect. (Variability is a function of r and is already included in the table and formula.)
3. Set α and β.

In Appendix 6C, look down the leftmost column of Table 6C for the effect size (r). Next, read across the table to the chosen values for α and β, yielding the total sample size required. Table 6C yields the appropriate sample size when the investigator wishes to reject the null hypothesis that there is no association between the predictor and outcome variables (e.g., $r = 0$). If the investigator wishes to determine whether the correlation coefficient in the study differs from a value other than zero (e.g., $r = 0.4$), she should see the text below Table 6C for the appropriate methodology.

Example 6.3 Calculating Sample Size When Using the Correlation Coefficient in a Cross-Sectional Study

Problem: The research question is whether urinary cotinine levels (a measure of the intensity of current cigarette smoking) are correlated with bone density in smokers. A previous study found a modest correlation ($r = -0.3$) between reported smoking (in cigarettes per day) and bone density; the investigator anticipates that

urinary cotinine levels will be at least as well correlated. How many smokers will need to be enrolled, at α (two-sided) = 0.05 and β = 0.10?
  Solution: The ingredients for the sample size calculation are as follows:

1. **Null Hypothesis:** *There is no correlation between urinary cotinine level and bone density in smokers.*
   Alternative Hypothesis: *There is a correlation between urinary cotinine level and bone density in smokers.*
2. *Effect size (r) = | − 0.3| = 0.3.*
3. *α (two-sided) = 0.05; β = 0.10.*

   Using Table 6C, reading across from r = 0.30 in the leftmost column and down from α (two-sided) = 0.05 and β = 0.10, 113 smokers will be required.

■ OTHER CONSIDERATIONS AND SPECIAL ISSUES

Dropouts
Each sampling unit must be available for analysis; subjects who are enrolled in a study but in whom outcome status cannot be ascertained (such as **dropouts**) do not count in the sample size. If the investigator anticipates that any of her subjects will not be available for follow-up, she should increase the size of the enrolled sample accordingly. If, for example, the investigator estimates that 20% of her sample will be lost to follow-up, then the sample size should be increased by a factor of $(1 \div [1 - 0.20])$, or 1.25.

Categorical Variables
Ordinal variables can often be treated as continuous variables, especially if the number of categories is relatively large (six or more) and if averaging the values of the variable makes sense. In other situations, the best strategy is to change the research hypothesis slightly by dichotomizing the categorical variable. As an example, suppose a researcher is studying whether the sex of a diabetic patient is associated with the number of times the patient visits a podiatrist in a year. The number of visits is unevenly distributed: many people will have no visits, some will make one visit, and only a few will make two or more visits. In this situation, the investigator could estimate the sample size as if the outcome were dichotomous (no visits versus one or more visits).

Survival Analysis
When an investigator wishes to compare which of two treatments is more effective in prolonging life or in reducing the symptomatic phase of a disease, survival analysis will be the appropriate technique for analyzing the data (2,3). Although the outcome variable, say weeks of survival, appears to be continuous, the *t* test is not appropriate because what is actually being assessed is not time (a continuous variable) but the proportion of subjects (a dichotomous variable) still alive at each point in time. A reasonable approximation can be made by dichotomizing the outcome variable at the end of the anticipated follow-up period (e.g., the proportion surviving for 6 months or more), and estimating the sample size with the chi-squared test.

Clustered Samples

Some research designs involve the use of **clustered samples,** in which subjects are sampled by groups (Chapter 11). Consider, for example, a study of whether an educational intervention directed at clinicians improves the rate of smoking cessation among their patients. Suppose that 20 physicians are randomly assigned to the group that receives the intervention and 20 physicians are assigned to a control group. One year later, the investigators plan to review the charts of a random sample of 50 patients who had been smokers at baseline in each practice to determine how many have quit smoking. Does the sample size equal 40 (the number of physicians) or 2,000 (the number of patients)? The answer, which lies somewhere in between those two extremes, depends upon how similar the patients within a physician's practice are (in terms of their likelihood of smoking cessation) compared with the similarity among all the patients. Estimating this quantity often requires obtaining pilot data, unless another investigator has previously done a similar study. There are several techniques for estimating the required sample size for a study using clustered samples (4–7), but they are challenging and usually require the assistance of a statistician.

Matching

For a variety of reasons (Chapter 9), an investigator may choose to use a matched design. The techniques in this chapter, which ignore any matching, nevertheless provide reasonable estimates of the required sample size. More precise estimates can be made using standard approaches (8) or an interactive Web-based program.

Multivariate Adjustment and Other Special Statistical Analyses

When designing an observational study, an investigator may decide that one or more variables will confound the association between the predictor and outcome (Chapter 9), and plan to use statistical techniques to adjust for these **confounders** when she analyzes her results. When this adjustment will be included in testing the primary hypothesis, the estimated sample size needs to take this into account.

Analytic approaches that adjust for confounding variables often increase the required sample size (9,10). The magnitude of that increase depends on several factors, including the prevalence of the confounder, the strength of the association between the predictor and the confounder, and the strength of the association between the confounder and the outcome. These effects are complex and no general rule covers all situations.

Statisticians have developed multivariate methods such as linear regression and logistic regression that allow the investigator to adjust for confounding variables. One widely used statistical technique, **Cox proportional hazards** analysis, can adjust both for confounders and for differences in length of follow-up. If one of these techniques is going to be used to analyze the data, there are corresponding approaches for estimating the required sample size (3,11–14). Sample size techniques are also available for other designs, such as studies of potential genetic risk factors or candidate genes (15–17), economic studies (18–20), dose–response studies (21), or studies that involve more than two groups (22). Again, the Internet is a useful resource for these more sophisticated approaches (e.g., search for "sample size" and "logistic regression").

It is usually easier, at least for novice investigators, to estimate the sample size assuming a simpler method of analysis, such as the chi-squared test or the t test. Suppose, for example, an investigator is planning a case–control study of whether serum cholesterol level (a continuous variable) is associated with the occurrence of brain tumors (a dichotomous variable). Even if the eventual plan is to analyze the data with the logistic regression technique, a ballpark sample size can be estimated with the t test. It turns out that the simplified approaches usually produce sample size estimates that are similar to those generated by more sophisticated techniques. An experienced statistician may need to be consulted, however, if a grant proposal that involves substantial costs is being submitted for funding: grant reviewers will expect you to use a sophisticated approach even if they accept that the sample size estimates are based on guesses about the risk of the outcome, the effect size, and so on.

Equivalence Studies

Sometimes the goal of a study is to show that the null hypothesis is correct and that there really is no substantial association between the predictor and outcome variables (23–26). A common example is a clinical trial to test whether a new drug is as effective as an established drug. This situation poses a challenge when planning sample size, because the desired effect size is zero (i.e., the investigator would like to show that the two drugs are equally effective).

One acceptable method is to design the study to have substantial power (say, 0.90 or 0.95) to reject the null hypothesis when the effect size is small enough that it would not be clinically important (e.g., a difference of 5 mg/dL in mean fasting glucose levels). If the results of such a well-powered study show "no effect" (i.e., the 95% confidence interval excludes the prespecified difference of 5 mg/dL), then the investigator can be reasonably sure that the two drugs have similar effects. One problem with equivalence studies, however, is that the additional power and the small effect size often require a very large sample size.

Another problem involves the loss of the usual safeguards that are inherent in the paradigm of the null hypothesis, which protects a conventional study, such as one that compares an active drug with a placebo, against Type I errors (falsely rejecting the null hypothesis). The paradigm ensures that many problems in the design or execution of a study, such as using imprecise measurements or inadequate numbers of subjects, make it harder to reject the null hypothesis. Investigators in a conventional study, who are trying to reject a null hypothesis, have a strong incentive to do the best possible study. The same is not true for an equivalence study, in which the goal is to find no difference, and the safeguards do not apply.

SAMPLE SIZE TECHNIQUES FOR DESCRIPTIVE STUDIES

Estimating the sample size for descriptive studies, including studies of diagnostic tests, is based on somewhat different principles. Such studies do not have predictor and outcome variables, nor do they compare different groups. Therefore the concepts of power and the null and alternative hypotheses do not apply. Instead, the investigator calculates descriptive statistics, such as means and proportions. Often, however, descriptive studies (*What is the prevalence of depression among elderly patients in a medical clinic?*) are also used to ask analytic questions (*What are the predictors of depression among these patients?*). In this situation, sample size should be estimated for the analytic study as well, to avoid the common problem of having inadequate power for what turns out to be the question of greater interest.

Descriptive studies commonly report **confidence intervals,** a range of values about the sample mean or proportion. A confidence interval is a measure of the precision of a sample estimate. The investigator sets the confidence level, such as

95% or 99%. An interval with a greater confidence level (say 99%) is wider, and therefore more likely to include the true population value, than an interval with a lower confidence level (90%).

The width of a confidence interval depends on the sample size. For example, an investigator might wish to estimate the mean score on the U.S. Medical Licensing Examination in a group of medical students. From a sample of 200 students, she might estimate that the mean score in the population of all students is 215, with a 95% confidence interval from 210 to 220. A smaller study, say with 50 students, might have about the same mean score but would almost certainly have a wider 95% confidence interval.

When estimating sample size for descriptive studies, the investigator specifies the desired level and width of the confidence interval. The sample size can then be determined from the tables or formulas in the appendix.

Continuous Variables
When the variable of interest is continuous, a confidence interval around the mean value of that variable is often reported. To estimate the sample size for that confidence interval, the investigator must

1. Estimate the standard deviation of the variable of interest.
2. Specify the desired precision (total width) of the confidence interval.
3. Select the confidence level for the interval (e.g., 95%, 99%).

To use Appendix 6D, standardize the total width of the interval (divide it by the standard deviation of the variable), then look down the leftmost column of Table 6D for the expected standardized width. Next, read across the table to the chosen confidence level for the required sample size.

Example 6.4 Calculating Sample Size for a Descriptive Study of a Continuous Variable

Problem: The investigator seeks to determine the mean IQ among third graders in an urban area with a 99% confidence interval of ±3 points. A previous study found that the standard deviation of IQ in a similar city was 15 points.
   Solution: The ingredients for the sample size calculation are as follows:

1. *Standard deviation of variable (SD) = 15 points.*
2. *Total width of interval = 6 points (3 points above and 3 points below). The standardized width of interval = total width ÷ SD = 6 ÷ 15 = 0.4.*
3. *Confidence level = 99%.*

   Reading across from a standardized width of 0.4 in the leftmost column of Table 6D and down from the 99% confidence level, the required sample size is 166 third graders.

Dichotomous Variables
In a descriptive study of a dichotomous variable, results can be expressed as a confidence interval around the estimated proportion of subjects with one of the values.

This includes studies of the **sensitivity** or **specificity** of a diagnostic test, which appear at first glance to be continuous variables but are actually dichotomous—proportions expressed as percentages (Chapter 12). To estimate the sample size for that confidence interval, the investigator must

1. Estimate the expected proportion with the variable of interest in the population. (If more than half of the population is expected to have the characteristic, then plan the sample size based on the proportion expected not to have the characteristic.)
2. Specify the desired precision (total width) of the confidence interval.
3. Select the confidence level for the interval (e.g., 95%).

   In Appendix 6E, look down the leftmost column of Table 6E for the expected proportion with the variable of interest. Next, read across the table to the chosen width and confidence level, yielding the required sample size.

   Example 6.5 provides a sample size calculation for studying the sensitivity of a diagnostic test, which yields the required number of subjects with the disease. When studying the specificity of the test, the investigator must estimate the required number of subjects who do *not* have the disease. There are also techniques for estimating the sample size for studies of receiver operating characteristic (ROC) curves (27), likelihood ratios (28), and reliability (29) (Chapter 12).

Example 6.5 Calculating Sample Size for a Descriptive Study of a Dichotomous Variable

Problem: The investigator wishes to determine the sensitivity of a new diagnostic test for pancreatic cancer. Based on a pilot study, she expects that 80% of patients with pancreatic cancer will have positive tests. How many such patients will be required to estimate a 95% confidence interval for the test's sensitivity of 0.80 ± 0.05?
Solution: The ingredients for the sample size calculation are as follows:

1. *Expected proportion = 0.20. (Because 0.80 is more than half, sample size is estimated from the proportion expected to have a negative result, that is, 0.20.)*
2. *Total width = 0.10 (0.05 below and 0.05 above).*
3. *Confidence level = 95%.*

Reading across from 0.20 in the leftmost column of Table 6E and down from a total width of 0.10, the middle number (representing a 95% confidence level) yields the required sample size of 246 patients with pancreatic cancer.

WHAT TO DO WHEN SAMPLE SIZE IS FIXED

Especially when doing secondary data analysis, the sample size may have been determined before you design your study. In this situation, or if the number of participants who are available or affordable for study is limited, the investigator must work backward from the fixed sample size. She estimates the effect size that can be detected at a given power (usually 80%) or, less commonly, the power to detect a given effect. The investigator can use the sample size tables in the chapter appendixes, interpolating when necessary, or use the sample size formulas in the appendixes for estimating the effect size.

A good general rule is that a study should have a power of 80% or greater to detect a reasonable effect size. It is often tempting to pursue research hypotheses that have less power if the cost of doing so is small, such as when doing an analysis of data that have already been collected. The investigator should keep in mind, however, that she might face the difficulty of interpreting (and publishing) a study that may have found no effect because of insufficient power; the broad confidence intervals will reveal the possibility of a substantial effect in the population from which the small study sample was drawn.

Example 6.6 Calculating the Detectable Effect Size When Sample Size is Fixed

Problem: An investigator determines that there are 100 patients with systemic lupus erythematosus (SLE) who might be willing to participate in a study of whether a 6-week meditation program affects disease activity, as compared with a control group that receives a pamphlet describing relaxation. If the standard deviation of the change in a validated SLE disease activity scale score is expected to be five points in both the control and the treatment groups, what size difference will the investigator be able to detect between the two groups, at α (two-sided) = 0.05 and β = 0.20?

Solution: In Table 6A, reading down from α (two-sided) = 0.05 and β = 0.20 (the rightmost column in the middle triad of numbers), 45 patients per group are required to detect a standardized effect size of 0.6, which is equal to three points (0.6 × 5 points). The investigator (who will have about 50 patients per group) will be able to detect a difference of a little less than three points between the two groups.

STRATEGIES FOR MINIMIZING SAMPLE SIZE AND MAXIMIZING POWER

When the estimated sample size is greater than the number of subjects that can be studied realistically, the investigator should proceed through several steps. First, the calculations should be checked, as it is easy to make mistakes. Next, the "ingredients" should be reviewed. Is the effect size unreasonably small or the variability unreasonably large? Could α or β, or both, be increased without harm? Would a one-sided alternative hypothesis be adequate? Is the confidence level too high or the interval unnecessarily narrow?

These technical adjustments can be useful, but it is important to realize that statistical tests ultimately depend on the information contained in the data. Many changes in the ingredients, such as reducing power from 90% to 80%, do not improve the quantity or quality of the data that will be collected. There are, however, several strategies for reducing the required sample size or for increasing power for a given sample size that actually increase the information content of the collected data. Many of these strategies involve modifications of the research hypothesis; the investigator should carefully consider whether the new hypothesis still answers the research question that she wishes to study.

Use Continuous Variables

When continuous variables are an option, they usually permit smaller sample sizes than dichotomous variables. Blood pressure, for example, can be expressed either as millimeters of mercury (continuous) or as the presence or absence of hypertension (dichotomous). The former permits a smaller sample size for a given power or a greater power for a given sample size.

In Example 6.7, the continuous outcome addresses the effect of nutrition supplements on muscle strength among the elderly. The dichotomous outcome is concerned with its effects on the proportion of subjects who have at least a minimal amount of strength, which may be a more valid surrogate for potential fall-related morbidity.

Example 6.7 Use of Continuous versus Dichotomous Variables

Problem: Consider a placebo-controlled trial to determine the effect of nutrition supplements on strength in elderly nursing home residents. Previous studies have established that quadriceps strength (as peak torque in newton-meters) is approximately normally distributed, with a mean of 33 N·m and a standard deviation of 10 N·m, and that about 10% of the elderly have very weak muscles (strength <20 N·m). Nutrition supplements for 6 months are anticipated to increase strength by 5 N·m as compared with the usual diet. This change in mean strength can be estimated, based on the distribution of quadriceps strength in the elderly, to correspond to a reduction in the proportion of the elderly who are very weak to about 5%.

One design might treat strength as a dichotomous variable: very weak versus not very weak. Another might use all the information contained in the measurement and treat strength as a continuous variable. How many subjects would each design require at α (two-sided) = 0.05 and β = 0.20? How does the change in design affect the research question?

*Solution: The ingredients for the sample size calculation using a **dichotomous outcome variable** (very weak versus not very weak) are as follows:*

1. **Null Hypothesis:** *The proportion of elderly nursing home residents who are very weak (peak quadriceps torque <20 N·m) after receiving 6 months of nutrition supplements is the same as the proportion who are very weak in those on a usual diet.*
   Alternative Hypothesis: *The proportion of elderly nursing home residents who are very weak (peak quadriceps torque <20 N·m) after receiving 6 months of nutrition supplements differs from the proportion in those on a usual diet.*
2. P_1 *(prevalence of being very weak on usual diet) = 0.10; P_2 (in supplement group) = 0.05. The smaller of these values is 0.05, and the difference between them ($P_1 - P_2$) is 0.05.*
3. *α (two-sided) = 0.05; β = 0.20.*

Using Table 6B.1, reading across from 0.05 in the leftmost column and down from an expected difference of 0.05, the middle number (for α [two-sided] = 0.05 and β = 0.20), this design would require 473 subjects per group.

*The ingredients for the sample size calculation using a **continuous outcome variable** (quadriceps strength as peak torque) are as follows:*

1. **Null Hypothesis:** *Mean quadriceps strength (as peak torque in N·m) in elderly nursing home residents after receiving 6 months of nutrition supplements is the same as mean quadriceps strength in those on a usual diet.*

Alternative Hypothesis: *Mean quadriceps strength (as peak torque in N·m) in elderly nursing home residents after receiving 6 months of nutrition supplements differs from mean quadriceps strength in those on a usual diet.*
2. *Effect size = 5 N·m*
3. *Standard deviation of quadriceps strength = 10 N·m*
4. *Standardized effect size = effect size ÷ standard deviation = 5 N·m ÷ 10 N·m = 0.5.*
5. *α (two-sided) 0.05; $\beta = 0.20$.*

Using Table 6A, reading across from a standardized effect size of 0.50, with α (two-sided) = 0.05 and β = 0.20, this design would require about 64 subjects in each group. (In this example, the shortcut sample size estimate from page 68 of $16 \div (standardized\ effect\ size)^2$, or $16 \div 0.5^2$ gives the same estimate of 64 subjects per group.) The bottom line is that the use of an outcome variable that was continuous rather than dichotomous meant that a substantially smaller sample size needed to study this research question

Use Paired Measurements

In some experiments or cohort studies with continuous outcome variables, paired measurements—one at baseline, another at the conclusion of the study—can be made in each subject. The outcome variable is the change between these two measurements. In this situation, a *t* test on the paired measurements can be used to compare the mean value of this change in the two groups. This technique often permits a smaller sample size because, by comparing each subject with herself, it removes the baseline between-subject part of the variability of the outcome variable. For example, the change in weight on a diet has less variability than the final weight, because final weight is highly correlated with initial weight. Sample size for this type of *t* test is estimated in the usual way, except that the standardized effect size (E/S in Table 6A) is the anticipated difference in the *change* in the variable divided by the standard deviation *of that change*.

Example 6.8 Use of the *t* Test with Paired Measurements

Problem: Recall Example 6.1, in which the investigator studying the treatment of asthma is interested in determining whether salbutamol can improve FEV_1 by 200 mL compared with ipratropium bromide. Sample size calculations indicated that 394 subjects per group are needed, more than are likely to be available. Fortunately, a colleague points out that asthmatic patients have great differences in their FEV_1 values before treatment. These between-subject differences account for much of the variability in FEV_1 after treatment, therefore obscuring the effect of treatment. She suggests using a paired t test to compare the changes in FEV_1 in the two groups. A pilot study finds that the standard deviation of the change in FEV_1 is only 250 mL. How many subjects would be required per group, at α (two-sided) = 0.05 and β = 0.20?

Solution: *The ingredients for the sample size calculation are as follows*:

1. **Null Hypothesis:** *Change in mean* FEV_1 *after 2 weeks of treatment is the same in asthmatic patients treated with salbutamol as it is in those treated with ipratropium bromide.*
   Alternative Hypothesis: *Change in mean* FEV_1 *after 2 weeks of treatment is different in asthmatic patients treated with salbutamol from what it is in those treated with ipratropium bromide.*
2. *Effect size = 200 mL.*
3. *Standard deviation of the outcome variable = 250 mL.*
4. *Standardized effect size = effect size ÷ standard deviation = 200 mL ÷ 250 mL = 0.8.*
5. *α (two-sided) = 0.05; β = 1 − 0.80 = 0.20.*

Using Table 6A, this design would require about 26 participants per group, a much more reasonable sample size than the 394 per group in "Example 6.1". In this example, the shortcut sample size estimate of 16 ÷ (standardized effect size)^2, or 16 ÷ 0.8^2 gives a similar estimate of 25 subjects per group.

A Brief Technical Note. This chapter always refers to **two-sample** t **tests,** which are used when comparing the mean values of an outcome variable in two groups of subjects. A two-sample t test can be **unpaired,** if the outcome variable itself is being compared between two groups (see "Example 6.1"), or **paired** if the outcome is the change in a pair of measurements, say before and after an intervention (see "Example 6.8").

A third type of t test, the *one-sample* **paired** t **test,** compares the mean change in a pair of measurements within a single group to zero change. This type of analysis is reasonably common in time series designs (Chapter 10), a before–after approach to examining treatments that are difficult to randomize (for example, the effect of elective hysterectomy, a decision few women are willing to leave to a coin toss, on quality of life). However, it is a fairly weak design because the absence of a comparison group makes it difficult to know what would have happened had the subjects been left untreated (Chapter 10). When planning a study that will be analyzed with a one-sample paired t test, the sample size in Appendix 6A represents the *total* number of subjects (because there is only one group). Appendix 6F presents additional information on the use and misuse of one- and two-sample t tests.

Use More Precise Variables

Because they reduce variability, more precise variables permit a smaller sample size in both analytic and descriptive studies. Even a modest change in precision can have a substantial effect on sample size. For example, when using the t test to estimate sample size, a 20% decrease in the standard deviation of the outcome variable results in a 36% decrease in the sample size. Techniques for increasing the precision of a variable, such as making measurements in duplicate, are presented in Chapter 4.

Use Unequal Group Sizes

Because an equal number of subjects in each of two groups usually gives the greatest power for a given total number of subjects, Tables 6A, 6B.1, and 6B.2 in the appendixes assume equal sample sizes in the two groups. Sometimes, however, the distribution of subjects is not equal in the two groups, or it is easier or less expensive to recruit study subjects for one group than the other. It may turn out, for example, that an investigator wants to estimate sample size based on the 30% of the subjects in a cohort who smoke cigarettes (compared with 70% who do not smoke). Or, in a case–control study, the number of persons with the disease may be small, but it may be possible to sample a much larger number of controls. In general, the gain in power when the size of one group is increased to twice the size of the other is considerable; tripling and quadrupling one of the groups provide progressively smaller gains. Sample sizes for unequal groups can be computed from the formulas found in the text to Appendixes 6A and 6B or from the Web.

Here is a useful approximation for estimating sample size for case–control studies of dichotomous risk factors and outcomes using c controls per case. If n represents the number of cases that would have been required for one control per case (at a given α, β, and effect size), then the approximate number of cases (n') with cn' controls that will be required is

$$n' = [(c+1) \div 2c] \times n.$$

For example, with $c = 2$ controls per case, then $[(2+1) \div (2 \times 2)] \times n = 3/4 \times n$, and only 75% as many cases are needed. As c gets larger, n' approaches 50% of n (when $c = 10$, for example, $n' = 11/20 \times n$).

Example 6.9 Use of Multiple Controls per Case in a Case–Control Study

Problem: An investigator is studying whether exposure to household insecticide is a risk factor for aplastic anemia. The original sample size calculation indicated that 25 cases would be required, using one control per case. Suppose that the investigator has access to only 18 cases. How should the investigator proceed?

Solution: The investigator should consider using multiple controls per case (after all, she can find many patients who do not have aplastic anemia). By using three controls per case, for example, the approximate number of cases that will be required is $[(3+1) \div (2 \times 3)] \times 25 = 17$.

Use a More Common Outcome

When the outcome is dichotomous, using a more frequent outcome, up to a frequency of 0.5, is usually one of the best ways to increase power: if an outcome occurs more often, there is more of a chance to detect its predictors. Power actually depends more on the number of subjects with a specified outcome than it does on the total number of subjects in the study. Studies with rare outcomes, like the occurrence of breast cancer in healthy women, require very large sample sizes to have adequate power.

One of the best ways to make an outcome more common is to enroll subjects at greater risk of developing that outcome (such as women with a family history of breast cancer). Others are to extend the follow-up period, so that there is more time to accumulate outcomes, or to loosen the definition of what constitutes an outcome (e.g., by including ductal carcinoma *in situ*). All these techniques, however, may change the research question, so they should be used with caution.

Example 6.10 Use of a More Common Outcome

Problem: *Suppose an investigator is comparing the efficacy of an antiseptic gargle versus a placebo gargle in preventing upper respiratory infections. Her initial calculations indicated that her anticipated sample of 200 volunteer college students was inadequate, in part because she expected that only about 20% of her subjects would have an upper respiratory infection during the 3-month follow-up period. Suggest a few changes in the study plan.*

Solution: *Here are two possible solutions: (a) study a sample of pediatric interns and residents, who are likely to experience a much greater incidence of upper respiratory infections than college students; or (b) follow the sample for a longer period of time, say 6 or 12 months. Both of these solutions involve modification of the research hypothesis, but neither change seems sufficiently large to affect the overall research question about the efficacy of antiseptic gargle.*

HOW TO ESTIMATE SAMPLE SIZE WHEN THERE IS INSUFFICIENT INFORMATION

Often the investigator finds that she is missing one or more of the ingredients for the sample size calculation and becomes frustrated in her attempts to plan the study. This is an especially frequent problem when the investigator is using an instrument of her design (such as a new questionnaire on quality of life in patients with urinary incontinence). How should she go about deciding what effect size or standard deviation to use?

The first strategy is an **extensive search** for previous and related findings on the topic and on similar research questions. Roughly comparable situations and mediocre or dated findings may be good enough. (For example, are there data on quality of life among patients with other urologic problems, or with related conditions like having a colostomy?) If the literature review is unproductive, she should contact other investigators about their judgment on what to expect, and whether they are aware of any unpublished results that may be relevant. If there is still no information available, she may consider doing a small **pilot study** or obtaining a data set for a secondary analysis to obtain the missing ingredients before embarking on the main study. (Indeed, a pilot study is highly recommended for almost all studies that involve new instruments, measurement methods, or recruitment strategies. They save time in the end by enabling investigators to do a much better job planning the main study). Pilot studies are useful for estimating the standard deviation of a measurement, or the proportion of subjects with a particular characteristic. Another trick is to recognize that for continuous variables that have a roughly bell-shaped distribution, the **standard deviation** can be estimated as one-quarter of the difference between the high and low ends of the range of values that occur commonly, ignoring extreme values. For example, if most subjects are likely to have a serum sodium level between 135 and 143 mEq/L, the standard deviation of serum sodium is about 2 mEq/L ($1/4 \times 8$ mEq/L).

Alternatively, the investigator can determine the detectable effect size based on a value that she considers to be **clinically meaningful.** For example, *suppose that an investigator is studying a new invasive treatment for severe refractory gastroparesis, a* *condition in which at most 5% of patients improve spontaneously. If the treatment is shown to be effective, she thinks that gastroenterologists would be willing to treat up to five patients to produce a sustained benefit in one of those patients (because the treatment has substantial side effects and is expensive, she doesn't think that the number would be more than 5). A number needed to treat (NNT) of 5 corresponds to a risk difference of 20% (NNT = 1/risk difference), so the investigator should estimate the sample size based on a comparison of P1 = 5% versus P2 = 25% (i.e., 59 subjects per group at a power of 0.80 and a two-sided α of 0.05).*

Another strategy, when the mean and standard deviation of a continuous or categorical variable are in doubt, is to **dichotomize** that variable. Categories can be lumped into two groups, and continuous variables can be split at their mean or median. For example, dividing quality of life into "better than the median" or "the median or less" avoids having to estimate its standard deviation in the sample, although one still has to estimate what proportions of subjects would be above the median in the two groups being studied. The chi-squared statistic can then be used to make a reasonable, albeit somewhat high, estimate of the sample size.

If all this fails, the investigator should just make an **educated guess** about the likely values of the missing ingredients. The process of thinking through the problem and imagining the findings will often result in a reasonable estimate, and that is what sample size planning is about. This is usually a better option than just deciding to design the study to have 80% power at a two-sided α of 0.05 to detect a standardized effect size of, say, 0.5 between the two groups ($n = 64$, per group, by the way). Very few grant reviewers will accept that sort of arbitrary decision.

COMMON ERRORS TO AVOID

Many inexperienced investigators (and some experienced ones!) make mistakes when planning sample size. A few of the more common ones follow:

1. The most common error is estimating the sample size **late** during the design of the study. Do it early in the process, when fundamental changes can still be made.

2. Dichotomous variables can appear to be continuous when they are expressed as a **percentage** or **rate.** For example, vital status (alive or dead) might be misinterpreted as continuous when expressed as percent alive. Similarly, in survival analysis a dichotomous outcome can appear to be continuous (e.g., median survival in months). For all of these, the outcome itself is actually dichotomous and the appropriate simple approach in planning sample size would be the chi-squared test.

3. The sample size estimates the number of subjects with outcome data, not the number who need to be enrolled. The investigator should always plan for **dropouts** and subjects with **missing data.**

4. The tables at the end of the chapter assume that the two groups being studied have equal sample sizes. Often that is not the case; for example, a cohort study of whether use of vitamin supplements reduces the risk of sunburn would probably not enroll equal numbers of subjects who used, or did not use, vitamins. If the sample sizes are **not equal,** then the formulas that follow the tables or the Web should be used.

5. When using the *t* test to estimate the sample size, what matters is the standard deviation of the outcome variable. Therefore if the outcome is **change** in a continuous variable, the investigator should use the standard deviation of that change rather than the standard deviation of the variable itself.

6. Be aware of **clustered** data. If there appear to be two "levels" of sample size (e.g., one for physicians and another for patients), clustering is a likely problem and the tables in the appendices do not apply.

SUMMARY

1. When estimating sample size for an **analytic study,** the following steps need to be taken: (a) state the **null** and **alternative hypotheses,** specifying the number of **sides;** (b) select a **statistical test** that could be used to analyze the data, based on the **types of predictor and outcome variables;** (c) estimate the **effect size** (and its **variability,** if necessary); and (d) specify appropriate values for α and β, based on the importance of avoiding **Type I** and **Type II errors.**

2. Other considerations in calculating sample size for analytic studies include adjusting for potential **dropouts,** and strategies for dealing with **categorical variables, survival analysis, clustered samples, multivariate adjustment,** and **equivalence studies.**

3. The steps for estimating sample size for **descriptive studies,** which do not have hypotheses, are to (a) estimate the **proportion** of subjects with a dichotomous outcome or the **standard deviation** of a continuous outcome; (b) specify the desired **precision** (width of the confidence interval); and (c) specify the **confidence level** (e.g., 95%).

4. When sample size is predetermined, the investigator can work backward to estimate the detectable **effect size** or, less commonly, the **power.**

5. Strategies **to minimize** the required sample size include using **continuous** variables, more **precise** measurements, **paired** measurements, **unequal group sizes,** and **more common outcomes.**

6. When there seems to be not enough information to estimate the sample size, the investigator should **review the literature** in related areas, do a small **pilot study** or choose an **effect size** that is clinically meaningful; **standard deviation** can be estimated as 1/4 of the range of commonly encountered values. If none of these is feasible, an educated guess can give a useful ballpark estimate.

APPENDIX 6A

Sample Size Required per Group When Using the *t* Test to Compare Means of Continuous Variables

TABLE 6A		Sample Size *per Group* for Comparing Two Means							
One-sided α =		**0.005**			**0.025**			**0.05**	
Two-sided α =		**0.01**			**0.05**			**0.10**	
E/S* β =	**0.05**	**0.10**	**0.20**	**0.05**	**0.10**	**0.20**	**0.05**	**0.10**	**0.20**
0.10	3,565	2,978	2,338	2,600	2,103	1,571	2,166	1,714	1,238
0.15	1,586	1,325	1,040	1,157	935	699	963	762	551
0.20	893	746	586	651	527	394	542	429	310
0.25	572	478	376	417	338	253	347	275	199
0.30	398	333	262	290	235	176	242	191	139
0.40	225	188	148	164	133	100	136	108	78
0.50	145	121	96	105	86	64	88	70	51
0.60	101	85	67	74	60	45	61	49	36
0.70	75	63	50	55	44	34	45	36	26
0.80	58	49	39	42	34	26	35	28	21
0.90	46	39	21	34	27	21	28	22	16
1.00	38	32	26	27	23	17	23	18	14

* E/S is the standardized effect size, computed as E (expected effect size) divided by S (SD of the outcome variable). To estimate the sample size, read across from the *standardized effect size*, and down from the specified values of α and β for the required sample size in each group.

Calculating Variability

Variability is usually reported as either the standard deviation or the standard error of the mean (SEM). For the purposes of sample size calculation, the standard deviation of the variable is most useful. Fortunately, it is easy to convert from one measure to another: the standard deviation is simply the standard error times the square root of N, where N is the number of subjects that makes up the mean. Suppose a study reported that the weight loss in 25 persons on a low-fiber diet was 10 ± 2 kg (mean $\pm$ SEM). The standard deviation would be $2 \times \sqrt{25} = 10$ kg.

General Formula for Other Values

The general formula for other values of E, S, α, and β, or for unequal group sizes, is as follows. Let:

z_α = the standard normal deviate for α (If the alternative hypothesis is two-sided, $z_\alpha = 2.58$ when $\alpha = 0.01$, $z_\alpha = 1.96$ when $\alpha = 0.05$, and $z_\alpha = 1.645$ when $\alpha = 0.10$. If the alternative hypothesis is one-sided, $z_\alpha = 1.645$ when $\alpha = 0.05$.)

z_β = the standard normal deviate for β ($z_\beta = 0.84$ when $\beta = 0.20$, and $z_\beta = 1.282$ when $\beta = 0.10$)

q_1 = proportion of subjects in group 1

q_2 = proportion of subjects in group 2

N = **total** number of subjects required

Then:

$$N = [(1/q_1 + 1/q_2)S^2(z_\alpha + z_\beta)^2] \div E^2.$$

Readers who would like to skip the work involved in hand calculations with this formula can get an instant answer from a calculator on our website (www.epibiostat.ucsf. edu/dcr/)(Because this formula is based on approximating the t statistic with a z statistic, it will slightly underestimate the sample size when N is less than about 30. Table 6A uses the t statistic to estimate sample size.)

APPENDIX 6B

Sample Size Required per Group When Using the Chi-Squared Statistic or Z Test to Compare Proportions of Dichotomous Variables

| TABLE 6B.1 | Sample Size *per Group* for Comparing Two Proportions |

Upper number: $\alpha = 0.05$ (one-sided) or $\alpha = 0.10$ (two-sided); $\beta = 0.20$
Middle number: $\alpha = 0.025$ (one-sided) or $\alpha = 0.05$ (two-sided); $\beta = 0.20$
Lower number: $\alpha = 0.025$ (one-sided) or $\alpha = 0.05$ (two-sided); $\beta = 0.10$

Smaller of P_1 and P_2*	\multicolumn{10}{c}{Difference Between P_1 and P_2}
	0.05	0.10	0.15	0.20	0.25	0.30	0.35	0.40	0.45	0.50
0.05	381	129	72	47	35	27	22	18	15	13
	473	159	88	59	43	33	26	22	18	16
	620	207	113	75	54	41	33	27	23	19
0.10	578	175	91	58	41	31	24	20	16	14
	724	219	112	72	51	37	29	24	20	17
	958	286	146	92	65	48	37	30	25	21
0.15	751	217	108	67	46	34	26	21	17	15
	944	270	133	82	57	41	32	26	21	18
	1,252	354	174	106	73	53	42	33	26	22
0.20	900	251	121	74	50	36	28	22	18	15
	1,133	313	151	91 ·	62	44	34	27	22	18
	1,504	412	197	118	80	57	44	34	27	23
0.25	1,024	278	132	79	53	38	29	23	18	15
	1,289	348	165	98	66	47	35	28	22	18
	1,714	459	216	127	85	60	46	35	28	23
0.30	1,123	300	141	83	55	39	29	23	18	15
	1,415	376	175	103	68	48	36	28	22	18
	1,883	496	230	134	88	62	47	36	28	23
0.35	1,197	315	146	85	56	39	29	23	18	15
	1,509	395	182	106	69	48	36	28	22	18
	2,009	522	239	138	90	62	47	35	27	22
0.40	1,246	325	149	86	56	39	29	22	17	14
	1,572	407	186	107	69	48	35	27	21	17
	2,093	538	244	139	90	62	46	34	26	21
0.45	1,271	328	149	85	55	38	28	21	16	13
	1,603	411	186	106	68	47	34	26	20	16
	2,135	543	244	138	88	60	44	33	25	19
0.50	1,271	325	146	83	53	36	26	20	15	—
	1,603	407	182	103	66	44	32	24	18	—
	2,135	538	239	134	85	57	42	30	23	—
0.55	1,246	315	141	79	50	34	24	18	—	—
	1,572	395	175	98	62	41	29	22	—	—
	2,093	522	230	127	80	53	37	27	—	—

TABLE 6B.1	(Continued)

Upper number: $\alpha=0.05$ (one-sided) or $\alpha=0.10$ (two-sided); $\beta=0.20$
Middle number: $\alpha=0.025$ (one-sided) or $\alpha=0.05$ (two-sided); $\beta=0.20$
Lower number: $\alpha=0.025$ (one-sided) or $\alpha=0.05$ (two-sided); $\beta=0.10$

Smaller of P_1 and P_2 *	Difference Between P_1 and P_2									
	0.05	0.10	0.15	0.20	0.25	0.30	0.35	0.40	0.45	0.50
0.60	1,197	300	132	74	46	31	22	—	—	—
	1,509	376	165	91	57	37	26	—	—	—
	2,009	496	216	118	73	48	33	—	—	—
0.65	1,123	278	121	67	41	27	—	—	—	—
	1,415	348	151	82	51	33	—	—	—	—
	1,883	459	197	106	65	41	—	—	—	—
0.70	1,024	251	108	58	35	—	—	—	—	—
	1,289	313	133	72	43	—	—	—	—	—
	1,714	412	174	92	54	—	—	—	—	—
0.75	900	217	91	47	—	—	—	—	—	—
	1,133	270	112	59	—	—	—	—	—	—
	1,504	354	146	75	—	—	—	—	—	—
0.80	751	175	72	—	—	—	—	—	—	—
	944	219	88	—	—	—	—	—	—	—
	1,252	286	113	—	—	—	—	—	—	—
0.85	578	129	—	—	—	—	—	—	—	—
	724	159	—	—	—	—	—	—	—	—
	958	207	—	—	—	—	—	—	—	—
0.90	381	—	—	—	—	—	—	—	—	—
	473	—	—	—	—	—	—	—	—	—
	620	—	—	—	—	—	—	—	—	—

The one-sided estimates use the z statistic.

* P_1 represents the proportion of subjects expected to have the outcome in one group; P_2 in the other group. (In a case–control study, P_1 represents the proportion of cases with the predictor variable; P_2 the proportion of controls with the predictor variable.) To estimate the sample size, read across from the smaller of P_1 and P_2, and down the expected *difference* between P_1 and P_2. The three numbers represent the sample size required in each group for the specified values of α and β.

Additional detail for P_1 and P_2 between 0.01 and 0.10 is given in Table 6B.2.

General Formula for Other Values

The general formula for calculating the *total* sample size (N) required for a study using the z statistic, where P_1 and P_2 are defined above, is as follows (see Appendix 6A for definitions of Z_α and Z_β). Let

$$q_1 = \text{proportion of subjects in group 1}$$
$$q_2 = \text{proportion of subjects in group 2}$$
$$N = total \text{ number of subjects}$$
$$P = q_1 P_1 + q_2 P_2$$

Then

$$N = \frac{[z_\alpha\sqrt{P(1-P)(1/q_1 + 1/q_2)} + z_\beta\sqrt{P_1(1-P_1)(1/q_1) + P_2(1-P_2)(1/q_2)}]^2}{(P_1 - P_2)^2}.$$

Readers who would like to skip the work involved in hand calculations with this formula can get an instant answer from a calculator on our website (www.epibiostat.ucsf.edu/dcr/) (This formula does not include the Fleiss-Tytun-Ury continuity correction and therefore underestimates the required sample size by up to about 10%. Tables 6B.1 and 6B.2 do include this continuity correction.)

TABLE 6B.2 Sample Size *per Group* for Comparing Two Proportions, the Smaller of Which Is Between 0.01 and 0.10

Upper number: $\alpha = 0.05$ (one-sided) or $\alpha = 0.10$ (two-sided); $\beta = 0.20$
Middle number: $\alpha = 0.025$ (one-sided) or $\alpha = 0.05$ (two-sided); $\beta = 0.20$
Lower number: $\alpha = 0.025$ (one-sided) or $\alpha = 0.05$ (two-sided); $\beta = 0.10$

Smaller of P_1 and P_2	Expected Difference Between P_1 and P_2									
	0.01	0.02	0.03	0.04	0.05	0.06	0.07	0.08	0.09	0.10
0.01	2,019	700	396	271	204	162	134	114	98	87
	2,512	864	487	332	249	197	163	138	120	106
	3,300	1,125	631	428	320	254	209	178	154	135
0.02	3,205	994	526	343	249	193	157	131	113	97
	4,018	1,237	651	423	306	238	192	161	137	120
	5,320	1,625	852	550	397	307	248	207	177	154
0.03	4,367	1,283	653	414	294	224	179	148	126	109
	5,493	1,602	813	512	363	276	220	182	154	133
	7,296	2,114	1,067	671	474	359	286	236	199	172
0.04	5,505	1,564	777	482	337	254	201	165	139	119
	6,935	1,959	969	600	419	314	248	203	170	146
	9,230	2,593	1,277	788	548	410	323	264	221	189
0.05	6,616	1,838	898	549	380	283	222	181	151	129
	8,347	2,308	1,123	686	473	351	275	223	186	159
	11,123	3,061	1,482	902	620	460	360	291	242	206
0.06	7,703	2,107	1,016	615	422	312	243	197	163	139
	9,726	2,650	1,272	769	526	388	301	243	202	171
	12,973	3,518	1,684	1,014	691	508	395	318	263	223
0.07	8,765	2,369	1,131	680	463	340	263	212	175	148
	11,076	2,983	1,419	850	577	423	327	263	217	183
	14,780	3,965	1,880	1,123	760	555	429	343	283	239
0.08	9,803	2,627	1,244	743	502	367	282	227	187	158
	12,393	3,308	1,562	930	627	457	352	282	232	195
	16,546	4,401	2,072	1,229	827	602	463	369	303	255
0.09	10,816	2,877	1,354	804	541	393	302	241	198	167
	13,679	3,626	1,702	1,007	676	491	377	300	246	207
	18,270	4,827	2,259	1,333	893	647	495	393	322	270
0.10	11,804	3,121	1,461	863	578	419	320	255	209	175
	14,933	3,936	1,838	1,083	724	523	401	318	260	218
	19,952	5,242	2,441	1,434	957	690	527	417	341	285

The one-sided estimates use the z statistic.

◼ APPENDIX 6C

Total Sample Size Required When Using the Correlation Coefficient (r)

TABLE 6C	Sample Size for Determining Whether a Correlation Coefficient Differs from Zero								
One-sided α =	0.005			0.025			0.05		
Two-sided α =	0.01			0.05			0.0101		
β =	0.05	0.10	0.20	0.05	0.10	0.20	0.05	0.10	0.20
r^*									
0.05	7,118	5,947	4,663	5,193	4,200	3,134	4,325	3,424	2,469
0.10	1,773	1,481	1,162	1,294	1,047	782	1,078	854	616
0.15	783	655	514	572	463	346	477	378	273
0.20	436	365	287	319	259	194	266	211	153
0.25	276	231	182	202	164	123	169	134	98
0.30	189	158	125	139	113	85	116	92	67
0.35	136	114	90	100	82	62	84	67	49
0.40	102	86	68	75	62	47	63	51	37
0.45	79	66	53	58	48	36	49	39	29
0.50	62	52	42	46	38	29	39	31	23
0.60	40	34	27	30	25	19	26	21	16
0.70	27	23	19	20	17	13	17	14	11
0.80	18	15	13	14	12	9	12	10	8

* To estimate the total sample size, read across from r (the expected correlation coefficient) and down from the specified values of α and β.

General Formula for Other Values

The general formula for other values of r, α, and β is as follows (see Appendix 6A for definitions of Z_α and Z_β). Let

$$r = \text{expected correlation coefficient}$$
$$C = 0.5 \times \ln[(1 + r)/(1 - r)]$$
$$N = \text{Total number of subjects required}$$

Then

$$N = [(z_\alpha + z_\beta) \div C]^2 + 3.$$

Estimating Sample Size for Difference between Two Correlations

If testing whether a correlation, r_1, is different from r_2 (i.e., the null hypothesis is that $r_1 = r_2$; the alternative hypothesis is that $r_1 \neq r_2$), let

$$C_1 = 0.5 \times \ln[(1 + r_1)/(1 - r_1)]$$
$$C_2 = 0.5 \times \ln[(1 + r_2)/(1 - r_2)]$$

Then

$$N = [(z_\alpha + z_\beta) \div (C_1 - C_2)]^2 + 3.$$

APPENDIX 6D

Sample Size for a Descriptive Study of a Continuous Variable

TABLE 6D	Sample Size for Common Values of W/S^*		
	Confidence Level		
W/S	**90%**	**95%**	**99%**
0.10	1,083	1,537	2,665
0.15	482	683	1,180
0.20	271	385	664
0.25	174	246	425
0.30	121	171	295
0.35	89	126	217
0.40	68	97	166
0.50	44	62	107
0.60	31	43	74
0.70	23	32	55
0.80	17	25	42
0.90	14	19	33
1.00	11	16	27

* W/S is the standardized width of the confidence interval, computed as W (desired total width) divided by S (standard deviation of the variable). To estimate the total sample size, read across from the *standardized width* and down from the specified confidence level.

General Formula for Other Values

For other values of W, S, and a confidence level of $(1 - \alpha)$, the total number of subjects required (N) is

$$N = 4z_\alpha^2 S^2 \div W^2$$

(see Appendix 6A for the definition of z_α).

APPENDIX 6E

Sample Size for a Descriptive Study of a Dichotomous Variable

TABLE 6E	Sample Size for Proportions

Upper number: 90% confidence level
Middle number: 95% confidence level
Lower number: 99% confidence level

Expected Proportion (P)*	Total Width of Confidence Interval (*W*)						
	0.10	0.15	0.20	0.25	0.30	0.35	0.40
0.10	98	44	—	—	—	—	—
	138	61	—	—	—	—	—
	239	106	—	—	—	—	—
0.15	139	62	35	22	—	—	—
	196	87	49	31	—	—	—
	339	151	85	54	—	—	—
0.20	174	77	44	28	19	14	—
	246	109	61	39	27	20	—
	426	189	107	68	47	35	—
0.25	204	91	51	33	23	17	13
	288	128	72	46	32	24	18
	499	222	125	80	55	41	31
0.30	229	102	57	37	25	19	14
	323	143	81	52	36	26	20
	559	249	140	89	62	46	35
0.40	261	116	65	42	29	21	16
	369	164	92	59	41	30	23
	639	284	160	102	71	52	40
0.50	272	121	68	44	30	22	17
	384	171	96	61	43	31	24
	666	296	166	107	74	54	42

* To estimate the sample size, read across the *expected proportion* (P) who have the variable of interest and down from the desired *total width* (*W*) of the confidence interval. The three numbers represent the sample size required for 90%, 95%, and 99% confidence levels.

General Formula for Other Values

The general formula for other values of P, W, and a confidence level of $(1 - \alpha)$, where P and W are defined above, is as follows. Let

Z_α = the standard normal deviate for a two-sided α, where $(1 - \alpha)$ is the confidence level (e.g., since $\alpha = 0.05$ for a 95% confidence level, $z_\alpha = 1.96$; therefore, for a 90% confidence level $z_\alpha = 1.65$, and for a 99% confidence level $z_\alpha = 2.58$).

Then the total number of subjects required is:

$$N = 4z_\alpha^2 P(1 - P) \div W^2$$

APPENDIX 6F

Use and Misuse of *t* Tests

Two-sample *t* tests, the primary focus of this chapter, are used when comparing the mean values of a variable in two groups of subjects. The two groups can be defined by a predictor variable—active drug versus placebo in a randomized trial, or presence versus absence of a risk factor in a cohort study—or they can be defined by an outcome variable, as in a case–control study. A two-sample *t* test can be **unpaired,** if measurements obtained on a single occasion are being compared between two groups, or **paired** if the change in measurements made at two points in time, say before and after an intervention, are being compared between the groups. A third type of *t* test, the **one-sample paired *t* test,** compares the mean change in measurements at two points in time within a single group to zero change.

Table 6F illustrates the misuse of one-sample paired *t* tests in a study designed for between-group comparisons—a randomized blinded trial of the effect of a new sleeping pill on quality of life. In situations like this, some investigators have performed (and published!) findings with two separate one-sample *t* tests—one each in the treatment and placebo groups.

In the table, the *P* values designated with a dagger (†) are from one-sample paired *t*-tests. The first *P* (0.05) shows a significant change in quality of life in the treatment group during the study; the second *P* value (0.16) shows no significant change in the control group. However, this analysis does not permit inferences about differences between the groups, and it would be wrong to conclude that there was a significant effect of the treatment.

The *P* values designated with a (*), represent the appropriate two-sample *t* test results. The first two *P* values (0.87 and 0.64) are two-sample unpaired *t* tests that show no statistically significant between-group differences in the initial or final measurements for quality of life. The last *P* value (0.17) is a two-sample paired *t* test; it is closer to 0.05 than the *P* value for the end of study values (0.64) because the paired mean differences have smaller standard deviations. However, the improved quality of life in the treatment group (1.3) was not significantly different from that in the placebo group (0.9), and the correct conclusion is that the study did not find the treatment to be effective.

TABLE 6F	Correct (and Incorrect) Ways to Analyze Paired Data		
	Quality of Life, as Mean ± SD		
Time of Measurement	**Treatment (*n* = 100)**	**Control (*n* = 100)**	***P* value**
Baseline	7.0 ± 4.5	7.1 ± 4.4	0.87*
End of study	8.3 ± 4.7	8.0 ± 4.6	0.64*
P value	0.05†	0.16†	
Difference	1.3 ± 2.1	0.9 ± 2.0	0.17*

REFERENCES

1. Lehr R. Sixteen S-squared over D-squared: a relation for crude sample size estimates. *Stat Med* 1992;11:1099–1102.
2. Lakatos E, Lan KK. A comparison of sample size methods for the logrank statistic. *Stat Med* 1992;11:179–191.
3. Shih JH. Sample size calculation for complex clinical trials with survival endpoints. *Control Clin Trials* 1995;16:395–407.
4. Donner A. Sample size requirements for stratified cluster randomization designs [published erratum appears in *Stat Med* 1997;30;16:2927]. *Stat Med* 1992;11:743–750.
5. Liu G, Liang KY. Sample size calculations for studies with correlated observations. *Biometrics* 1997;53:937–947.
6. Kerry SM, Bland JM. Trials which randomize practices II: sample size. *Fam Pract* 1998;15:84–87.
7. Hayes RJ, Bennett S. Simple sample size calculation for cluster-randomized trials. *Int J Epidemiol* 1999;28:319–326.
8. Edwardes MD. Sample size requirements for case-control study designs. *BMC Med Res Methodol* 2001;1:11.
9. Drescher K, Timm J, Jöckel KH. The design of case-control studies: the effect of confounding on sample size requirements. *Stat Med* 1990;9:765–776.
10. Lui KJ. Sample size determination for case-control studies: the influence of the joint distribution of exposure and confounder. *Stat Med* 1990;9:1485–1493.
11. Vaeth M, Skovlund E. A simple approach to power and sample size calculations in logistic regression and Cox regression models. *Stat Med* 2004;23:1781–1792.
12. Dupont WD, Plummer WD Jr. Power and sample size calculations for studies involving linear regression. *Control Clin Trials* 1998;19:589–601.
13. Hsieh FY, Bloch DA, Larsen MD. A simple method of sample size calculation for linear and logistic regression. *Stat Med* 1998;17:1623–1634.
14. Hsieh FY, Lavori PW. Sample-size calculations for the Cox proportional hazards regression model with nonbinary covariates. *Control Clin Trials* 2000;21:552–560.
15. Sasieni PD. From genotypes to genes: doubling the sample size. *Biometrics* 1997;53:1253–1261.
16. Elston RC, Idury RM, Cardon LR, et al. The study of candidate genes in drug trials: sample size considerations. *Stat Med* 1999;18:741–751.
17. García-Closas M, Lubin JH. Power and sample size calculations in case-control studies of gene-environment interactions: comments on different approaches. *Am J Epidemiol* 1999;149:689–692.
18. Torgerson DJ, Ryan M, Ratcliffe J. Economics in sample size determination for clinical trials. *QJM* 1995;88:517–521.
19. Laska EM, Meisner M, Siegel C. Power and sample size in cost-effectiveness analysis. *Med Decis Making* 1999;19:339–343.
20. Willan AR, O'Brien BJ. Sample size and power issues in estimating incremental cost-effectiveness ratios from clinical trials data. *Health Econ* 1999;8:203–211.
21. Patel HI. Sample size for a dose-response study [published erratum appears in *J Biopharm Stat* 1994;4:127]. *J Biopharm Stat* 1992;2:1–8.
22. Day SJ, Graham DF. Sample size estimation for comparing two or more treatment groups in clinical trials. *Stat Med* 1991;10:33–43.
23. Nam JM. Sample size determination in stratified trials to establish the equivalence of two treatments. *Stat Med* 1995;14:2037–2049.
24. Bristol DR. Determining equivalence and the impact of sample size in anti-infective studies: a point to consider. *J Biopharm Stat* 1996;6:319–326.
25. Tai BC, Lee J. Sample size and power calculations for comparing two independent proportions in a "negative" trial. *Psychiatry Res* 1998;80:197–200.

26. Hauschke D, Kieser M, Diletti E, et al. Sample size determination for proving equivalence based on the ratio of two means for normally distributed data. *Stat Med* 1999;18:93–105.

27. Obuchowski NA. Computing sample size for receiver operating characteristic studies. *Invest Radiol* 1994;29:238–243.

28. Simel DL, Samsa GP, Matchar DB. Likelihood ratios with confidence: sample size estimation for diagnostic test studies. *J Clin Epidemiol* 1991;44:763–770.

29. Walter SD, Eliasziw M, Donner A. Sample size and optimal designs for reliability studies. *Stat Med* 1998;17:101–110.

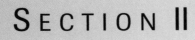

Study Designs

Steven R. Cummings, Thomas B. Newman,
and Stephen B. Hulley

Cohort studies involve following groups of subjects over time. There are two primary purposes: **descriptive**, typically to describe the occurrence of certain outcomes over time; and **analytic**, to analyze associations between predictors and those outcomes. This chapter begins with a description of the classic **prospective cohort** study, in which the investigator defines the sample and measures predictor variables before undertaking a follow-up period to observe outcomes. We then review **retrospective cohort** studies, which save time and money because the follow-up period and outcomes have already occurred when the study takes place, and include highly efficient **nested case–control** and **case–cohort** options. The chapter concludes by describing **multiple-cohort** studies and reviewing the methods for optimizing a key ingredient for all cohort designs, **cohort retention** during follow-up.

PROSPECTIVE COHORT STUDIES

Structure

Cohort was the Roman term for a group of soldiers that marched together, and in clinical research a cohort is a group of subjects followed over time. In a **prospective cohort study**, the investigator begins by assembling a sample of subjects (Fig. 7.1). She measures characteristics in each subject that might predict the subsequent outcomes, and follows these subjects with periodic measurements of the outcomes of interest.

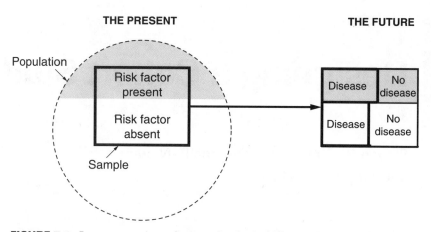

THE PRESENT   THE FUTURE

FIGURE 7.1. In a prospective cohort study, the investigator (a) selects a sample from the population (the dotted line signifies its large and undefined size) (b) measures the predictor variables (in this case whether a dichotomous risk factor is present [shaded]), and (c) measures the outcome variables during follow-up (in this case whether a disease occurs [outlined in bold]).

Example 7.1 Prospective Cohort Study

The Nurses' Health Study examines incidence and risk factors for common diseases in women. The basic steps in performing the study were to:

1. **Assemble the Cohort.** *In 1976, the investigators obtained lists of registered nurses aged 25 to 42 in the 11 most populous states and mailed them an invitation to participate in the study; those who agreed became the cohort.*
2. **Measure Predictor Variables and Potential Confounders.** *They mailed a questionnaire about weight, exercise and other potential risk factors and obtained completed questionnaires from 121,700 nurses. They send questionnaires periodically to ask about additional risk factors and update the status of some risk factors that had been measured previously.*
3. **Follow-up the Cohort and Measure Outcomes.** *The periodic questionnaires also included questions about the occurrence of a variety of disease outcomes.*

The prospective approach allowed investigators to make measurements at baseline, and collect data on subsequent outcomes. The large size of the cohort and long period of follow-up have provided substantial statistical power to study risk factors for cancers and other diseases.

For example, the investigators examined the hypothesis that gaining weight increases a woman's risk of breast cancer after menopause (1). The women reported their weight at age 18 in an early questionnaire, and their current weights in later questionnaires. The investigators succeeded in following 95% of the women and 1,517 cases of breast cancer were confirmed during the next 12 years. Heavier women had a higher risk of breast cancer after menopause, and those who gained more than 20 kg since age 18 had a twofold increased risk of developing breast cancer (relative risk = 2.0; 95% confidence interval, 1.4 to 2.8). Adjusting for potential confounding factors did not change the result.

Strengths and Weaknesses

The **prospective cohort design** is a powerful strategy for assessing incidence (the number of new cases of a condition in a specified time interval), and it is helpful in investigating the potential causes of the condition. Measuring levels of the predictor before the outcome occurs establishes the time sequence of the variables and prevents the predictor measurements from being influenced by knowledge of the outcome. The prospective approach also allows the investigator to measure variables more completely and accurately than is possible retrospectively. This is important for predictors such as dietary habits that are difficult for a subject to remember accurately. When fatal diseases are studied retrospectively, predictor variables about the decedent can only be reconstructed from indirect sources such as medical records or friends and relatives.

All cohort studies share the general disadvantage of observational studies (relative to clinical trials) that causal inference is challenging and interpretation often muddied by the influences of confounding variables (Chapter 9). A particular weakness of the prospective design is its expense and inefficiency for studying rare outcomes. Even diseases we think of as relatively common, such as breast cancer, happen so infrequently in any given year that large numbers of people must be followed for long periods of time to observe enough outcomes to produce meaningful results. Cohort designs become more efficient as the outcomes become more common and immediate; a prospective study of risk factors for progression after treatment of patients with breast cancer will be smaller and less time consuming than a prospective study of risk factors for the occurrence of breast cancer in a healthy population.

■ RETROSPECTIVE COHORT STUDIES

Structure

The design of a **retrospective cohort** study (Fig. 7.2) differs from that of a prospective one in that the assembly of the cohort, baseline measurements, and follow-up have

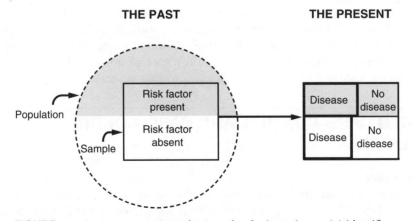

FIGURE 7.2. In a retrospective cohort study, the investigator (a) identifies a cohort that has been assembled in the past, (b) collects data on predictor variables (measured in the past), and (c) collects data on outcome variables (measured in the present).

all happened in the past. This type of study is only possible if adequate data about the risk factors and outcomes are available on a cohort of subjects that has been assembled for other purposes.

Example 7.2 Retrospective Cohort Study

To describe the natural history of thoracic aortic aneurysms and risk factors for rupture of these aneurysms, Clouse et al. analyzed data from the medical records of 133 patients who had aneurysms (2). The basic steps in performing the study were to

1. **Identify a Suitable Cohort.** *The investigators used the residents of Olmsted County, Minnesota. They searched a database of diagnoses made between 1980 and 1995 and found 133 residents who had a diagnosis of aortic aneurysm.*
2. **Collect Data about Predictor Variables.** *They reviewed patients' records to collect gender, age, size of aneurysm, and risk factors for cardiovascular disease at the time of diagnosis.*
3. **Collect Data about Subsequent Outcomes.** *They collected data from the medical records of the 133 patients to determine whether the aneurysm ruptured or was surgically repaired.*

The investigators found that the 5-year risk of rupture was 20% and that women were 6.8 times more likely to suffer a rupture than men (95% confidence interval, 2.3 to 20). They also found that 31% of aneurysms with diameters of more than 6 cm ruptured, compared with none with diameters of less than 4 cm.

Strengths and Weaknesses

Retrospective cohort studies have many of the same strengths as prospective cohort studies, and they have the advantage of being much less costly and time consuming. The subjects are already assembled, baseline measurements have already been made, and the follow-up period has already taken place. The main disadvantages are the limited control the investigator has over the approach to sampling the population, and over the nature and the quality of the predictor variables. The existing data may be incomplete, inaccurate, or measured in ways that are not ideal for answering the research question.

■ NESTED CASE–CONTROL AND CASE–COHORT STUDIES[1]

Structure

A **nested case–control** design has a case–control study "nested" within a cohort study (Fig. 7.3). It is an excellent design for predictor variables that are expensive to measure and that can be assessed at the end of the study on subjects who

---

[1]These terms are used inconsistently in the literature; the definitions provided here are the simplest. For a detailed discussion, see Szklo and Nieto (3).

**MEASUREMENTS IN THE PRESENT OF
SPECIMENS FROM THE PAST**   **THE PRESENT**

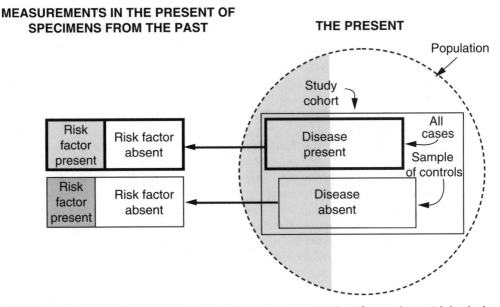

FIGURE 7.3. In a nested case–control study, the investigator (a) identifies a cohort with banked specimens, images, or information; (b) identifies those participants who developed the outcome during follow-up (the cases); (c) selects a sample from the rest of the cohort (the controls); and (d) measures predictor variables in cases and controls.

develop the outcome during the study (the cases), and on a sample of those who do not (the controls). The investigator begins with a suitable cohort with enough cases by the end of follow-up to provide adequate power to answer the research question. At the end of the study she applies criteria that define the outcome of interest to identify all those who have developed the outcome (the cases). Next, she selects a random sample of the subjects who have not developed the outcome (the controls); she can increase power by selecting two or three controls for each case, and by matching on constitutional determinants of outcome such as age and sex (see Chapter 9 for the pros and cons of matching). She then retrieves specimens, images or records that were collected before the outcomes had occurred, measures the predictor variables, and compares the levels in cases and controls.

The **nested case–cohort** approach is the same design except that the controls are a random sample of all the members of the cohort regardless of outcomes. This means that there will be some cases among those sampled for the comparison group, who will also appear among the cases and be analyzed as such (removing them from the cohort sample for purposes of analysis is a negligible problem provided that the outcome is uncommon). This approach has the advantage that the controls represent the cohort in general, and therefore provide a basis for estimating incidence and prevalence in the population from which it was drawn. More important, it means that this cohort sample can be used as the comparison group for more than one type of outcome provided that it is not too common. In Example 7.3, for instance, a single set of sex hormone levels from the baseline exam measured in a random sample of the cohort could be compared with levels from baseline in cases with breast cancer in one analysis, and in cases with fractures in another.

Example 7.3 Nested Case–Control Design

Cauley et al. carried out a nested case–control study of whether higher levels of sex hormones were risk factors for breast cancer, (4). The basic steps in this study were to

1. **Identify a Cohort with Banked Samples**. *The investigators used serum and data from the Study of Osteoporotic Fractures, a prospective cohort of 9,704 women age 65 and older.*
2. **Identify Cases at the End of Follow-up**. *Based on responses to follow-up questionnaires and review of death certificates, the investigators identified 97 subjects with a first occurrence of breast cancer during 3.2 years of follow-up.*
3. **Select Controls**. *The investigators selected a random sample of 244 women in the cohort who did not develop breast cancer during that follow-up period.*
4. **Measure Predictors on Baseline Samples from Cases and Controls**. *Levels of estradiol and testosterone were measured in serum specimens from the baseline examination that had been stored at $-190°$ C by laboratory staff who were blinded to case–control status.*

Women who had high levels of either estradiol or testosterone had a threefold increase in the risk of a subsequent diagnosis of breast cancer compared with women who had very low levels of these hormones.

Strengths and Weaknesses

Nested case–control and **case–cohort** studies are especially useful for costly measurements on serum, electronic images, hospital charts, etc. that have been archived at the beginning of the study and preserved for later analysis. In addition to the cost savings of not making the measurements on the entire cohort, the design allows the investigator to introduce novel measurements that were not available at the outset of the study. The design preserves all the advantages of cohort studies that result from collecting predictor variables before the outcomes have happened, and it avoids the potential biases of conventional case–control studies that draw cases and controls from different populations and cannot make measurements on cases and controls who have died.

The chief disadvantage of this design is that many research questions and circumstances are not amenable to the strategy of storing materials for later analysis on a sample of the study subjects. Also, when data are available for the entire cohort at no additional cost, nothing is gained by studying only a sample of controls—the whole cohort should be used.

These are such great designs that an investigator planning a prospective study should always consider preserving biologic samples and storing images or records that involve expensive measurements for subsequent nested case–control or case–cohort analyses. She should ensure that the conditions of storage will preserve substances of interest for many years, and consider setting aside specimens for periodic measurements to confirm that the components have remained stable. She may also find it useful to collect new samples or information during the follow-up period that can be used in the case–control comparisons.

MULTIPLE-COHORT STUDIES AND EXTERNAL CONTROLS

Structure

Multiple-cohort studies begin with two or more separate samples of subjects: typically, one group with exposure to a potential risk factor and one or more other groups with no exposure or a lower level of exposure (Fig. 7.4). After defining suitable cohorts with different levels of exposure to the predictor of interest, the investigator measures predictor variables, follows up the cohorts, and assesses outcomes as in any other type of cohort study.

The use of two different samples of subjects in a double-cohort design should not be confused with the use of two samples in the case–control design (Chapter 8). In a double-cohort study the two groups of subjects are chosen based on the level of a predictor variable, whereas in a case–control study the two groups are chosen based on the presence or absence of the outcome.

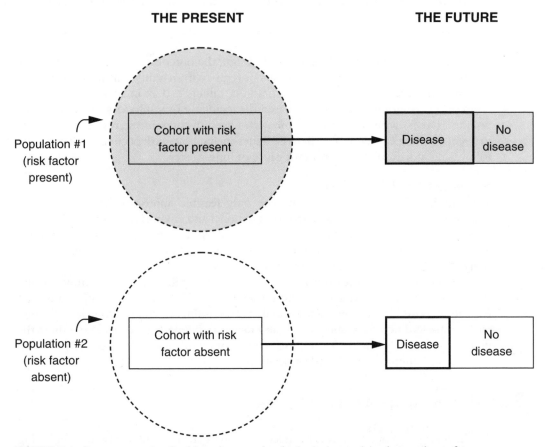

FIGURE 7.4. In a prospective double-cohort study, the investigator (a) selects cohorts from two populations with different levels of the predictor, and (b) measures outcome variables during follow-up. (Double-cohort studies can also be conducted retrospectively.)

Example 7.4 Multiple-Cohort Design

To determine whether significant neonatal jaundice or dehydration has any significant adverse effects on neurodevelopment, investigators from UCSF and the Northern California Kaiser Permanente Medical Care Program (5) undertook a triple- cohort study. The basic steps in performing the study were to

1. **Identify Cohorts with Different Exposures**. *The investigators used electronic databases to identify term and near-term newborns who (1) had a total serum bilirubin level of $\geq$ 25 mg/dL, or (2) were readmitted for dehydration with a serum sodium of $\geq$ 150 mEq/L or weight loss of $\geq$ 12% from birth, or (3) were randomly selected from the birth cohort.*
2. **Determine Outcomes**: *The investigators used electronic databases to search for diagnoses of neurological disorders and did full neurodevelopmental examinations at the age of 5 for consenting participants.*

With few exceptions, neither hyperbilirubinemia nor dehydration was associated with adverse outcomes.

In a variation on the multiple-cohort design, the outcome rate in a cohort can be compared with outcome rates in a census or registry from a different population. For example, in a classic study of whether uranium miners had an increased incidence of lung cancer, Wagoner et al. (6) compared the incidence of respiratory cancer in 3,415 uranium miners with that of white men who lived in the same states. The increased incidence of lung cancer observed in the miners helped establish occupational exposure to ionizing radiation as an important cause of lung cancer.

Strengths and Weaknesses

The multiple-cohort design may be the only feasible approach for studying rare exposures, and exposures to potential occupational and environmental hazards. Using data from a census or registry as the external control group has the additional advantage of being population based and economical. Otherwise, the strengths of this design are similar to those of other cohort studies.

The problem of **confounding** is accentuated in a multiple-cohort study because the cohorts are assembled from different populations that can differ in important ways (besides exposure to the predictor variable) that influence the outcomes. Although some of these differences, such as age and race, can be matched or used to adjust the findings statistically, other characteristics may not be measurable and create problems in the interpretation of observed associations.

■ OTHER COHORT STUDY ISSUES

The hallmark of a cohort study is the need to define a group of subjects at the beginning of a period of follow-up. The subjects should be appropriate to the research question and available for follow-up. They should sufficiently resemble the population to which the results will be generalized. The number of subjects should provide adequate power.

The quality of the study will depend on the precision and accuracy of the measurements of predictor and outcome variables. The ability to draw inferences about cause and effect will also depend on the degree to which the investigator has identified and **measured all potential confounders** and sources of effect modification (Chapter 9). Predictor variables may change during the study; whether and how frequently measurements should be repeated depends on cost, how much the variable is likely to change, and the importance to the research question of observing these changes. Outcomes should be assessed using standardized criteria and **blindly**— without knowing the values of the predictor variables.

Follow-up of the entire cohort is important, and prospective studies should take a number of steps to achieve this goal. Loss of subjects can be minimized in several ways (Table 7.1). Those who plan to move out of reach during the study or who will be difficult to follow for other reasons should be excluded at the outset. The investigator should collect information early on that she can use to find subjects if they move or die. This includes the address, telephone number and e-mail address of the subject, personal physician and one or two close friends or relatives who do not live in the same house. It is useful to obtain the social security number and (for those over

---

TABLE 7.1   Strategies for Minimizing Losses during Follow-up

During enrollment

1. Exclude those likely to be lost
   a. Planning to move
   b. Uncertainty about willingness to return
   c. Ill health or fatal disease unrelated to research question
2. Obtain information to allow future tracking
   a. Address, telephone number(s), and e-mail address of subject
   b. Social Security/Medicare numbers
   c. Name, address, telephone number, and e-mail addresses for one or two close friends or relatives who do not live with the subject
   d. Name, e-mail, address, and telephone number of physician(s)

During follow-up

1. Periodic contact with subjects to collect information, provide results, express care, and so on.
   a. By telephone: may require calls during weekends and evenings
   b. By mail: repeated mailings by e-mail or with stamped, self-addressed return cards
   c. Other: newsletters, token gifts
2. For those who are not reached by phone or mail:*
   a. Contact friends, relatives, or physicians
   b. Request forwarding addresses from postal service
   c. Seek address through other public sources, such as telephone directories and the Internet, and ultimately a credit bureau search.
   d. For subjects receiving Medicare, collect data about hospital discharges from Social Security Administration
   e. Determine vital status from state health department or National Death Registry

At all times

1. Treat study subjects with appreciation, kindness and respect, helping them to understand the research question so they will want to join as partners in making the study successful

---

* This assumes that participants in the study have given informed consent to collect the tracking information and for follow-up contact.

65) the medicare number. This information will allow the investigator to determine the vital status of subjects who are lost to follow-up using the National Death Index and to obtain hospital discharge information from the Social Security Administration for subjects who receive Medicare. Periodic contact with the subjects once or twice a year helps in keeping track of them, and may improve the timeliness and accuracy of recording the outcomes of interest. Finding subjects for follow-up assessments sometimes requires persistent and repeated efforts by mail, e-mail, telephone, house calls, or professional tracking.

SUMMARY

1. In **cohort studies**, subjects are followed over time to **describe the incidence** or natural history of a condition and to **analyze predictors** (risk factors) for various outcomes. Measuring the predictor before the outcome occurs establishes the sequence of events and helps control bias in that measurement.

2. **Prospective cohort** studies begin at the outset of follow-up and may require large numbers of subjects followed for long periods of time. This disadvantage can sometimes be overcome by identifying a **retrospective cohort** in which measurements of predictor variables have already occurred.

3. Another efficient variant is the **nested case–control** design. A bank of specimens, images, or records is collected at baseline; measurements are made on the stored materials for all subjects who have developed an outcome, and for a subset of those who have not. In the **nested case–cohort strategy**, a single random sample of the cohort can serve as the comparison group for several case–control studies.

4. The **multiple-cohort** design, which compares the incidence of outcomes in cohorts that differ in level of a predictor variable, is useful for studying the effects of rare and occupational exposures.

5. Inferences about **cause and effect** are strengthened by measuring all potential confounding variables at baseline. Bias in the assessment of outcomes is prevented by **standardizing** the measurements and **blinding** those assessing the outcome to the predictor variable values.

6. The strengths of a cohort design can be undermined by incomplete **follow-up** of subjects. Losses can be minimized by **excluding subjects** who may not be available for follow-up, collecting **baseline information** that facilitates tracking, **staying in touch** with all subjects regularly, and involving subjects as **partners in the research**.

REFERENCES

1. Huang Z, Hankinson SE, Colditz GA, et al. Dual effect of weight and weight gain on breast cancer risk. *JAMA* 1997;278:1407–1411.
2. Clouse WD, Hallett JW Jr, Schaff HV, et al. Improved prognosis of thoracic aortic aneurysms: a population-based study. *JAMA* 1998;280:1926–1929.

3. Szklo M, Nieto FJ. *Epidemiology: beyond the basics*. Gaithersburg, MD: Aspen, 2000:33–38.
4. Cauley JA, Lucas FL, Kuller LH, et al. Study of Osteoporotic Fractures Research Group. Elevated serum estradiol and testosterone concentrations are associated with a high risk for breast cancer. *Ann Intern Med* 1999;130:270–277.
5. Newman TB, Liljestrand P, Jeremy RJ, et al. Outcomes of newborns with total serum bilirubin levels of 25 mg/dL or more. *N Engl J Med* 2006;354:1889–900.
6. Wagoner JK, Archer VE, Lundin FE, et al. Radiation as the cause of lung cancer among uranium miners. *N Engl J Med* 1965;273:181–187.

8

Designing Cross-sectional and Case–Control Studies

Thomas B. Newman, Warren S. Browner, Steven R. Cummings, and Stephen B. Hulley

Chapter 7 dealt with cohort studies, in which the sequence of the measurements is the same as the chronology of cause and effect: first the predictor, then (after an interval of follow-up) the outcome. In this chapter we turn to two kinds of observational studies that are not guided by this logical time sequence.

In a **cross-sectional** study, the investigator makes all of her measurements on a single occasion or within a short period of time. She draws a sample from the population and looks at distributions of variables within that sample, sometimes designating predictor and outcome variables based on biologic plausibility and information from other sources. In a **case–control** study, the investigator works backward. She begins by choosing one sample from a population of patients with the outcome (the cases) and another from a population without it (the controls); then she compares the distribution levels of the predictor variables in the two samples to see which ones are associated with and might cause the outcome.

CROSS-SECTIONAL STUDIES

Structure
The structure of a cross-sectional study is similar to that of a cohort study except that all the measurements are made at about the same time, with no follow-up period (Fig. 8.1). Cross-sectional designs are very well suited to the goal of describing variables and their distribution patterns. In the National Health and Nutrition Examination Survey (NHANES), for example, a sample designed to represent the US population is interviewed and examined. NHANES surveys have been carried out periodically, and an NHANES follow-up (cohort) study has been added to the original cross-sectional design. Each cross-sectional study is a major source of information about the health and habits of the US population in the year it is carried out, providing estimates of such things as the prevalence of smoking in various demographic groups. All NHANES datasets are available for public use.

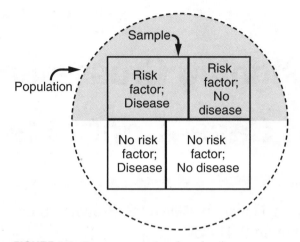

FIGURE 8.1. In a cross-sectional study, the investigator (a) selects a sample from the population and (b) measures predictor and outcome variables (e.g., presence or absence of a risk factor and disease).

Cross-sectional studies can also be used for examining associations, although the choice of which variables to label as predictors and which as outcomes depends on the cause-and-effect hypotheses of the investigator rather than on the study design. This choice is easy for constitutional factors such as age and race; these cannot be altered by other variables and therefore are predictors. For other variables, however, the choice can go either way. For example, a cross-sectional finding in NHANES III is an association between childhood obesity and hours spent watching television (1). Whether to label obesity or TV-watching as the outcome depends on the question of interest to the investigator.

Unlike cohort studies, which have a longitudinal time dimension and can be used to estimate **incidence** (the proportion who *get* a disease or condition over time), cross-sectional studies can generally provide information only about **prevalence,** the proportion who *have* a disease or condition at one point in time (Table 8.1). Prevalence is useful to health planners who want to know how many people have certain diseases so that they can allocate enough resources to care for them, and it is useful to the clinician who must estimate the likelihood that the patient sitting in her office has a particular disease. When analyzing cross-sectional studies, the prevalence

TABLE 8.1	Statistics for Expressing Disease Frequency in Observational Studies	
Type of Study	**Statistic**	**Definition**
Cohort	Incidence rate	$\dfrac{\text{Number of people who } get \text{ a disease or condition}}{\text{Number of people at risk } \times \text{ Time period at risk}}$
Cross-sectional	Prevalence	$\dfrac{\text{Number of people who } have \text{ a disease or condition}}{\text{Number of people at risk}}$
Both	Cumulative incidence	$\dfrac{\text{Number of people who get (cohort) or report ever having acquired (cross-sectional) a disease or condition}}{\text{Number of people at risk}}$

of the outcome is compared in those with and without an exposure, giving the relative prevalence of the outcome, the cross-sectional equivalent of relative risk. An example calculation of prevalence and relative prevalence is provided in Appendix 8A.

Sometimes cross-sectional studies describe the prevalence of ever having done something or ever having had a disease or condition. In that case, the prevalence is the same as the **cumulative incidence,** and it is important to make sure that follow-up time is the same in those exposed and unexposed. This is illustrated in Example 8.1, in which the prevalence of ever having tried smoking was studied in a cross-sectional study of children with differing levels of exposure to movies in which the actors smoke. Of course, children who had seen more movies were also older, and therefore had longer to try smoking, so it was very important to adjust for age in analyses (multivariate adjustment is discussed in Chapter 9).

Example 8.1 Cross-sectional Study

To determine whether exposure to movies in which the actors smoke is associated with smoking initiation, Sargent et al. (2):

1. **Selected the Sample:** *They did a random-digit-dial survey of 6,522 children aged 10 to 14 years.*
2. **Measured the Variables:** *They quantified smoking in 532 popular movies and for each subject asked which of a randomly selected subset of 50 movies they had seen. Subjects were also asked about a variety of covariates such as age, race, gender, parental smoking and education, sensation-seeking (e.g., "I like to do dangerous things") and self-esteem (e.g., "I wish I were someone else.") The outcome variable was whether the child had ever tried smoking a cigarette.*

   The prevalence of ever having tried smoking varied from 2% in the lowest quartile of movie smoking exposure to 22% in the highest quartile. After adjusting for age and other confounders, odds ratios were much lower but still significant: 1.7, 1.8, and 2.6 for the second, third, and highest quartiles of movie smoking exposure, compared with the lowest quartile. Based on the adjusted odds ratios, the authors estimated that 38% of smoking initiation was attributable to exposure to movies in which the actors smoke.

Strengths and Weaknesses of Cross-sectional Studies

A major strength of cross-sectional studies over cohort studies and clinical trials is that there is no waiting for the outcome to occur. This makes them fast and inexpensive, and it means that there is no loss to follow-up. A cross-sectional study can be included as the first step in a cohort study or experiment at little or no added cost. The results define the demographic and clinical characteristics of the study group at baseline and can sometimes reveal cross-sectional associations of interest.

A weakness of cross-sectional studies is the difficulty of establishing causal relationships from observational data collected in a cross-sectional time frame. Cross-sectional studies are also impractical for the study of rare diseases if the design involves collecting data on a sample of individuals from the general population. A cross-sectional study of stomach cancer in a general population of 45- to 59-year-old men, for example, would need about 10,000 subjects to find just one case.

Cross-sectional studies can be done on rare diseases if the sample is drawn from a population of diseased patients rather than from the general population. A **case series** of this sort is better suited to describing the characteristics of the disease than to analyzing differences between these patients and healthy people, although informal comparisons with prior experience can sometimes identify very strong risk factors. Of the first 1,000 patients with AIDS, for example, 727 were homosexual or bisexual males and 236 were injection drug users (3). It did not require a formal control group to conclude that these groups were at increased risk. Furthermore, within a sample of persons with a disease there may be associations of interest (e.g., the higher risk of Kaposi's sarcoma among patients with AIDS who were homosexual than among those who were injection drug users).

When cross-sectional studies measure only prevalence and not cumulative incidence it limits the information they can produce on prognosis, natural history, and disease causation. To show causation, investigators need to demonstrate that the incidence of disease differs in those exposed to a risk factor. Because prevalence is the product of disease incidence and disease duration, a factor that is associated with higher prevalence of disease may be a cause of the disease but could also be associated with prolonged duration of the disease. For example, the prevalence of severe depression is affected not just by its incidence, but by the duration of episodes, the suicide rate and the responsiveness to medication of those affected. Therefore, cross-sectional studies may show increased relative prevalence either because the condition occurs more frequently in those with the exposure, or because the condition lasts longer in those with the exposure.

Serial Surveys

A series of cross-sectional studies of a single population observed at several points in time is sometimes used to draw inferences about changing patterns over time. For example, Zito et al. (4), using annual cross-sectional surveys, reported that the prevalence of prescription psychotropic drug use among youth (<20 years old) increased more than threefold between 1987 and 1996 in a mid-Atlantic Medicaid population. This is not a cohort design because it does not follow a single group of people over time; there are changes in the population over time due to births, deaths, aging, migration, and eligibility changes.

CASE–CONTROL STUDIES

Structure

To investigate the causes of all but the most common diseases, both cohort and cross-sectional studies of general population samples are expensive: each would require thousands of subjects to identify risk factors for a rare disease like stomach cancer. A case series of patients with the disease can identify an obvious risk factor (such as, for AIDS, injection drug use), using prior knowledge of the prevalence of the risk factor in the general population. For most risk factors, however, it is necessary to assemble a reference group, so that the prevalence of the risk factor in subjects with the disease (cases) can be compared with the prevalence in subjects without the disease (controls).

The **retrospective** structure of a case–control study is shown in Fig. 8.2. The study identifies one group of subjects with the disease and another without it, then

THE PAST OR PRESENT **THE PRESENT**

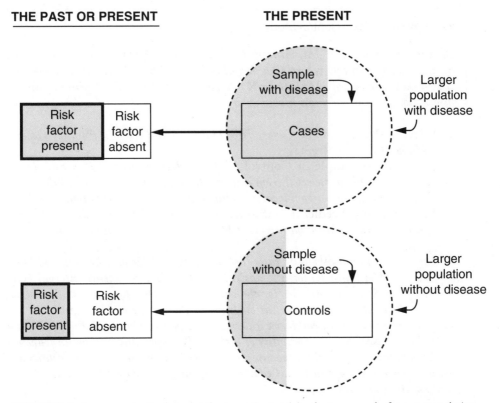

FIGURE 8.2. In a case–control study, the investigator (a) selects a sample from a population with the disease (cases), (b) selects a sample from a population at risk that is free of the disease (controls), and (c) measures predictor variables.

looks backward to find differences in predictor variables that may explain why the cases got the disease and the controls did not.

Case–control studies began as epidemiologic studies to try to identify risk factors for diseases. Therefore the outcome traditionally used to determine case–control status has been the presence or absence of a disease. For this reason and because it makes the discussion easier to follow, we generally refer to "cases" as those with the disease. However, the case–control design can also be used to look at other outcomes, such as disability among those who already have a disease. In addition, when undesired outcomes are the rule rather than the exception, the cases in a case–control study may be the rare patients who have had a good outcome, such as recovery from a usually fatal disease.

Case–control studies are the "house red" on the research design wine list: more modest and a little riskier than the other selections but much less expensive and sometimes surprisingly good. The design of a case–control study is challenging because of the increased opportunities for bias, but there are many examples of well-designed case–control studies that have yielded important results. These include the links between maternal diethylstilbestrol use and vaginal cancer in daughters (a classic study that provided a definitive conclusion based on just seven cases!) (5), and prone sleeping position to prevent sudden infant death syndrome (6), a simple result that has saved thousands of lives.

Example 8.2 Case–Control Study

Because intramuscular (IM) vitamin K is given routinely to newborns in the United States, a pair of studies reporting a doubling in the risk of childhood cancer among those who had received IM vitamin K caused quite a stir (7,8). To investigate this association further, German investigators (9)

1. **Selected the Sample of Cases.** *107 children with leukemia from the German Childhood Cancer Registry.*
2. **Selected the Sample of Controls.** *107 children matched by sex and date of birth and randomly selected from children living in the same town as the case at the time of diagnosis (from local government residential registration records).*
3. **Measured the Predictor Variable.** *Reviewed medical records to determine which cases and controls had received IM vitamin K in the newborn period.*

The authors found 69 of 107 cases (64%) and 63 of 107 controls (59%) had been exposed to IM vitamin K, for an odds ratio of 1.2 (95% confidence interval [CI], 0.7 to 2.3). (See Appendix 8A for the calculation.) Therefore, this study did not confirm the existence of an association between the receipt of IM vitamin K as a newborn and subsequent childhood leukemia. The point estimate and upper limit of the 95% CI leave open the possibility of a clinically important increase in leukemia in the population from which the samples were drawn, but several other studies and an analysis using an additional control group in the example study also failed to confirm the association (10,11).

Case–control studies cannot yield estimates of the incidence or prevalence of a disease because the proportion of study subjects who have the disease is determined by how many cases and how many controls the investigator chooses to sample, rather than by their proportions in the population. What case–control studies do provide is descriptive information on the characteristics of the cases and, more important, an estimate of the strength of the association between each predictor variable and the presence or absence of the disease. These estimates are in the form of the odds ratio, which approximates the relative risk if the prevalence of the disease is relatively low (about 10% or less) (Appendix 8B).

Strengths of Case–Control Studies

Efficiency for Rare Outcomes.   One of the major strengths of case–control studies is their rapid, high yield of information from relatively few subjects. Consider a study of the effect of circumcision on subsequent carcinoma of the penis. This cancer is very rare in circumcised men but is also rare in uncircumcised men: their lifetime cumulative incidence is about 0.16% (12). To do a cohort study with a reasonable chance (80%) of detecting even a very strong risk factor (say a relative risk of 50) would require more than 6,000 men, assuming that roughly equal proportions were circumcised and uncircumcised. A randomized clinical trial of circumcision at birth would require the same sample size, but the cases would occur at a median of 67 years after entry into the study—it would take three generations of epidemiologists to follow the subjects!

Now consider a case–control study of the same question. For the same chance of detecting the same relative risk, only 16 cases and 16 controls (and not much investigator time) would be required. For diseases that are either rare or have long latent periods between exposure and disease, case–control studies are far more efficient than the other designs. In fact, they are often the only feasible option.

Usefulness for Generating Hypotheses.   The retrospective approach of case–control studies, and their ability to examine a large number of predictor variables makes them useful for generating hypotheses about the causes of a new outbreak of disease. For example, a case–control study of an epidemic of acute renal failure in Haitian children found an odds ratio of 53 for ingestion of locally manufactured acetaminophen syrup. Further investigation revealed that the renal failure was due to poisoning by diethylene glycol, which was found to contaminate the glycerine solution used to make the acetaminophen syrup (13).

Weaknesses of Case–Control Studies

Case–control studies have great strengths, but they also have major limitations. The information available in case–control studies is limited: unless the population and time period from which the cases arose are known, there is no direct way to estimate the incidence or prevalence of the disease, nor the attributable or excess risk. There is also the problem that only one outcome can be studied (the presence or absence of the disease that was the criterion for drawing the two samples), whereas cohort and cross-sectional studies (and clinical trials) can study any number of outcome variables. But the biggest weakness of case–control studies is their **susceptibility to bias.** This bias comes chiefly from two sources: the separate sampling of the cases and controls, and the retrospective measurement of the predictor variables. These two problems and the strategies for dealing with them are the topic of the next two sections.

Sampling Bias and How to Control It

The sampling in a case–control study begins with the cases. Ideally, the sample of cases would be a complete or a random sample of everyone who develops the disease under study. An immediate problem comes up, however. How do we know who has developed the disease and who has not? In cross-sectional and cohort studies the disease is systematically sought in all the study participants, but in case–control studies the cases must be sampled from patients in whom the disease has already been diagnosed and who are available for study. This sample may not be representative of all patients who develop the disease because those who are undiagnosed, misdiagnosed, unavailable for study or dead are less likely to be included (Fig. 8.3).

In general, sampling bias is important when the sample of cases is unrepresentative with respect to the risk factor being studied. Diseases that almost always require hospitalization and are relatively easy to diagnose, such as hip fracture and traumatic amputations, can be safely sampled from diagnosed and accessible cases. On the other hand, conditions that may not come to medical attention are not well suited to retrospective studies because of the selection that precedes diagnosis. For example, women seen in a gynecologic clinic with first-trimester spontaneous abortions would probably differ from the entire population of women experiencing spontaneous abortions because those with greater access to gynecologic care or with complications would be overrepresented. If a predictor variable of interest is associated with gynecologic care in the population (such as past use of an intrauterine device [IUD]), sampling cases from the clinic could be an important source of bias. If, on the other

New cases of the diseases

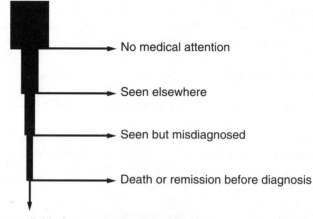

No medical attention

Seen elsewhere

Seen but misdiagnosed

Death or remission before diagnosis

Cases available for case-control study

FIGURE 8.3. Some reasons that the cases in a case–control study may not be representative of all cases of the disease.

hand, a predictor is unrelated to gynecologic care (such as blood type) there would be less likelihood of a clinic-based sample being unrepresentative.

Although it is important to think about these issues, in actual practice the selection of cases is often straightforward because the accessible sources of subjects are limited. The sample of cases may not be entirely representative, but it may be all that the investigator has to work with. The more difficult decisions faced by an investigator designing a case–control study then relates to the more open-ended task of selecting the controls. The general goal is to sample controls from a population at risk for the disease that is otherwise similar to the cases. Four strategies for sampling controls follow:

- *Hospital- or clinic-based controls.* One strategy to compensate for the possible selection bias caused by obtaining cases from a hospital or clinic is to select controls from the same facilities. For example, in a study of past use of an IUD as a risk factor for spontaneous abortion, controls could be sampled from a population of women seeking care for vaginitis at the same gynecologic clinic. Compared with a random sample of women from the same area, these controls would presumably better represent the population of women who, had they developed a spontaneous abortion, would have come to the clinic and become a case.

    However, selection of an unrepresentative sample of controls to compensate for an unrepresentative sample of cases can be problematic. If the risk factor of interest also causes diseases for which the controls seek care, the prevalence of the risk factor in the control group will be falsely high, biasing the study results toward the null. If, for example, many women in the control group had vaginitis and use of an IUD increased the risk of vaginitis, there would be an excess of IUD users among the controls, masking a possible real association between IUD use and spontaneous abortion.

    Because hospital-based and clinic-based control subjects are usually unwell and because their diseases may be associated with the risk factors being studied, the use of hospital- or clinic-based controls can produce misleading findings. For this reason, the added convenience of hospital- or clinic-based controls is not often worth the possible threat to the validity of the study.

- *Matching.* Matching is a simple method of ensuring that cases and controls are comparable with respect to major factors that are related to the disease but not of interest to the investigator. So many risk factors and diseases are related to age and sex, for example, that the study results may be unconvincing unless the cases and controls are comparable with regard to these two variables. One approach to avoiding this problem is to choose controls that match the cases on these constitutional predictor variables. For example, in a study that matched on sex and age (say, within 2 years), for a 44-year-old male case the investigators would choose a male control between the ages of 42 and 46 years. Alternatively, the investigators can try to make sure that the overall proportions of men in each age-group are the same in the cases and controls (a process known as frequency matching). Matching does have its adverse consequences, however, particularly when modifiable predictors such as income or serum cholesterol level are matched. The reasons for this and the alternatives to matching are discussed in Chapter 9.

- *Using a population-based sample of cases.* Population-based case–control studies are now possible for many diseases, because of a rapid increase in the use of disease registries, both in geographically defined populations and within health maintenance organizations. Because cases obtained from such registries are generally representative of the general population of patients in the area with the disease, the choice of a control group is simplified: it should be a representative sample from the population covered by the registry. In Example 8.2, all residents of the town were registered with the local government, making selection of such a sample straightforward.

  When registries are available, population-based case–control studies are clearly the most desirable. As the disease registry approaches completeness and the population it covers approaches stability (no migration in or out), the population-based case–control study approaches a case–control study that is nested within a cohort study or clinical trial (Chapter 7). When information on the cases and controls can come from previously recorded sources, (thereby not requiring consent of the subject and the selection bias likely to accompany such consent) this design has the potential for eliminating sampling bias, because both cases and controls are selected from the same population. When designing the sampling approach for a case–control study, the **nested case–control** design is useful to keep in mind as the model to emulate.

- *Using two or more control groups.* Because selection of a control group can be so tricky, particularly when the cases are not a representative sample of those with disease, it is sometimes advisable to use two or more control groups selected in different ways. The Public Health Service study of Reye's syndrome and medications (14), for example, used four types of controls: emergency room controls (seen in the same emergency room as the case), inpatient controls (admitted to the same hospital as the case), school controls (attending the same school or day care center as the case), and community controls (identified by random-digit dialing). The odds ratios for salicylate use in cases compared with each of these control groups (in the order listed) were 39, 66, 33, and 44, and each was statistically significant. The consistent finding of a strong association using control groups that would have a variety of sampling biases makes a convincing case for the inference that there is a real association in the population.

  Unfortunately, many causal factors have odds ratios that are much closer to unity, and the biases associated with different strategies for selecting controls can endanger causal inference. What happens if the control groups give conflicting results? This is actually helpful, revealing inherent fragility to the case–control method for the research question at hand. If possible, the investigator should seek additional information to try to determine the magnitude of potential biases from each of the control groups. In any case, it is better to have inconsistent results and conclude that the answer is not known than to have just one control group and draw the wrong conclusion.

Differential Measurement Bias and How to Control It

The second particular problem of case–control studies is bias due to **measurement error** caused by the retrospective approach to measuring the predictor variables, particularly when it occurs to a different extent in cases than in controls. Case–control studies of birth defects, for example, are susceptible to **recall bias:** parents of babies with birth defects may be more likely to recall drug exposures than parents of normal babies, because they will already have been worrying about what caused the defect. Recall bias cannot occur in a cohort study because the parents are asked about exposures before the baby is born.

In addition to the strategies set out in Chapter 4 for controlling biased measurements (standardizing the operational definitions of variables, choosing objective approaches, supplementing key variables with data from several sources, etc.), there are two specific strategies for avoiding bias in measuring risk factors in case–control studies:

- *Use data recorded before the outcome occurred.* It may be possible, for example, to examine prenatal records in a case–control study of IM vitamin K as a risk factor for cancer. This excellent strategy is limited to the extent that recorded information about the risk factor of interest is available and of satisfactory reliability. For example, information about vitamin K administration was often missing from medical records, and how that missing information was treated affected results of some studies of vitamin K and subsequent cancer risk (10).
- *Use blinding.* The general approach to blinding was discussed in Chapter 4, but there are some issues that are specific to designing interviews in case–control studies. Because both observers and study subjects could be blinded both to the case–control status of each subject and to the risk factor being studied, four types of blinding are possible (Table 8.2).

TABLE 8.2	Approaches to Blinding Interview Questions in a Case–Control Study	
Person Blinded	**Blinding Case–Control Status**	**Blinding Risk Factor Measurement**
Subject	Possible if both cases and controls have diseases that could plausibly be related to the risk factor	Include "dummy" risk factors and be suspicious if they differ between cases and controls
		May not work if the risk factor for the disease has already been publicized
Observer	Possible if cases are not externally distinguishable from controls, but subtle signs and statements, volunteered by the subjects make it difficult	Possible if interviewer is not the investigator, but may be difficult to maintain

Ideally, neither the study subjects nor the observers should know which subjects are cases and which are controls. If this can be done successfully, differential bias in measuring the predictor variable is eliminated. In practice, this is often difficult. The subjects know whether they are sick or well, so they can be blinded to case–control status only if controls are also ill with diseases that they believe might be related to the risk factors being studied. (Of course, if the controls are selected for a disease that *is* related to the risk factor being studied, it will cause sampling bias.) Efforts to blind interviewers are hampered by the obvious nature of some diseases (an interviewer can hardly help noticing if the subject is jaundiced or has had a laryngectomy), and by the clues that interviewers may discern in the subject's responses.

Blinding to specific risk factors being studied is usually easier than blinding to case–control status. Case–control studies are often first steps in investigating an illness, so there may not be one risk factor of particular interest. When there is, the study subjects and the interviewer can be kept in the dark about the study hypotheses by including "dummy" questions about plausible risk factors not associated with the disease. For example, if the specific hypothesis to be tested is whether honey intake is associated with increased risk of infant botulism, equally detailed questions about jelly, yogurt, and bananas could be included in the interview. This type of blinding does not actually prevent differential bias, but it allows an estimate of whether it is a problem: if the cases report more exposure to honey but no increase in the other foods, then differential measurement bias is less likely. This strategy would not work if the association between infant botulism and honey had previously been widely publicized or if some of the dummy risk factors turned out to be real risk factors.

Blinding the observer to the case–control status of the study subject is a particularly good strategy for **laboratory measurements** such as blood tests and x-rays. Blinding under these circumstances is easy and should always be done: someone other than the individual who will make the measurement simply applies coded identification labels to each specimen. The importance of blinding was illustrated by 15 case–control studies comparing measurements of bone mass between hip fracture patients and controls; much larger differences were found in the studies that used unblinded measurements than in the blinded studies (15).

Case-Crossover Studies

A variant of the case–control design, useful for studying the short-term effects of intermittent exposures, is the case-crossover design (16). As with regular case–control studies, these are retrospective studies that begin with a group of cases: people who have had the outcome of interest. However, unlike traditional case–control studies, in which the exposures of the cases are compared with exposures of a group of controls, in case-crossover studies each case serves as his or her own control. Exposures of the cases at the time (or right before) the outcome occurred are compared with exposures of those same cases at one or more other points in time.

For example, McEvoy et al. (17) studied cases who were injured in car crashes and reported owning or using a mobile phone. Using phone company records, they compared mobile phone usage in the 10 minutes before the crash with usage when the subjects were driving at the same time of day 24 hours, 72 hours, and 7 days before the crash. They found that mobile phone usage was more likely in the 10 minutes before a crash than in the comparison time periods, with an odds ratio of about 4. The analysis of a case-crossover study is like that of a matched case–control study, except that the control exposures are exposures of the case at different time periods,

TABLE 8.3	Advantages and Disadvantages of the Major Observational Designs

Design	Advantages	Disadvantages*
Cohort		
All	Establishes sequence of events	Often requires large sample sizes
	Multiple predictors and outcomes	Less feasible for rare outcomes
	Number of outcome events grows over time	
	Yields incidence, relative risk, excess risk	
Prospective	More control over subject selection and measurements	Follow-up can be lengthy Often expensive
	Avoids bias in measuring predictors	
Retrospective	Follow-up is in the past Relatively inexpensive	Less control over subject selection and measurements
Multiple cohort	Useful when distinct cohorts have different or rare exposures	Bias and confounding from sampling several populations
Cross-sectional		
	Relatively short duration A good first step for a cohort study or clinical trial Yields prevalence of multiple predictors and outcomes	Does not establish sequence of events Not feasible for rare predictors or rare outcomes Does not yield incidence
Case–Control		
	Useful for rare outcomes Short duration, small sample size Relatively inexpensive Yields odds ratio (resembles relative risk for uncommon outcomes)	Bias and confounding from sampling two populations Differential measurement bias Limited to one outcome variable Sequence of events unclear Does not yield prevalence, incidence, or excess risk
Combination Designs		
Nested case–control	Advantages of a retrospective cohort design, only much more efficient	Suitable cohort and specimens many not be available
Nested case–cohort	Can use a single control group for multiple case–control studies	Suitable cohort and specimens many not be available
Case-crossover	Cases serve as their own controls, reducing random error and confounding	Requires special circumstances

* All these observational designs have the disadvantage (compared with randomized trials) of being susceptible to the influence of confounding variables—See Chapter 9.

rather than exposures of the matched control. This is illustrated in "Case-crossover Study" in Appendix 8A. Other examples of use of the case-crossover design include a series of studies of possible triggers of myocardial infarction, including episodes of anger (18), and use of marijuana (19) and of sildenafil (Viagra) (20).

CHOOSING AMONG OBSERVATIONAL DESIGNS

The pros and cons of the main observational designs presented in the last two chapters are summarized in Table 8.3. We have already described these issues in detail and will make only one final point here. Among all these designs, none is best and none is worst; each has its place and purpose, depending on the research question and the circumstances.

SUMMARY

1. In a **cross-sectional** study, the variables are all measured at a single point in time, with no structural distinction between predictors and outcomes. Cross-sectional studies are valuable for providing **descriptive** information about **prevalence;** they also have the advantage of **avoiding the time, expense,** and **dropout problems** of a follow-up-design.

2. Cross-sectional studies yield **weaker evidence for causality** than cohort studies, because the predictor variable is not shown to precede the outcome. A further weakness is the need for a large sample size (compared with that of a case–control study) when studying uncommon diseases. The cross-sectional design can be used for an uncommon disease in a **case series** of patients with that disease, and it often serves as the first step of a cohort study or experiment.

3. In a **case–control study,** the prevalence of risk factors in a sample of subjects who have a disease or other outcome of interest (the cases) is compared with that in a separate sample who do not (the controls). This design is relatively **inexpensive** and uniquely **efficient** for studying **rare diseases.**

4. One problem with case–control studies is their susceptibility to **sampling bias.** Four approaches to reducing sampling bias are (a) to sample controls and cases in the **same** (admittedly unrepresentative) **way;** (b) to **match** the cases and controls; (c) to do a **population-based** study; and (d) to use **several** control groups sampled in different ways.

5. The other major problem with case–control studies is their retrospective design, which makes them susceptible to **measurement bias** that affects cases and controls differentially. Such bias can be reduced by **measuring the predictor prior to the outcome** and by **blinding** the subjects and observers.

6. **Case-crossover studies** are a variation on the matched case–control design in which observations at two points in time allow each case to serve as his or her own control.

APPENDIX 8A

Calculating Measures of Association

1. *Cross-sectional study.* Reijneveld (21) did a cross-sectional study of maternal smoking as a risk factor for infant colic. Partial results are shown below:

Predictor Variable	Outcome Variable:		
	Infant Colic	No Infant Colic	Total
Mother smokes 15–50 cigarettes/day	15 (a)	167 (b)	182 ($a + b$)
Mother does not smoke	111 (c)	2,477 (d)	2,588 ($c + d$)
Total	126 ($a + c$)	2,644 ($b + d$)	2,770 ($a + b + c + d$)

Prevalence of colic with smoking mothers = $a/(a + b) = 15/182 = 8.2\%$.
Prevalence of colic with nonsmoking mothers = $c/(c + d) = 111/2,588 = 4.3\%$.
Prevalence of colic overall = $(a + c)/(a + b + c + d) = 126/2,770 = 4.5\%$.

$$\text{Relative prevalence}^1 = \frac{8.2\%}{4.3\%} = 1.9$$
$$\text{Excess prevalence}^1 = 8.2\% - 4.3\% = 3.9\%$$

2. *Case–control study.* The research question for Example 8.2 was whether there is an association between IM vitamin K and risk of childhood leukemia. The findings were that 69/107 leukemia cases and 63/107 controls had received IM vitamin K. A two-by-two table of these findings is as follows:

Predictor Variable: Medication History	Outcome Variable: Diagnosis	
	Childhood Leukemia	Control
IM vitamin K	69(a)	63(b)
No IM vitamin K	38(c)	44(d)
Total	107	107

$$\text{Relative risk} \approx \textit{odds ratio} = \frac{ad}{bc} = \frac{69 \times 44}{63 \times 38} = 1.27$$

Because the disease (leukemia in this instance) is rare, the odds ratio provides a good estimate of the relative risk.[2]

3. *Matched case–control study*

(To illustrate the similarity between analysis of a matched case–control study and a case-crossover study, we will use the same example for both.) The

---

[1] Relative prevalence and excess prevalence are the cross-sectional analogs of relative risk and excess risk.
[2] The authors actually did a multivariate, matched analysis, as was appropriate for the matched design, but in this case the simple, unmatched odds ratio was almost the same as the one reported in the study.

research question is whether mobile telephone use increases the risk of car crashes among mobile telephone owners. A traditional matched case–control study might consider self-reported frequency of using a mobile telephone while driving as the risk factor. Then the cases would be people injured in crashes and they could be matched to controls who had not been in crashes by age, sex, and mobile telephone prefix. The cases and controls would be asked whether they ever use a mobile telephone while driving. (To simplify, for this example, we dichotomize the exposure and consider people as either "users' or "nonusers" of mobile telephones while driving.) We then classify each case/control pair according to whether both are users, neither is a user, or the case was a user but not the control, or the control was a user but not the case. If we had 300 pairs, the results might look like this:

Matched Controls	Cases (with crash injuries)		
	User	Nonuser	Total
User	110	40	150
Nonuser	90	60	150
Total	200	100	300

The table above shows that there were 90 pairs where the case ever used a mobile phone while driving, but not the matched control, and 40 pairs where the matched control but not the case was a "user." Note that this 2×2 table is different from the 2×2 table from the unmatched vitamin K study above, in which each cell in the table is the number of people in that cell. In the 2×2 table for a *matched* case–control study the number in each cell is the number of *pairs* of subjects in that cell; the total N in the table above is therefore 600 (300 cases and 300 controls). The odds ratio for such a table is simply the ratio of the two types of discordant pairs; in the table above the OR $= 90/40 = 2.25$.

4. *Case-crossover study*

   Now consider the case-crossover study of the same question. Data from the study by McEvoy et al. are shown below.

Seven Days Before Crash	Crash Time Period		
	Driver Using Phone	Not Using	Total
Driver using phone	5	6	11
Not using	27	288	315
Total	32	294	326

For the case-crossover study, each cell in the table is a number of subjects, not a number of pairs, but *each cell represents two time periods* for that one subject: the time period just before the crash and a comparison time period 7 days before. Therefore the 5 in the upper left cell means there were 5 drivers involved in crashes who were using a mobile phone just before they crashed, and also using a mobile phone during the comparison period 7 days before, while the 27 just below indicates that there were 27 drivers involved in crashes who were using a phone just before crashing, but *not* using a phone during the comparison period 7 days before. The odds ratio is the ratio of the numbers of discordant time periods, in this example $27/6 = 4.5$.

APPENDIX 8B

Why the Odds Ratio Can Be Used as an Estimate for Relative Risk in a Case–Control Study

The data in a case–control study represent two samples: the cases are drawn from a population of people who have the disease and the controls from a population of people who do not have the disease. The predictor variable is measured, and the following two-by-two table produced:

	Disease	No Disease
Risk factor present	a	b
Risk factor absent	c	d

If this two-by-two table represented data from a cohort study, then the incidence of the disease in those with the risk factor would be $a/(a + b)$ and the relative risk would be simply $[a/(a + b)]/[c/(c + d)]$. However, it is not appropriate to compute either incidence or relative risk in this way in a case–control study because the two samples are not drawn from the population in the same proportions. Usually, there are roughly equal numbers of cases and controls in the study samples but many fewer cases than controls in the population. Instead, relative risk in a case–control study can be approximated by the odds ratio, computed as the cross-product of the two-by-two table, ad/bc.

This extremely useful fact is difficult to grasp intuitively but easy to demonstrate algebraically. Consider the situation for the full population, represented by a', b', c', and d'.

	Disease	No Disease
Risk factor present	a'	b'
Risk factor absent	c'	d'

Here it is appropriate to calculate the risk of disease among people with the risk factor as $a'/(a' + b')$, the risk among those without the risk factor as $c'/(c' + d')$, and the relative risk as $[a'/(a' + b')]/[c'/(c' + d')]$. We have already discussed the fact that $a'/(a' + b')$ is not equal to $a/(a + b)$. However, if the disease is relatively uncommon (as most are), then a' is much smaller than b', and c' is much smaller than d'. This means that $a'/(a' + b')$ is closely approximated by a'/b' and that $c'/(c' + d')$ is closely approximated by c'/d'. Therefore the relative risk of the population can be approximated as follows:

$$\frac{a'/(a' + b')}{c'/(c' + d')} \approx \frac{a'/b'}{c'/d'}$$

The latter term is the odds ratio of the population (literally, the ratio of the odds of disease in those with the risk factor, a'/b', to the odds of disease in those without the risk factor, c'/d'). This can be rearranged as the cross-product:

$$\left(\frac{a'}{b'}\right)\left(\frac{d'}{c'}\right) = \left(\frac{a'}{c'}\right)\left(\frac{d'}{b'}\right)$$

However, a'/c' in the population equals a/c in the sample if the cases are representative of all cases in the population (i.e., have the same prevalence of the risk factor). Similarly, b'/d' equals b/d if the controls are representative.

Therefore the population parameters in this last term can be replaced by the sample parameters, and we are left with the fact that the odds ratio observed in the sample, ad/bc, is a close approximation of the relative risk in the population, $[a'/(a' + b')]/[c'/(c' + d')]$, provided that the disease is rare and sampling error (systematic as well as random) is small.

REFERENCES

1. Andersen RE, Crespo CJ, Bartlett SJ, et al. Relationship of physical activity and television watching with body weight and level of fatness among children: results from the Third National Health and Nutrition Examination Survey. *JAMA* 1998;279(12):938–942.
2. Sargent JD, Beach ML, Adachi-Mejia AM, et al. Exposure to movie smoking: its relation to smoking initiation among US adolescents. *Pediatrics* 2005;116(5):1183–1191.
3. Jaffe HW, Bregman DJ, Selik RM. Acquired immune deficiency syndrome in the United States: the first 1,000 cases. *J Infect Dis* 1983;148(2):339–345.
4. Zito JM, Safer DJ, DosReis S, et al. Psychotropic practice patterns for youth: a 10-year perspective. *Arch Pediatr Adolesc Med* 2003;157(1):17–25.
5. Herbst AL, Ulfelder H, Poskanzer DC. Adenocarcinoma of the vagina. Association of maternal stilbestrol therapy with tumor appearance in young women. *N Engl J Med* 1971;284(15):878–881.
6. Beal SM, Finch CF. An overview of retrospective case-control studies investigating the relationship between prone sleeping position and SIDS. *J Paediatr Child Health* 1991;27(6):334–339.
7. Golding J, Paterson M, Kinlen LJ. Factors associated with childhood cancer in a national cohort study. *Br J Cancer* 1990;62(2):304–308.
8. Golding J, Greenwood R, Birmingham K, et al. Childhood cancer, intramuscular vitamin K, and pethidine given during labour. *BMJ* 1992;305(6849):341–346.
9. von Kries R, Gobel U, Hachmeister A, et al. Vitamin K and childhood cancer: a population based case-control study in Lower Saxony, Germany. *BMJ* 1996;313(7051):199–203.
10. Roman E, Fear NT, Ansell P, et al. Vitamin K and childhood cancer: analysis of individual patient data from six case-control studies. *Br J Cancer* 2002;86(1):63–69.
11. Fear NT, Roman E, Ansell P, et al. Vitamin K and childhood cancer: a report from the United Kingdom Childhood Cancer Study. *Br J Cancer* 2003;89(7):1228–1231.
12. Kochen M, McCurdy S. Circumcision and the risk of cancer of the penis. A life-table analysis. *Am J Dis Child* 1980;134:484–486.
13. O'Brien KL, Selanikio JD, Hecdivert C. et al. Epidemic of pediatric deaths from acute renal failure caused by diethylene glycol poisoning. Acute Renal Failure Investigation Team. *JAMA* 1998;279(15):1175–1180.
14. Hurwitz ES, Barrett MJ, Bregman D, et al. Public Health Service study of Reye's syndrome and medications. Report of the main study. *JAMA* 1987;257(14):1905–1911.
15. Cummings SR. Are patients with hip fractures more osteoporotic? Review of the evidence. *Am J Med* 1985;78:487–494.
16. Maclure M, Mittleman MA. Should we use a case-crossover design? *Annu Rev Public Health* 2000;21:193–221.
17. McEvoy SP, Stevenson MR, McCartt AT, et al. Role of mobile phones in motor vehicle crashes resulting in hospital attendance: a case-crossover study. *BMJ* 2005;331(7514):428.
18. Mittleman MA, Maclure M, Sherwood JB, et al. Determinants of Myocardial Infarction Onset Study Investigators. Triggering of acute myocardial infarction onset by episodes of anger. *Circulation* 1995;92(7):1720–1725.

19. Mittleman MA, Lewis RA, Maclure M, et al. Triggering myocardial infarction by marijuana. *Circulation* 2001;103(23):2805–2809.

20. Mittleman MA, Maclure M, Glasser DB. Evaluation of acute risk for myocardial infarction in men treated with sildenafil citrate. *Am J Cardiol* 2005;96(3):443–446.

21. Reijneveld SA, Brugman E, Hirasing RA. Infantile colic: maternal smoking as potential risk factor. *Arch Dis Child* 2000;83(4):302–303.

Enhancing Causal

Inference in Observational

Studies

Thomas B. Newman, Warren S. Browner, and Stephen B. Hulley

For many research questions, the inference that an association represents a **cause–effect** relation is important. (Exceptions are studies of diagnostic and prognostic tests, discussed in Chapter 12.) The ability to make that inference depends upon decisions made during both the design and analysis phases of a study. Although this text is concerned primarily with *designing* clinical research, in this chapter we discuss ways to strengthen causal inference in both phases, because knowledge of analysis phase options can help inform decisions about study design. We begin with a discussion of how to avoid **spurious associations** and then concentrate on ruling out **real associations** that do not represent cause–effect, especially those due to confounding.

Suppose that a study reveals an association between coffee drinking and myocardial infarction (MI). One possibility is that coffee drinking is a cause of MI. Before reaching this conclusion, however, four rival explanations must be considered (Table 9.1). The first two of these, **chance** (random error) and **bias** (systematic error), represent spurious associations: coffee drinking and MI are associated only in the study findings, not in the population.

Even if the association is real, however, it may not represent a cause–effect relationship. Two rival explanations must be considered. One is the possibility of **effect–cause**—that having an MI makes people drink more coffee. (This is just cause and effect in reverse.) The other is the possibility of **confounding**, in which a third factor (such as cigarette smoking) is both associated with coffee drinking and a cause of MI.

SPURIOUS ASSOCIATIONS

Ruling Out Spurious Associations Due to Chance

Imagine that there is no association between coffee drinking and MI in the population, and that 60% of the entire population drinks coffee, whether or not they have had an MI. If we were to select a random sample of 20 patients with MI, we would expect

127

| TABLE 9.1 | The Five Explanations When an Association between Coffee Drinking and Myocardial Infarction (MI) is Observed in a Sample |

Explanation	Type of Association	What's Really Going on in the Population?	Causal Model
1. Chance (random error)	Spurious	Coffee drinking and MI are not related	–
2. Bias (systematic error)	Spurious	Coffee drinking and MI are not related	–
3. Effect–cause	Real	MI is a cause of coffee drinking	Coffee drinking ← MI
4. Confounding	Real	Coffee drinking is associated with a third, extrinsic factor that is a cause of MI	Factor X / Coffee drinking MI
5. Cause–effect	Real	Coffee drinking is a cause of MI	Coffee drinking → MI

about 12 of them to drink coffee. But by chance alone we might happen to get 19 coffee drinkers in a sample of 20 patients with MI. In that case, unless we were lucky enough to get a similar chance excess of coffee drinkers among the controls, a spurious association between coffee consumption and MI would be observed. Such an association due to **random error** (chance), if statistically significant, is called a **type I error** (Chapter 5).

Strategies for addressing random error are available in both the design and analysis phases of research (Table 9.2). The design strategies of increasing the **precision of measurements** and increasing the **sample size** are important ways to reduce random error that are discussed in Chapters 4 and 6. The analysis strategy of calculating **P values** helps the investigator quantify the magnitude of the observed association in comparison with what might have occurred by chance alone. For example, a P value of 0.10 indicates that the observed value of the test statistic (or larger) would occur by chance alone about one time in ten. **Confidence intervals** show a range of values for the parameter being estimated (e.g., risk ratio) that are consistent with that estimate, based on the study's results.

Ruling Out Spurious Associations Due to Bias

Associations that are spurious because of bias are trickier. To understand bias it is helpful to distinguish between the research question and the question actually answered by the study (Chapter 1). The research question is what the investigator really wishes to answer, while the question answered by the study reflects the compromises the investigator needed to make for the study to be feasible. Bias can be thought of as a systematic difference between the research question and the actual question answered by the study that causes the study to give the wrong answer to the research question. Strategies for minimizing these **systematic errors** are available in both the design and analysis phases of research (Table 9.2).

- *Design Phase.* Many kinds of bias have been identified, and dealing with some of them has been a major topic of this book. To the specific strategies noted in

TABLE 9.2	Strengthening the Inference that an Association has a Cause–Effect Basis: Ruling Out Spurious Associations	
Type of Spurious Association	Design Phase (How to Prevent the Rival Explanation)	Analysis Phase (How to Evaluate the Rival Explanation)
Chance (due to random error)	Increase sample size and other strategies to increase precision (Chapters 4 and 6)	Calculate P values and confidence intervals
		Interpret them in the context of prior evidence (Chapter 5)
Bias (due to systematic error)	Carefully consider the potential consequences of each difference between the research question and the study plan (see Fig. 1.6):	Obtain additional data to see if potential biases have actually occurred
	population/subjects phenomena/measurements	Check consistency with other studies (especially those using different methods)

Chapters 3, 4, 7, and 8 we now add a general approach to minimizing sources of bias. Write down the research question and the study plan side by side, as in Figure 9.1. Then carefully think through the following three concerns as they pertain to this particular research question:

a. Do the **samples** of study subjects (e.g., cases and controls or exposed and unexposed subjects) represent the population(s) of interest?

b. Do the **measurements of the predictor variables** represent the predictors of interest?

c. Do the **measurements of the outcome variables** represent the outcomes of interest?

For each question, answered "No" or "Maybe not," consider whether the bias applies similarly to one or both groups studied (e.g., cases and controls or exposed and unexposed) and whether it is large enough to affect the answer to the research question.

To illustrate this with our coffee and MI example, consider the implications of drawing the sample of control subjects from a population of hospitalized patients. If many of these patients have chronic illnesses that have caused them to reduce their coffee intake, the sample of controls will not represent the target population from which the patients with MI arose; there will be a shortage of coffee drinkers. Furthermore, if coffee drinking is measured by questionnaire, the answers on the questionnaire may not accurately represent actual coffee drinking, the predictor of interest. And if esophageal spasm, which can be exacerbated by coffee, is misdiagnosed as MI, a spurious association between coffee and MI could be found because the measured outcome (diagnosis of MI) did not accurately represent the outcome of interest (actual MI).

The next step is to think about possible strategies for preventing each potential bias. For example, as discussed in Chapter 8, selecting more than one control group in a case–control study is one approach to addressing sampling bias. In Chapter 4

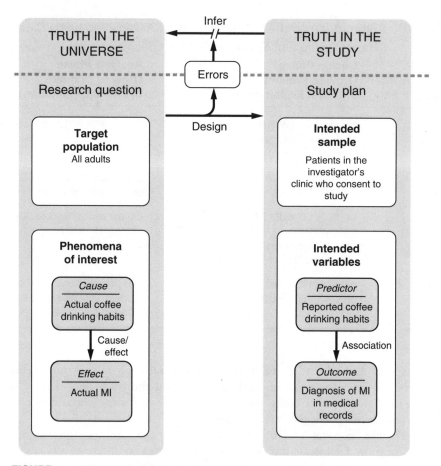

FIGURE 9.1. Minimizing bias by comparing the research question and the study plan.

we suggested strategies for reducing measurement bias. In each case, judgments are required about the likelihood of bias, and how easily it could be prevented with changes in the study plan. If the bias is easily preventable, revise the study plan and ask the three questions again. If the bias is not easily preventable, decide whether the study is still worth doing by making a judgment on the likelihood of the potential bias and the degree to which it will compromise the conclusions.

- *Analysis Phase.* The investigator is often faced with one or more potential biases after the data have been collected. Some may have been anticipated but too difficult to prevent, and others may not have been suspected until it was too late to avoid them.

In either situation, one approach is to obtain **additional information** to estimate the magnitude of the potential bias. Suppose, for example, the investigator is concerned that the hospitalized control subjects do not represent the target population of people free of MI because they have decreased their coffee intake due to chronic illness. The magnitude of this sampling bias could be estimated by reviewing the diagnoses of the control subjects and separating them into two groups: those with illnesses that might alter coffee habits and those with illnesses that would not. If both types of controls drank less coffee than the MI cases, then sampling bias would be a less likely explanation for the findings. Similarly, if the investigator is concerned that a questionnaire does not accurately capture coffee drinking (perhaps because of poorly worded questions), she could assign a blinded interviewer to question a subset of the cases and controls to determine the agreement with their questionnaire responses. Finally, if it is the outcome measure that is in doubt, the investigator could specify objective electrocardiographic and serum enzyme changes needed for the diagnosis, and reanalyze the data excluding the subset of cases that do not meet these criteria.

The investigator can also look at the results of **other studies**. If the conclusions are consistent, the association is less likely to be due to bias. This is especially true if the other studies have used different methods and are therefore unlikely to share the same biases. In many cases, potential biases turn out not to be a major problem. The decision on how vigorously to pursue additional information and how best to discuss these issues in reporting the study are matters of judgment for which it is helpful to seek advice from colleagues.

■ REAL ASSOCIATIONS OTHER THAN CAUSE–EFFECT

In addition to chance and bias, the two types of associations that are real but do not represent cause–effect must be considered (Table 9.3).

Effect–Cause

One possibility is that the cart has come before the horse—the outcome has caused the predictor. Effect–cause is often a problem in cross-sectional and case–control studies, especially when the predictor variable is a laboratory test for which no previous values are available, and in case-crossover studies if the timing of events is uncertain. For example, in the study of mobile phone use and motor vehicle accidents described in

TABLE 9.3	Strengthening the Inference that an Association has a Cause–Effect Basis: Ruling Out Other Real Associations	
Type of Real Association	**Design Phase (How to Prevent the Rival Explanation)**	**Analysis Phase (How to Evaluate the Rival Explanation)**
Effect–cause (the outcome is actually the cause of the predictor)	Do a longitudinal study	Consider biologic plausibility
	Obtain data on the historic sequence of the variables	Consider findings of other studies with different designs
	(Ultimate solution: do a randomized trial)	
Confounding (another variable is associated with the predictor and a cause of the outcome)	See Table 9.4	See Table 9.5

Chapter 8, a car crash could cause a mobile phone call (to report the crash right after it happened), rather than vice versa. To address this possibility, the investigators asked drivers who had been involved in a crash about phone use both before and after the crash, and verified the responses using phone records and the estimated time of the crash (1).

Effect–cause is less commonly a problem in cohort studies because risk factor measurements can be made in a group of people who do not yet have the disease. Even in cohort studies, however, effect–cause is possible if the disease has a long latent period and those with subclinical disease cannot be identified at baseline. For example, type 2 diabetes is associated with subsequent risk of pancreatic cancer. Some of this association is almost certainly effect–cause, because pancreatic cancer can cause diabetes, and the association between diabetes and pancreatic cancer diminishes with follow-up time (2). However, some association persists (a relative risk of about 1.5) even when pancreatic cancer cases diagnosed within 4 years of the onset of diabetes are excluded, leaving open the possibility that part of the relationship might be cause–effect.

This example illustrates a general approach to ruling out effect–cause: drawing inferences from assessments of the variables at different points in time. In addition, effect–cause is often unlikely on the grounds of biologic implausibility. For example, it is unlikely that incipient lung cancer causes cigarette smoking.

Confounding

The other rival explanation in Table 9.3 is confounding, which occurs when there is a third factor involved in the association that is the real cause of the outcome. The word confounding usually means something that confuses interpretation, but in clinical research the term has a more specific definition.

> **A confounding variable is one that is associated with the predictor variable, and a cause of the outcome variable.**

Cigarette smoking is a likely confounder in the coffee and MI example because smoking is associated with coffee drinking and is a cause of MI. If this is the actual explanation, then the association between coffee and MI does not represent cause–effect although it is still real; the coffee is an innocent bystander. Appendix 9A gives a numeric example of how cigarette smoking could cause an apparent association between coffee drinking and MI.

Aside from bias, confounding is often the only likely alternative explanation to cause–effect and the most important one to try to rule out. It is also the most challenging; much of the rest of this chapter is devoted to strategies for coping with confounders.

COPING WITH CONFOUNDERS IN THE DESIGN PHASE

In observational studies, most strategies for coping with confounding variables require that an investigator be aware of and able to measure them. It is helpful to list the variables (like age and sex) that may be associated with the predictor variable of interest and that may also be a cause of the outcome. The investigator must then choose among **design** and **analysis** strategies for controlling the influence of these potential confounding variables.

TABLE 9.4	Design Phase Strategies for Coping with Confounders	
Strategy	**Advantages**	**Disadvantages**
Specification	• Easily understood • Focuses the sample of subjects for the research question at hand	• Limits generalizability • May make it difficult to acquire an adequate sample size
Matching	• Can eliminate the influence of strong constitutional confounders like age and sex • Can eliminate the influence of confounders that are difficult to measure • Can increase precision (power) by balancing the number of cases and controls in each stratum • May be a sampling convenience, making it easier to select the controls in a case–control study	• May be time consuming and expensive; less efficient than increasing the number of subjects • Decision to match must be made at the outset of the study and can have an irreversible adverse effect on the analysis and conclusions • Requires an early decision about which variables are predictors and which are confounders • Eliminates the option of studying matched variables as predictors or as intervening variables • Requires a matched analysis • Creates the danger of overmatching (i.e., matching on a factor that is not a confounder, thereby reducing power) • Only feasible for case–control and multiple-cohort studies
"Opportunistic" study designs	• Can provide great strength of causal inference • May be a lower cost and elegant alternative to a randomized trial	• Only possible in select circumstances where the predictor variable is randomly or virtually randomly assigned, and an instrumental variable exists

The first two design phase strategies (Table 9.4), **specification** and **matching**, involve changes in the sampling scheme. Cases and controls (in a case–control study) or exposed and unexposed subjects (in a cohort study) are sampled in such a way that they have comparable values of the confounding variable. This removes the confounder as an explanation for any association that is observed between predictor and outcome. The third design phase strategy, use of what we call **opportunistic study designs**, is only applicable to selected research questions for which the right conditions exist. However, when applicable, these designs resemble randomized trials in their ability to reduce or eliminate confounding not only by measured variables, but by unmeasured variables as well.

Specification
The simplest strategy is to design inclusion criteria that **specify** a value of the potential confounding variable and exclude everyone with a different value. For example, the investigator studying coffee and MI could specify that only nonsmokers be included

in the study. If an association were then observed between coffee and MI, it obviously could not be due to smoking.

Specification is an effective strategy, but, as with all restrictions in the sampling scheme, it has disadvantages. First, even if coffee does not cause MI in nonsmokers, it may cause them in smokers. (This phenomenon—an effect of coffee on MI that is different in smokers from that in nonsmokers—is called **effect modification** or **interaction**.) Therefore, specification limits the generalizability of information available from a study, in this instance compromising our ability to generalize to smokers. Second, if smoking is highly prevalent among the patients available for the study, the investigator may not be able to recruit a large enough sample of nonsmokers.

These problems can become serious if specification is used to control too many confounders or to control them too narrowly. Sample size and generalizability would be major problems if a study were restricted to lower-income, nonsmoking, 70- to 75-year-old men.

Matching

In a case–control study, **matching** involves selecting cases and controls with matching values of the confounding variable(s). Matching and specification are both sampling strategies that prevent confounding by allowing comparison only of cases and controls that share comparable levels of the confounder. Matching differs from specification, however, in preserving generalizability because subjects at all levels of the confounder can be studied.

Matching is usually done individually (**pairwise matching**). In the study of coffee drinking as a predictor of MI, for example, each case (a patient with an MI) could be individually matched to one or more controls that smoked roughly the same amount as the case (e.g., 10 to 20 cigarettes/day). The coffee drinking of each case would then be compared with the coffee drinking of the matched control(s).

An alternative approach to pairwise matching is to match in groups (**frequency matching**). For each level of smoking, the number of cases with that amount of smoking could be counted, and an appropriate number of controls with the same level of smoking could be selected. If the study called for two controls per case and there were 20 cases that had smoked 10 to 20 cigarettes/day, the investigators would select 40 controls that smoked this amount, matched as a group to the 20 cases.

Matching is most commonly used in case–control studies, but it can also be used with multiple-cohort designs. For example, to investigate the effects of service in the 1990 to 1991 Gulf War on subsequent fertility in male veterans, Maconochie et al. compared 51,581 men deployed to the Gulf region during the war with 51,688 men who were not deployed, but were frequency-matched by service, age, fitness to be deployed, serving status and rank (3). There was a slightly higher risk of reported infertility and a longer time to conception in the Gulf War veterans.

There are four main **advantages** to matching (Table 9.4). The first three relate to the control of confounding variables; the last is a matter of logistics.

- Matching is an effective way to prevent confounding by **constitutional factors** like age and sex that are strong determinants of outcome, not susceptible to intervention, and unlikely to be an intermediary in a causal pathway.
- Matching can be used to control confounders that cannot be measured and controlled in any other way. For example, matching siblings (or, better yet, twins) with one another can control for a whole range of genetic and familial factors that would be impossible to measure, and matching for clinical center in a multicenter

study can control for unspecified differences among the populations seen at the centers.

- Matching may increase the precision of comparisons between groups (and therefore the power of the study to find a real association) by balancing the number of cases and controls at each level of the confounder. This may be important if the available number of cases is limited or if the cost of studying the subjects is high. However, the effect of matching on precision is modest and not always favorable (see "overmatching," below). In general, the desire to enhance precision is a less important reason to match than the need to control confounding.

- Finally, matching may be used primarily as a sampling convenience, to narrow down an otherwise impossibly large number of potential controls. For example, in a nationwide study of toxic shock syndrome, victims were asked to identify friends to serve as controls (6). This convenience, however, also runs the risk of overmatching.

There are a number of **disadvantages** to matching (Table 9.4).

- Matching sometimes requires additional **time and expense** to identify a match for each subject. In case–control studies, for example, the more matching criteria there are, the larger the pool of controls that must be searched to match each case. Cases for which no match can be found will need to be discarded. The possible increase in statistical power from matching must therefore be weighed against the potential loss of otherwise eligible cases or controls.

- Because matching is a sampling strategy, the decision to match must be made at the beginning of the study and is irreversible. This precludes further analysis of the effect of the matched variables on the outcome. It also can create a serious error if the matching variable is not a fixed (constitutional) variable like age or sex, but a variable intermediate in the causal pathway between the predictor and outcome. For example, if an investigator wishing to investigate the effects of alcohol intake on risk of MI matched on serum high-density lipoprotein (HDL) levels, she would miss any beneficial effects of alcohol that are mediated through an increase in HDL. Although the same error can occur with the analysis phase strategies discussed later, matching builds the error into the study in a way that cannot be undone; with the analysis phase strategies the error can be avoided simply by appropriately altering the analysis.

- Correct analysis of pair-matched data requires special analytic techniques that compare each subject only with the individual(s) with whom she has been matched, and not with subjects who have differing levels of confounders. The use of ordinary statistical analysis techniques on matched data can lead to incorrect results (generally biased toward no effect) because the assumption that the groups are sampled independently is violated. This sometimes creates a problem because the appropriate matched analyses, especially multivariate techniques, are less familiar to most investigators and less readily available in packaged statistical programs than are the usual unmatched techniques.

- A final disadvantage of matching is the possibility of **overmatching**, which occurs when the matching variable is not a confounder because it is not associated with the outcome. Overmatching can reduce the power of a case–control study, making it more difficult to find an association that really exists in the population. In the study of toxic shock syndrome that used friends for controls, for example, matching may have inappropriately controlled for regional differences in tampon marketing, making it more probable that cases and controls would use the same brand of tampon. It is important to note, however, that overmatching will not distort the estimated relative risk (provided that a matched analysis is used); it will only reduce its statistical significance.[1] Therefore when the findings of the study are statistically significant (as was the case in the toxic shock example), overmatching is not a problem.

Opportunistic Studies

Under certain conditions or for certain research questions, there may be opportunities to control for confounding variables in the design phase, even without measuring them. Because these designs are not generally available, we call them "**opportunistic**" designs. One example for short-term exposures with immediate effects is the case-crossover study (Chapter 8)—all potential confounding variables that are constant over the time (e.g., sex, race, social class, genetic factors) are controlled because each subject is compared only to herself in a different time period.

Occasionally, investigators discover a **natural experiment**, in which subjects are either exposed or not exposed through a process that in effect randomly allocates them to have or not have a risk factor or intervention. For example, Lofgren et al. (4) studied the effects of discontinuity of care on test ordering and length of stay by taking advantage of the fact that patients admitted after 5:00 PM to their institution were alternately assigned to senior residents that either maintained care of the patients or transferred them to another team the following morning. They found that patients whose care was transferred had 38% more laboratory tests ($P = 0.01$) and 2-day longer median length of stay ($P = 0.06$) than those kept on the same team. Similarly, Bell and Redelmeier (5) studied effects of nursing staffing by comparing outcomes for patients with selected diagnoses who were admitted on weekends to those admitted on weekdays. They found higher mortality from all three conditions hypothesized to be sensitive to staffing ratios, but not for other conditions.

As genetic differences in susceptibility to an exposure are elucidated, a strategy called **Mendelian randomization** (6) becomes an option. Mendelian randomization takes advantage of the fact that for common genetic polymorphisms, the allele a person receives is determined at random within families, and usually not linked to relevant confounding variables. Therefore, if people with alleles expected to confer increased susceptibility to a risk factor do indeed have a higher rate of disease than those who are either unexposed, or exposed but less susceptible, the study can provide strong evidence for causality.

For example, some farmers who dip sheep in insecticides (to kill ticks, lice, etc.) have health complaints that might or might not be due to their occupational exposures. Investigators at the University of Manchester took advantage of a polymorphism in the paraoxonase-1 gene, which leads to enzymes with differing ability to hydrolyze the organophosphate sheep dip diazinonoxon. They hypothesized that if sheep dip was a cause of ill health in exposed farmers, that farmers with ill health would be more likely to have alleles associated with reduced paraoxonase-1 activity. They asked farmers who believed that sheep dip had adversely affected their health to suggest control farmers

---

[1]The reason that overmatching reduces power can be seen with a matched pairs analysis of a case–control study. In the matched analysis, only case–control pairs that are discordant for exposure to the risk factor are analyzed (Appendix 8A). Matching on a variable associated with the risk factor will lead to fewer discordant pairs, and hence smaller effective sample size and less power. Of course, this happens to some extent any time matching is used, not just with overmatching. The difference with overmatching is that this cost comes with no benefit, because the matching was not necessary to control confounding. If a matched analysis is not used, then the estimate of the effect size will be distorted, because the matching causes the cases and controls to be more likely to have the same value of the risk factor.

who were similarly exposed to sheep dip, but in good health. Their finding that exposed farmers with health complaints had a higher frequency of alleles associated with reduced paraoxonase-1 activity than similarly exposed but asymptomatic farmers provided strong evidence of a causal relationship between exposure to sheep dip and ill health (7).

Natural experiments and Mendelian randomization are examples of a more general approach to enhancing causal inference in observational studies, use of **instrumental variables**. These are variables associated with the predictor of interest, but *not* independently associated with outcome. Whether someone is admitted on a weekend, for example, is associated with staffing levels, but was thought not to be independently associated with mortality risk (for the diagnoses studied), so admission on a weekend can be considered an instrumental variable. Similarly, activity of the paraoxonase-1 enzyme is associated with possible toxicity due to dipping sheep, but not otherwise associated with ill health. Other examples of instrumental variables are draft lottery number (used to investigate delayed effects of military service during the Vietnam War era (8)) and the distance of residence from a facility that does coronary revascularization procedures (used to investigate the effects of these procedures on mortality (9)).

COPING WITH CONFOUNDERS IN THE ANALYSIS PHASE

Design phase strategies require deciding at the outset of the study which variables are predictors and which are confounders. An advantage of analysis phase strategies is that they allow the investigator to defer that decision until she has examined the data for evidence as to which variables may be confounders (i.e., associated with the predictor of interest and a cause of the outcome).

Sometimes there are several predictor variables, each of which may act as a confounder to the others. For example, although coffee drinking, smoking, male sex, and personality type are associated with MI, they are also associated with each other. The goal is to determine which of these predictor variables are independently associated with MI and which are associated with MI only because they are associated with other (causal) risk factors. In this section, we discuss analytic methods for assessing the **independent** contribution of predictor variables in observational studies. These methods are summarized in Table 9.5.

Stratification

Like specification and matching, **stratification** ensures that only cases and controls (or exposed and unexposed subjects) with similar levels of a potential confounding variable are compared. It involves segregating the subjects into strata (subgroups) according to the level of a potential confounder and then examining the relation between the predictor and outcome separately in each stratum. Stratification is illustrated in Appendix 9A. By considering smokers and nonsmokers separately ("stratifying on smoking"), the confounding effects of smoking can be removed.

Appendix 9A also illustrates **interaction**, in which stratification reveals that the association between predictor and outcome varies with the level of a third factor. Because the third factor (smoking in this example) modifies the effect of the predictor (coffee drinking) on outcome (MI), interaction is sometimes also called **effect modification**. By chance alone the estimates of association in different strata

TABLE 9.5	Analysis Phase Strategies for Coping with Confounders	
Strategy	**Advantages**	**Disadvantages**
Stratification	• Easily understood • Flexible and reversible; can choose which variables to stratify upon after data collection	• Number of strata limited by sample size needed for each stratum • Few covariables can be considered • Few strata per covariable leads to incomplete control of confounding • Relevant covariables must have been measured

Statistical adjustment	• Multiple confounders can be controlled simultaneously
	• Information in continuous variables can be fully used
	• Flexible and reversible
		• Model may not fit:
		  • Incomplete control of confounding (if model does not fit confounder-outcome relationship)
		  • Inaccurate estimates of strength of effect (if model does not fit predictor-outcome relationship)
		• Results may be hard to understand. (Many people do not readily comprehend the meaning of a regression coefficient.)
		• Relevant covariables must have been measured

Propensity scores	• Multiple confounders can be controlled simultaneously • Information in continuous variables can be fully used • Enhances control for confounding when more people receive the treatment than get the outcome • If a stratified or matched analysis is used, does not require model assumptions • Flexible and reversible	• Results may be hard to understand • Relevant covariables must have been measured • Can only be done for exposed and unexposed subjects with overlapping propensity scores, reducing sample size

will rarely be precisely the same, and interaction introduces additional complexity, because a single measure of association no longer can summarize the relationship between predictor and outcome. For this reason, before concluding that an interaction is present, it is necessary to assess its biological plausibility and statistical significance (using a formal test for interaction, or, as a shortcut, checking to see whether the confidence intervals in the different strata overlap). The issue of interaction also arises for subgroup analyses of clinical trials (Chapter 11), and for meta-analyses when homogeneity of studies is being considered (Chapter 13).

Stratification resembles matching and specification in being easily understood. An advantage of stratification is its flexibility: by performing several stratified analyses, the investigators can decide which variables appear to be confounders and ignore the remainder. (This is done by determining whether the results of stratified analyses substantially differ from those of unstratified analyses; see Appendix 9A.) Stratification also has the advantage over design phase strategies of being reversible: no choices need be made at the beginning of the study that might later be regretted.

The principal disadvantage of stratified analysis is the limited number of variables that can be controlled simultaneously. For example, possible confounders in the coffee and MI study might include age, systolic blood pressure, serum cholesterol, cigarette smoking, and alcohol intake. To stratify on these five variables, with three strata for each, would require $3^5(= 243)$ strata! With this many strata there will be some with no cases or no controls, and these strata cannot be used.

To maintain a sufficient number of subjects in each stratum, a variable is often divided into just two strata. When the strata are too broad, however, the confounder may not be adequately controlled. For example, if the preceding study stratified using only two age strata (e.g., age < 50 and age ≥50), some residual confounding would still be possible if within each stratum the subjects drinking the most coffee were older and therefore at higher risk of MI.

Adjustment

Several statistical techniques are available to **adjust** for confounders. These techniques **model** the nature of the associations among the variables to isolate the effects of predictor variables and confounders. For example, a study of the effect of lead levels on IQ in children might examine parental education as a potential confounder. Statistical adjustment might model the relation between parents' years of schooling and the child's IQ as a straight line, in which each year of parent education is associated with a fixed increase in child IQ. The IQs of children with different lead levels could then be adjusted to remove the effect of parental education using the approach described in Appendix 9B. Similar adjustments can be made for several confounders simultaneously, using software for multivariate analysis.

One of the great **advantages of multivariate adjustment** techniques is the capacity to adjust for the influence of many confounders simultaneously. Another advantage is their use of all the information in continuous variables. It is easy, for example, to adjust for a parent's education level in 1-year intervals, rather than stratifying into just two categories.

There are, however, two **disadvantages of multivariate adjustment**. First, the model may not fit. Computerized statistical packages have made these models so accessible that the investigator may not stop to consider whether their use is appropriate for the predictor and outcome variables in the study. Taking the example in Appendix 9B, the investigator should examine whether the relation between the parents' years of schooling and the child's IQ is actually linear. If the pattern is very different (e.g., the slope of the line becomes steeper with increasing education) then attempts to adjust IQ for parental education using a linear model will be imperfect and the estimate of the independent effect of lead will be incorrect.

Second, the resulting highly derived statistics are difficult to understand intuitively. This is particularly a problem if a simple model does not fit and transformations (e.g., parental education squared) or interaction terms (used when the effect of one variable is modified by another) are needed.

Propensity Scores

Propensity scores are a relatively new analytic technique that can be useful in observational studies of treatment efficacy. They are a tool for controlling **confounding by indication**—the problem that patients for whom a treatment is indicated (and hence prescribed) are often at higher risk or otherwise intrinsically different from those who do not get the treatment. Recall that in order to be a confounder, a variable must be associated with both the predictor and outcome. Instead of adjusting for all other factors that predict outcome, use of propensity scores involves creating a multivariate (usually logistic) model to predict receipt of the treatment. Each subject can then be assigned a predicted probability of treatment—a propensity score. This single score can be used as the only confounding variable in stratified or multivariate analysis. Alternatively, subjects who did and did not receive the treatment can be matched by propensity score, and outcomes compared between matched pairs.

Example 9.1 Propensity analysis

Gum et al. (10) prospectively studied 6,174 consecutive adults undergoing stress echocardiography, 2,310 of whom (37%) were taking aspirin and 276 of whom died in the 3.1-year follow-up period. In unadjusted analyses, aspirin use was not associated with mortality (4.5% in both groups). However, when 1,351 patients who had received aspirin were matched to 1,351 patients with the same propensity to receive aspirin but who did not, mortality was 47% lower in those treated (P = 0.002).

Analysis using propensity scores has three distinct **advantages**. First, the number of potential confounding variables that can be modeled as predictors of the intervention in the propensity score is greater than if one is modeling the predictors of outcome because the number of people treated is generally much greater than the number who develop the outcome (2,310 compared with 276 in Example 9.1).[2] Second, because the potential confounding variables are reduced to a single score, the primary analysis of the relationship between the main predictor and outcome can be a stratified or matched analysis, which does not require assumptions about the form of the relationship between predictor, outcome, and confounding variables. Finally, if the predictor variable is receipt of a prescribed treatment, investigators might be more confident in understanding determinants of treatment than determinants of outcome, because after all, treatment decisions are made by clinicians based on a limited and potentially knowable number of patient characteristics.

Of course, like other multivariate techniques, use of propensity scores still requires that potential confounding variables be identified and measured. A **limitation** of this technique is that it does not provide information about the relationship between any of the confounding variables and outcome—the only result is for the treatment that was modeled with the propensity score. However, because this is an analysis phase strategy, it does not preclude doing more traditional multivariate analyses as well, and both types of analysis are usually done. The main disadvantages of this technique are that it requires an additional step and is less intuitive, less familiar and less well understood by journals and reviewers than traditional multivariate analyses.

---

[2]Another reason that more confounders can be included is that there is no danger of "overfitting" the propensity model—interaction terms, quadratic terms, and multiple indicator variables can all be included (11).

UNDERESTIMATION OF CAUSAL EFFECTS

To this point, we have focused on determining whether observed associations are causal. The emphasis has been on whether alternative bases for an association exist, that is, on avoiding a false conclusion that an association is real and causal when it is not. However, another type of error is also possible—underestimation of causal effects. It is important to remember that chance, bias and confounding can all be reasons why a real association might be missed or underestimated.

We discussed **chance** as a reason for missing an association in Chapter 5, when we reviewed type II errors and the need to make sure the sample size will provide adequate **power** to find real associations. After a study has been completed, however, the power calculation is no longer the best way to quantify uncertainty due to random error. At this stage estimating the probability of finding an effect of a specified size is less relevant than the actual findings, expressed as the observed estimate of association (e.g., risk ratio) and its 95% **confidence interval**.

Bias can also distort estimates of association toward no effect. In Chapter 8, the need for blinding in ascertaining risk factor status among cases and controls was to avoid **differential measurement bias**, for example, differences between the cases and controls in the way questions were asked or answers interpreted that might lead observers to get the answers they desire. Because observers might desire results in either direction, differential measurement bias can bias results in either direction.

Confounding can also lead to attenuation of real associations. For example, suppose coffee drinking actually protected against MI, but was more common in smokers. If smoking were not controlled for, the beneficial effects of coffee might be missed—coffee drinkers might appear to have the same risk of MI as those who did not drink coffee, when (based on their greater smoking) one would have expected their risk to be higher. This type of confounding, in which the effects of a beneficial factor are hidden by its association with a cause of the outcome, is sometimes called **suppression** (12). It is a common problem for observational studies of treatments, because treatments are often most indicated in those at higher risk of a bad outcome. The result, noted earlier, is **confounding by indication** in which a beneficial treatment can appear to be useless (as aspirin did in Example 9.1) or even harmful.

CHOOSING A STRATEGY

What general guidelines can be offered for deciding whether to cope with confounders during the design or analysis phases, and how best to do it? The use of **specification** to control confounding is most appropriate for situations in which the investigator is chiefly interested in specific subgroups of the population; this is really just a special form of the general process in every study of establishing criteria for selecting the study subjects (Chapter 3).

An important decision to make in the design phase of the study is whether to **match**. Matching is most appropriate for case–control studies and fixed constitutional factors such as age, race, and sex. Matching may also be helpful when the sample size is small compared with the number of strata necessary to control for known confounders, and when the confounders are more easily matched than measured. However, because matching can permanently compromise the investigator's ability to observe real associations, it should be used sparingly, particularly for variables that may be in the causal chain. In many situations the analysis phase strategies (stratification, adjustment, and propensity scores) are just as good for controlling confounding, and have the great advantage of being **reversible**—they allow the investigator to add or subtract covariates to the statistical model in her efforts to infer causal pathways.

The decision to **stratify, adjust** or use **propensity scores** can wait until after the data are collected; in many cases the investigator may wish to do all of the above. However, it is important at the time the study is designed to consider which factors may later be used for adjustment, in order to know which variables to measure. Also, because strategies to adjust for the influence of a specific confounding variable can only succeed to the degree that the confounder is well measured, it is important to design measurement approaches that have adequate precision and accuracy (Chapter 4).

Evidence Favoring Causality

The approach to enhancing causal inference has largely been a negative one thus far—how to rule out the four rival explanations in Table 9.1. A complementary strategy is to seek characteristics of associations that provide positive evidence for causality, of which the most important are the consistency and strength of the association, the presence of a dose–response relation, and biologic plausibility.

When the results are **consistent** in studies of various designs, it is less likely that chance or bias is the cause of an association. Real associations that represent effect–cause or confounding, however, will also be consistently observed. For example, if cigarette smokers drink more coffee and have more MIs in the population, studies will consistently observe an association between coffee drinking and MI.

The **strength** of the association is also important. For one thing, stronger associations give more significant P values, making chance a less likely explanation. Stronger associations also provide better evidence for causality by reducing the likelihood of confounding. Associations due to confounding are indirect (i.e., via the confounder) and therefore are generally weaker than direct cause–effect associations. This is illustrated in Appendix 9A: the strong associations between coffee and smoking (odds ratio = 16) and between smoking and MI (odds ratio = 4) led to a much weaker association between coffee and MI (odds ratio = 2.25).

A **dose–response** relation provides positive evidence for causality. The association between cigarette smoking and lung cancer is an example: moderate smokers have higher rates of cancer than do nonsmokers, and heavy smokers have even higher rates. Whenever possible, predictor variables should be measured continuously or in several categories, so that any dose–response relation that is present can be observed. Once again, however, a dose–response relation can be observed with effect–cause associations or with confounding. For example, if heavier coffee drinkers also were heavier smokers, their MI risk would be greater than that of moderate coffee drinkers.

Finally, **biologic plausibility** is an important consideration for drawing causal inference—if a causal mechanism that makes sense biologically can be proposed, evidence for causality is enhanced, whereas associations that do not make sense given our current understanding of biology are less likely to represent cause–effect. It is important not to overemphasize biologic plausibility, however. Investigators seem to be able to come up with a plausible mechanism for virtually any association.

SUMMARY

1. The design of **observational studies** should anticipate the need to interpret **associations**. The inference that the association represents a **cause–effect** relationship (often the goal of the study) is strengthened by strategies that reduce the likelihood of the **four rival explanations—chance, bias, effect–cause**, and **confounding**.

2. The role of **chance** can be minimized by designing a study with **adequate sample size and precision** to assure a low **type I error** rate. Once the study is completed, the likelihood that chance is the basis of the association can be judged from the *P* **value** and the consistency of the results with **previous evidence**.

3. **Bias** arises from differences between the population and phenomena addressed by the research question and the actual subjects and measurements in the study. Bias can be avoided by basing design decisions on a **judgment** as to whether these differences will lead to a wrong answer to the research question.

4. **Effect–cause** is made less likely by designing a study that permits assessment of **temporal sequence**, and by considering **biologic plausibility**.

5. **Confounding** is made less likely by the following strategies, most of which require potential confounders to be anticipated and measured:
   a. **Specification** or **matching** in the design phase, which alters the sampling strategy to ensure that only groups with similar levels of the confounder are compared. These strategies should be used sparingly because they can irreversibly limit the information available from the study.
   b. **Stratification, adjustment or propensity analysis** in the analysis phase, which accomplish the same goal statistically and preserve more options for inferring causal pathways. **Stratification** is the easiest to grasp intuitively, and **adjustment** can permit many factors to be controlled simultaneously. **Propensity scores** are particularly helpful for addressing **confounding by indication** in studies of treatment efficacy.

6. Investigators should be on the lookout for **opportunistic** observational designs, including **natural experiments, Mendelian randomization** and other **instrumental variable** designs, that offer a strength of causal inferences that can approach that of a randomized clinical trial.

7. In addition to serving as rival explanations for observed associations, chance, bias, and confounding can also lead to **suppression** (underestimation) of real causal associations.

8. Causal inference can be enhanced by positive evidence, notably the **consistency and strength of the association**, the presence of a **dose–response** relation, and prior evidence on **biologic plausibility**.

APPENDIX 9A

Hypothetical Example of Confounding and Interaction

The entries in these tables are numbers of subjects. Therefore, the top left entry means that there were 90 subjects with MI who drank coffee.

1. If we look at the entire group of study subjects, there appears to be an association between coffee drinking and MI (odds ratio = 2.25):

	Smokers and Nonsmokers Combined	
	MI	No MI
Coffee	90	60
No coffee	60	90

Odds ratio for MI associated with coffee:

$$\text{in smokers and non smokers combined} = \frac{90 \times 90}{60 \times 60}$$
$$= 2.25 \ (P = 0.0005; 95\% \text{ CI } 1.4, 3.7)$$

2. However, this could be due to **confounding**, as shown by the tables stratified on smoking below. These tables show that coffee drinking is not associated with MI in either smokers or nonsmokers:

	Smokers		Nonsmokers	
	MI	No MI	MI	No MI
Coffee	80	40	10	20
No coffee	20	10	40	80

Odds ratio for MI associated with coffee:

$$\text{in smokers} = \frac{80 \times 10}{20 \times 40} = 1 \ (95\% \text{ CI } 0.4, 2.5)$$
$$\text{in nonsmokers} = \frac{10 \times 80}{40 \times 20} = 1 \ (95\% \text{ CI } 0.4, 2.5)$$

Smoking is a confounder because it is strongly associated with coffee drinking (below, left panel) and with MI (below, right panel):

	MI and No MI Combined	
	Coffee	No Coffee
Smokers	120	30
Nonsmokers	30	120

	Coffee and No Coffee Combined	
	MI	No MI
Smokers	100	50
Nonsmokers	50	100

Odds ratio for coffee drinking associated

$$\text{with smoking} = \frac{120 \times 120}{30 \times 30} = 16$$

Odds ratio for MI associated with

$$\text{smoking} = \frac{100 \times 100}{50 \times 50} = 4$$

3. A more complicated situation is **interaction**. In that case, the association between coffee drinking and MI differs in smokers and nonsmokers. (In this example, the association between coffee drinking and MI in the whole study is due entirely to a strong association in smokers). When interaction is present, the odds ratios in different strata are different, and must be reported separately:

Smokers		
	MI	**No MI**
Coffee	50	15
No Coffee	10	33

$$OR = \frac{50 \times 33}{15 \times 10} = 11 \ (95\% \ CI, \ 4.1, \ 30.6)$$

Nonsmokers		
	MI	**No MI**
Coffee	40	45
No Coffee	50	57

$$OR = \frac{40 \times 57}{45 \times 50} = 1.0 \ (95\% \ CI, \ 0.55, \ 1.9)$$

APPENDIX 9B

A Simplified Example of Adjustment

Suppose that a study finds two major predictors of the IQ of children: the parental education level and the child's blood lead level. Consider the following hypothetical data on children with normal and high lead levels:

	Average Years of Parental Education	Average IQ of Child
High lead level	10.0	95
Normal lead level	12.0	110

Note that the parental education level is also associated with the child's blood lead level. The question is, "Is the difference in IQ more than can be accounted for on the basis of the difference in parental education?" To answer this question we look at how much difference in IQ the difference in parental education levels would be expected to produce. We do this by plotting parental educational level versus IQ in the children with normal lead levels (Fig. 9.2).[3]

The dotted line in Figure 9.2 shows the relationship between the child's IQ and parental education in children with normal lead levels; there is an increase in the child's IQ of five points for each 2 years of parental education. Therefore, we can adjust the IQ of the normal lead group to account for the difference in mean parental education by sliding down the line from point A to point A'. (Because the group with normal lead levels had 2 more years of parental education on the average, we adjust their IQs downward by five points to make them comparable in mean parental education to the high lead group.) This still leaves a 10-point difference in IQ between points A and B, suggesting that lead has an independent effect on IQ of this magnitude. Therefore, of the 15-point difference in IQ of children with low and high lead levels, five points can be accounted for by their parents' different education levels and the remaining ten are attributable to the lead exposure.

[3] This description of analysis of covariance (ANCOVA) is simplified. Actually, parental education is plotted against the child's IQ in both the normal and high lead groups, and the single slope that fits both plots the best is used. The model for this form of adjustment therefore assumes linear relationships between education and IQ in both groups, and that the slopes of the lines in the two groups are the same.

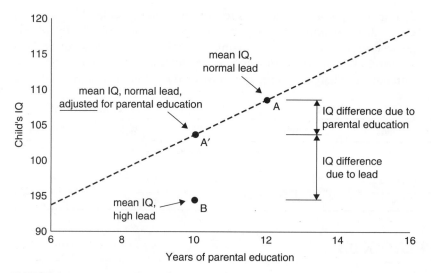

FIGURE 9.2. Hypothetical graph of child's IQ as a linear function (*dotted line*) of years of parental education.

REFERENCES

1. McEvoy SP, Stevenson MR, McCartt AT, et al. Role of mobile phones in motor vehicle crashes resulting in hospital attendance: a case-crossover study. *BMJ* 2005;331(7514):428.
2. Huxley R, Ansary-Moghaddam A, Berrington de Gonzalez A, et al. Type-II diabetes and pancreatic cancer: a meta-analysis of 36 studies. *Br J Cancer* 2005;92(11):2076–2083.
3. Maconochie N, Doyle P, Carson C. Infertility among male veterans of the 1990–1991 Gulf war: reproductive cohort study. *BMJ* 2004;329:196–201. Erratum in *BMJ* 2004;329:323.
4. Lofgren RP, Gottlieb D, Williams RA, et al. Post-call transfer of resident responsibility: its effect on patient care [see comments]. *J Gen Intern Med* 1990;5(6):501–505.
5. Bell CM, Redelmeier DA. Mortality among patients admitted to hospitals on weekends as compared with weekdays. *N Engl J Med* 2001;345(9):663–668.
6. Davey Smith G, Ebrahim S. 'Mendelian randomization': can genetic epidemiology contribute to understanding environmental determinants of disease? *Int J Epidemiol* 2003;32(1):1–22.
7. Cherry N, Mackness M, Durrington P, et al. Paraoxonase (PON1) polymorphisms in farmers attributing ill health to sheep dip. *Lancet* 2002;359(9308):763–764.
8. Hearst N, Newman TB, Hulley SB. Delayed effects of the military draft on mortality. A randomized natural experiment. *N Engl J Med* 1986;314(10):620–624.
9. McClellan M, McNeil BJ, Newhouse JP. Does more intensive treatment of acute myocardial infarction in the elderly reduce mortality? Analysis using instrumental variables. *JAMA* 1994;272(11):859–866.
10. Gum PA, Thamilarasan M, Watanabe J, et al. Aspirin use and all-cause mortality among patients being evaluated for known or suspected coronary artery disease: a propensity analysis. *JAMA* 2001;286(10):1187–1194.
11. Klungel OH, Martens EP, Psaty BM, et al. Methods to assess intended effects of drug treatment in observational studies are reviewed. *J Clin Epidemiol* 2004;57(12):1223–1231.
12. Katz M. *Multivariable analysis: a practical guide for clinicians*. Cambridge: Cambridge University Press, 1999.

10 Designing a Randomized Blinded Trial

Steven R. Cummings, Deborah Grady, and Stephen B. Hulley

In clinical trials, the investigator applies an **intervention** and observes the effect on **outcomes.** The major advantage of a trial over an observational study is the ability to demonstrate causality. In particular, **randomly assigning** the intervention can eliminate the influence of confounding variables, and **blinding** its administration can eliminate the possibility that the observed effects of the intervention are due to differential use of other treatments in the treatment and control groups or to biased ascertainment or adjudication of the outcome.

However, clinical trials are generally expensive, time consuming, address narrow clinical questions, and sometimes expose participants to potential harm. For these reasons, trials are best reserved for relatively **mature research questions,** when observational studies and other lines of evidence suggest that an intervention might be effective and safe but stronger evidence is required before it can be approved or recommended. Not every research question is amenable to the clinical trial design—it is not feasible to study whether drug treatment of high LDL-cholesterol in children will prevent heart attacks many decades later. But clinical trial evidence on clinical interventions should be obtained whenever possible.

This chapter focuses on **designing** the classic **randomized blinded trial** (Fig. 10.1), addressing the choice of **intervention and control**, defining **outcomes,** selecting **participants,** measuring **baseline variables,** and approaches to **randomizing** and **blinding.** In the next chapter we will cover alternative trial designs and implementation and analysis issues.

SELECTING THE INTERVENTION AND CONTROL CONDITIONS

In a clinical trial, the investigator compares the outcome in groups of participants that receive different interventions. **Between-group designs** always include a group

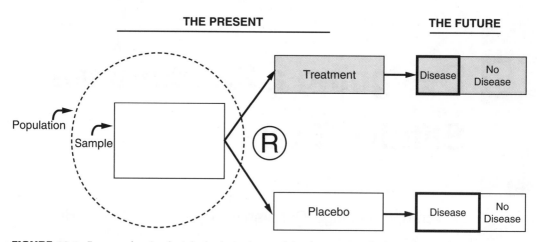

THE PRESENT

THE FUTURE

Population

Sample

Treatment → Disease | No Disease

Placebo → Disease | No Disease

FIGURE 10.1. In a randomized trial, the investigator (a) selects a sample from the population, (b) measures baseline variables, (c) randomizes the participants (R), (d) applies interventions (one should be a blinded placebo, if possible), (e) measures outcome variables during follow-up (blinded to randomized group assignment).

that receives an intervention to be tested, and another that receives either no active treatment (preferably a placebo) or a comparison treatment.

Choice of Intervention

The choice of intervention is the critical first step in designing a clinical trial. Investigators should consider several issues as they design their interventions, including the intensity, duration and frequency of the intervention that best balances effectiveness and safety. It is also important to consider the feasibility of blinding, whether to treat with one or a combination of interventions, and generalizability to the way the treatment will be used in practice. If important decisions are uncertain, such as which dose best balances effectiveness and safety, it is generally best to postpone major or costly trials until pilot studies have been completed to help resolve the issue. Choosing the best treatment can be especially difficult in studies that involve years of follow-up because a treatment that reflects current practice at the outset of the study may have become outmoded by the end, transforming a pragmatic test into an academic exercise.

The best balance between **effectiveness** and **safety** depends on the condition being studied. On the one hand, effectiveness is generally the paramount consideration in designing interventions to treat illnesses that cause severe symptoms and a high risk of death. Therefore, it may be best to choose the "highest tolerable dose" for treatment of metastatic cancer. On the other hand, safety should be the primary criterion for designing interventions to treat less severe conditions or to prevent illness. Preventive therapy in healthy people should meet stringent tests of safety: if it is effective, the treatment will prevent the condition in a few persons, but everyone treated will be at risk of the adverse effects of the drug. In this case, it is generally best to choose the "lowest effective dose." If the best dose is not certain based on prior animal and human research findings, there may be a need for additional **trials** that compare the effects of multiple doses on surrogate outcomes (see phase II trials, Chapter 11).

Sometimes an investigator may decide to compare **several promising doses** with a single control group in a major disease endpoint trial. For example, at the time the Multiple Outcomes of Raloxifene Evaluation Trial was designed, it was not clear which dose of raloxifene (60 or 120 mg) was best, so the trial tested two doses of raloxifene for preventing fractures (1). This is sometimes a reasonable strategy, but it has its costs: a larger and more expensive trial, and the complexity of dealing with multiple hypotheses (Chapter 5).

Trials to test **single interventions** are generally much easier to plan and implement than those testing combinations of treatments. However, many medical conditions, such as HIV infection or congestive heart failure, are treated with **combinations** of drugs or therapies. The most important disadvantage of testing combinations of treatments is that the result cannot provide clear conclusions about any one of the interventions. In the first Women's Health Initiative trial, for example, postmenopausal women were treated with estrogen plus progestin therapy or placebo. The intervention increased the risk of several conditions, such as breast cancer; however, it was unclear whether the effect was due to the estrogen or the progestin (2). In general, it is preferable to design trials that have only one major difference between any two study groups.

The investigator should consider how well the intervention can be incorporated in practice. **Simple interventions** are generally better than complicated ones (patients are more likely to take a pill once a day than two or three times). Complicated interventions, such as multifaceted counseling about changing behavior, may not be feasible to incorporate in general practice because they require rare expertise or are too time consuming or costly. Such interventions are less likely to have clinical impact, even if a trial proves that they are effective.

Some treatments are generally given in doses that vary from patient to patient. In these instances, it may be best to design an intervention so that the **active drug is titrated** to achieve a clinical outcome such as reduction in the hepatitis C viral load. To maintain blinding, corresponding changes should be made (by someone not otherwise involved in the trial) in the "dose" of placebo for a randomly selected or matched participant in the placebo group.

Choice of Control

The best control group receives **no active treatment** in a way that can be **blinded,** which for medications generally requires a **placebo** that is indistinguishable from active treatment. This strategy compensates for any placebo effect of the active intervention (i.e., through suggestion and other nonpharmacologic mechanisms) so that any outcome difference between study groups can be ascribed to a biological effect.

The cleanest comparison between the intervention and control groups occurs when there are no **cointerventions**—medications, therapies or behaviors (other than the study intervention) that reduce the risk of developing the outcome of interest. If participants use effective cointerventions, power will be reduced and the sample size will need to be larger or the trial longer. In the absence of effective blinding, the trial protocol must include plans to obtain data to allow statistical adjustment for differences between the groups in the rate of use of such cointerventions during the trial. However, adjusting for such postrandomization differences violates the intention-to-treat principle and should be viewed as a secondary or explanatory analysis (Chapter 11).

Often it is not possible to withhold treatments other than the study intervention. For example, in a trial of a new drug to reduce the risk of myocardial infarction in persons with known coronary heart disease (CHD), the investigators cannot ethically prohibit or discourage participants from taking medical treatments that are indicated for persons with known CHD, including aspirin, statins and beta-blockers. One solution is to **give standard care drugs to all** participants in the trial; although this approach reduces the event rate and therefore increases the required sample size, it minimizes the potential for differences in cointerventions between the groups and tests whether the new intervention improves outcome when given in addition to standard care.

When the treatment to be studied is a new drug that is believed to be a good alternative to standard care, one option is to design an **equivalence trial** in which new treatments are compared with those already proven effective (see Chapter 11). When the treatment to be studied is a surgery or other procedure that is so attractive that prospective participants are reluctant to be randomized to something different, an excellent approach may be randomization to immediate intervention versus a **wait-list control.** This design requires an outcome that can be assessed within a few months of starting the intervention. It provides an opportunity for a randomized comparison between the immediate intervention and wait-list control groups during the first several months, and also for a within-group comparison before and after the intervention in the wait-list control group (see Chapter 11 for **time-series** and **cross-over designs**).

CHOOSING OUTCOME MEASUREMENTS

The definition of the specific outcomes of the trial influences many other design components, as well as the cost and even the feasibility of answering the question. Trials should include several outcome measurements to increase the richness of the results and possibilities for secondary analyses. However, a single outcome must be chosen that reflects the main question, allows calculation of the sample size and sets the priority for efforts to implement the study.

Clinical outcomes provide the best evidence about whether and how to use treatments. However for outcomes that are uncommon, such as the occurrence of cancer, trials must generally be large, long, and expensive. As noted in Chapter 6, outcomes measured as continuous variables, such as quality of life, can generally be studied with fewer subjects and shorter follow-up times than rates of a dichotomous clinical outcome, such as recurrence of treated breast cancer.

Intermediate markers, such as bone density, are measurements that are related to the clinical outcome. Trials that use intermediate outcomes can further our understanding of pathophysiology and provide information to design the best dose or frequency of treatment for use in trials with clinical outcomes. The clinical relevance of trials with intermediate outcomes depends in large part on how accurately changes in these markers, especially changes that occur due to treatment, represent changes in the risk or natural history of clinical outcomes. Intermediate markers can be considered **surrogate markers** for the clinical outcome to the extent that treatment-induced changes in the marker consistently predict how treatment changes the clinical outcome (3). Generally, a good surrogate measures changes in an intermediate factor in the main pathway that determines the clinical outcome.

HIV viral load is a good surrogate marker because treatments that reduce the viral load consistently reduce morbidity and mortality in patients with HIV infection. In contrast, bone mineral density (BMD) is considered a poor surrogate marker (3). It reflects the amount of mineral in a section of bone, but treatments that improve

BMD sometimes have little or no effect on fracture risk, and the magnitude of change in BMD can substantially underestimate how much the treatment reduces fracture risk (4). The best evidence that a biological marker is a good surrogate comes from randomized trials of the clinical outcome (*fractures*) that also measure change in the marker (*BMD*) in all participants. If the marker is a good surrogate, then statistical adjustment for changes in the marker will account for much of the effect of treatment on the outcome (3).

Number of Outcome Variables

It is often desirable to have **several outcome variables** that measure different aspects of the phenomena of interest. In the Heart and Estrogen/progestin Replacement Study (HERS), CHD events were chosen as the primary endpoint. Nonfatal myocardial infarction, coronary revascularization, hospitalization for unstable angina or congestive heart failure, stroke and transient ischemic attack, venous thromboembolic events, and all-cause mortality were all assessed and adjudicated to provide a more detailed description of the cardiovascular effects of hormone therapy (5). However, a **single primary endpoint** (*CHD events*) was designated for the purpose of planning the sample size and duration of the study and to avoid the problems of interpreting tests of multiple hypotheses (Chapter 5).

Adverse Effects

The investigator should include outcome measures that will detect the occurrence of **adverse effects** that may result from the intervention. Revealing whether the beneficial effects of an intervention outweigh the adverse ones is a major goal of most clinical trials, even those that test apparently innocuous treatments like a health education program. Adverse effects may range from relatively minor symptoms such as a mild or transient rash, to serious and fatal complications. The investigator should consider the problem that the rate of occurrence, the effect of treatment and the sample size requirements for detecting adverse effects will generally be different from those for detecting benefits. Unfortunately, rare side effects will usually be impossible to detect no matter how large the trial and are discovered (if at all) only after an intervention is in widespread clinical use.

In the early stages of testing a new treatment when potential adverse effects are unclear, investigators should ask broad, open-ended questions about all types of potential adverse effects. In large trials, assessment and coding of all potential adverse events can be very expensive and time consuming, often with a low yield of important results. Investigators should consider strategies for minimizing this burden while preserving an adequate assessment of potential harms of the intervention. For example, in very large trials, common and minor events, such as upper respiratory infections and gastrointestinal upset, might be recorded in a subset of the participants. Important potential adverse events or effects that are expected because of previous research or clinical experience should be ascertained by specific queries. For example, because rhabdomyolysis is a reported side effect of treatment with statins, the signs and symptoms of myositis should be queried in any trial of a new statin.

When data from a trial is used to apply for regulatory approval of a new drug, the trial design must satisfy regulatory expectations for reporting adverse events (see "Good Clinical Practices" on the U.S. Food and Drug Administration [FDA] website). Certain disease areas, such as cancer, have established methods for classifying adverse events (see "NCI Common Toxicity Criteria" on the National Cancer Institute website).

SELECTING THE PARTICIPANTS

Chapter 3 discussed how to specify entry criteria defining a target population that is appropriate to the research question and an accessible population that is practical to study, how to design an efficient and scientific approach to selecting participants, and how to recruit them. Here we cover issues that are especially relevant to clinical trials.

Define Entry Criteria

In a clinical trial, inclusion and exclusion criteria have the joint goal of identifying a population in which it is feasible, ethical and relevant to study the impact of the intervention on outcomes. **Inclusion criteria** should produce a sufficient number of enrollees who have a high enough rate of the primary outcome to achieve adequate power to find an important effect on the outcome. On the other hand, criteria should also maximize the generalizability of findings from the trial and ease of recruitment. For example, if the outcome of interest is a rare event, such as breast cancer, it is usually necessary to recruit participants who have a high risk of the outcome to reduce the sample size and follow-up time to feasible levels. On the other hand, narrowing the inclusion criteria to higher-risk women limits the generalizability of the results and makes it more difficult to recruit participants into the trial.

To plan the right **sample size,** the investigator must have reliable estimates of the rate of the primary outcome in people who might be enrolled. These estimates can be based on data from vital statistics, longitudinal observational studies, or rates observed in the untreated group in trials with outcomes similar to those in the planned trial. For example, expected rates of breast cancer in postmenopausal women can be estimated from cancer registry data. The investigator should keep in mind, however, that screening and healthy volunteer effects generally mean that event rates among those who qualify and agree to enter clinical trials are lower than in the general population; it may be preferable to obtain rates of breast cancer from the placebo group of other trials with similar inclusion criteria.

Including participants with a **high risk** of the outcome can decrease the number of subjects needed for the trial. If risk factors for the outcome have been established, then the selection criteria can be designed to include participants who have a minimum estimated risk of the outcome of interest. The Raloxifene Use for The Heart trial, designed to test the effect of raloxifene for prevention of cardiovascular disease (CVD) and breast cancer, enrolled women who were at increased risk of CVD based on a combination of risk factors (6). Another way to increase the rate of events is to limit enrollment to people who already have the disease. The Heart and Estrogen/Progestin Replacement Study included 2,763 women who already had CHD to test whether estrogen plus progestin reduced the risk of new CHD events (5). This approach was much less costly than the Women's Health Initiative trial of the same research question in women without CHD, which required about 17,000 participants (7).

Additionally, a trial can be smaller and shorter if it includes people who are likely to have the **greatest benefit** from the treatment. For example, tamoxifen blocks the binding of estradiol to its receptor and decreases the risk of breast cancer that is estrogen receptor positive but not that of cancer that is estrogen receptor negative (8). Therefore, a trial testing the effect of tamoxifen on the risk of breast cancer would be somewhat smaller and shorter if the selection criteria specify participants at high risk of estrogen receptor–positive breast cancer.

Although probability samples of general populations confer advantages in observational studies, this type of sampling is generally not feasible and has limited value for randomized trials. Inclusion of participants with diverse characteristics will increase the confidence that the results of a trial apply broadly. However, setting aside issues of adherence to randomized treatment, it is generally true that results of a trial done in a convenience sample (e.g., *women with CHD who respond to advertisements*) will be similar to results obtained in probability samples of eligible people (*all women with CHD*).

Stratification by a characteristic, such as racial group, allows investigators to enroll a desired number of participants with a characteristic that may have an influence on the effect of the treatment or its generalizability. Recruitment to a stratum is generally closed when the goal for participants with that characteristic has been reached.

Exclusion criteria should be parsimonious because unnecessary exclusions may diminish the generalizability of the results, make it more difficult to recruit the necessary number of participants, and increase the complexity and cost of recruitment. There are five reasons for excluding people from a clinical trial (Table 10.1).

The treatment may be unsafe in people who are susceptible to known or suspected adverse effects of the active treatment. For example, myocardial infarction is a rare adverse effect of treatment with sildenafil (Viagra). Therefore, trials of Viagra to treat painful vasospasm in patients with Raynaud's disease should exclude patients who have CHD (9). Conversely receiving placebo may be considered unsafe for some participants. For example, bisphosphonates are known to be so beneficial in women with vertebral fractures that it would be unacceptable to enter them in a placebo-controlled trial of a new treatment for osteoporosis unless bisphosphonates could also be provided for all trial participants. Persons in whom the active treatment

TABLE 10.1	Reasons for Excluding People from a Clinical Trial
Reason	**Example (A trial of raloxifene vs. placebo to prevent heart disease)**
1. A study treatment would be harmful	
• Unacceptable risk of adverse reaction to active treatment	Prior venous thromboembolic event (raloxifene increases risk of venous thromboembolic events)
• Unacceptable risk of assignment to placebo	Recent estrogen receptor–positive breast cancer (treatment with an anti-estrogen is an effective standard of care)
2. Active treatment is unlikely to be effective	
• At low risk for the outcome	Low coronary heart disease risk factors
• Has a type of disease that is not likely to respond to treatment	
• Taking a treatment that is likely to interfere with the intervention	Taking estrogen therapy (which competes with raloxifene)
3. Unlikely to adhere to the intervention	Poor adherence during run-in
4. Unlikely to complete follow-up	Plans to move before trial ends
	Short life expectancy because of a serious illness
	Unreliable participation in visits before randomization
5. Practical problems with participating in the protocol	Impaired mental state that prevents accurate answers to questions

is unlikely to be effective should be excluded, as well as those who are unlikely to be adherent to the intervention or unlikely to complete follow-up. It is wise to exclude people who are not likely to contribute a primary outcome to the study (e.g., *because they will move during the period of follow-up*). Occasionally, practical problems such as impaired mental status that makes it difficult to follow instructions justify exclusion. Investigators should carefully weigh potential exclusion criteria that apply to many people (e.g., *diabetes or upper age limits*) as these may have a large impact on the feasibility and costs of recruitment and the generalizability of results.

Design an Adequate Sample Size and Plan the Recruitment Accordingly

Trials with too few participants to detect substantial effects are wasteful, unethical, and may produce misleading conclusions (10). Estimating the sample size is one of the most important early parts of planning a trial (Chapter 6). Outcome rates in clinical trials are commonly lower than estimated, primarily due to screening and volunteer bias. Recruitment for a trial is usually more difficult than recruitment for an observational study. For these reasons, the investigator should plan an adequate sample from a large accessible population, and enough time and money to get the desired sample size when (as usually happens) the barriers to doing so turn out to be greater than expected.

MEASURING BASELINE VARIABLES

To facilitate contacting participants who are lost to follow-up, it is important to record the names, phone numbers, addresses, and e-mail addresses of two or three friends or relatives who will always know how to reach the participant. It is also valuable to record Social Security numbers or other national I.D. numbers. These can be used to determine the vital status of participants (through the National Death Index) or to detect key outcomes using health records (e.g., health insurance systems). However, this is confidential "protected personal health information" that must be kept confidential and should not accompany data that are sent to a coordinating center or sponsoring institution.

Describe the Participants

Investigators should collect enough information (e.g., age, gender, and measurements of the severity of disease) to help others judge the generalizability of the findings. These measurements also provide a means for checking on the comparability of the study groups at baseline; the first table of the final report of a clinical trial typically compares the levels of baseline characteristics in the study groups. The goal is to make sure that differences in these levels do not exceed what might be expected from the play of chance, which might suggest a technical error or bias in carrying out the randomization.

Measure Variables that are Risk Factors for the Outcome or can be Used to Define Subgroups

It is a good idea to measure baseline variables that are likely to be strong predictors of the outcome (e.g., *smoking habits of the spouse* in a trial of a smoking intervention). This allows the investigator to study secondary research questions, such as predictors of the outcomes. In small trials where randomization is more prone to produce chance maldistributions of baseline characteristics, measurement of important predictors of the outcome permits statistical adjustment of the primary randomized comparison to reduce the influence of these chance maldistributions on the outcome of the trial. Baseline measurements of potential predictors of the outcome also allow the investigator to examine whether the intervention has different effects in **subgroups** classified by baseline variables, an uncommon but important phenomenon termed **effect modification** or **interaction** (Chapter 9). For example, bone density measured at baseline in the Fracture Intervention Trial led to the finding that treatment with alendronate significantly decreased the risk of nonspine fractures in women with very low bone density (osteoporosis) but had no effect in women with higher bone density (11). Importantly, a specific test for the interaction was of bone density and treatment effect was statistically significant ($P = 0.02$).

Measure Baseline Value of the Outcome Variable

If outcomes include change in a variable, the outcome variable must be measured at the beginning of the study in the same way that it will be measured at the end. In studies that have a dichotomous outcome (*incidence of CHD*, for example) it may be important to demonstrate by history and electrocardiogram that the disease is not present at the outset. In studies that have a continuous outcome variable (*effects of antihypertensive drugs on blood pressure*) the best measure is generally a change in the outcome over the course of the study. This approach usually minimizes the variability in the outcome between study participants and offers more power than simply comparing blood pressure values at the end of the trial. Similarly, it may also be useful to measure secondary outcome variables, and outcomes of planned ancillary studies, at baseline.

Be Parsimonious

Having pointed out all these uses for baseline measurements, we should stress that the design of a clinical trial does not require that *any* be measured, because randomization eliminates the problem of confounding by factors that are present at the outset. Making a lot of measurements adds expense and complexity. In a randomized trial that has a limited budget, time and money are usually better spent on things that are vital to the integrity of the trial, such as the adequacy of the sample size, the success of randomization and blinding, and the completeness of follow-up. Yusuf et al. have promoted the use of large trials with very few measurements (12).

Establish Banks of Materials

Storing images, sera, DNA, and other biologic specimens at baseline will allow subsequent measurement of biological effects of the treatment, biological markers that predict the outcome, and factors (such as genotype) that might identify people who respond well or poorly to the treatment. Stored specimens can also be a rich resource to study other research questions not directly related to the main outcome.

■ RANDOMIZING AND BLINDING

The third step in Figure 10.1 is to randomly assign the participants to two or more groups. In the simplest design, one group receives an active treatment intervention and the other receives a placebo. The random allocation of participants to one or another of the study groups establishes the basis for testing the statistical significance of differences between these groups in the measured outcome. Random assignment provides that age, sex, and other prognostic baseline characteristics that could confound an observed association (even those that are unknown or unmeasured) will be distributed equally, except for chance variation, among the randomized groups.

Do a Good Job of Random Assignment

Because randomization is the cornerstone of a clinical trial, it is important that it be done correctly. The two most important features are that the procedure truly **allocates treatments randomly** and that the assignments are **tamperproof** so that neither intentional nor unintentional factors can influence the randomization.

Ordinarily, the participant completes the baseline examinations, is found eligible for inclusion, and gives consent to enter the study before randomization. He is then randomly assigned by computerized algorithm or by applying a set of random numbers, which are typically computer-generated. Once a list of the random order of assignment to study groups is generated, it must be applied to participants in strict sequence as they enter the trial.

It is essential to design the random assignment procedure so that members of the research team who have any contact with the study participants cannot influence the allocation. For example, random treatment assignments can be placed in advance in a set of sealed envelopes by someone who will not be involved in opening the envelopes. Each envelope must be numbered (so that all can be accounted for at the end of the study), opaque (to prevent transillumination by a strong light), and otherwise tamperproof. When a participant is randomized, his name and the number of the next unopened envelope are first recorded in the presence of a second staff member and both staff sign the envelope; *then* the envelope is opened and the randomization number contained therein assigned to the participant.

Multicenter trials typically use a separate tamperproof randomization facility that the trial staff contact when an eligible participant is ready to be randomized. The staff member provides the name and study ID of the new participant. This information is recorded and the treatment group is then randomly assigned by providing a treatment assignment number linked to the interventions. Treatment can also be randomly assigned by computer programs at a single research site as long as these programs are tamperproof. Rigorous precautions to prevent tampering with randomization are needed because investigators sometimes find themselves under pressure to influence the randomization process (e.g., for an individual who seems particularly suitable for an active treatment group in a placebo-controlled trial).

Consider Special Randomization Techniques

The preferred approach is typically simple randomization of individual participants in an equal ratio to each intervention group. Trials of small to moderate size will have a small gain in power if special randomization procedures are used to balance the study groups in the numbers of participants they contain (blocked randomization) and in the distribution of baseline variables known to predict the outcome (stratified blocked randomization).

Blocked randomization is a commonly used technique to ensure that the number of participants is equally distributed among the study groups. Randomization is done in "blocks" of predetermined size. For example, if the block size is six, randomization proceeds normally within each block until the third person is randomized to one group, after which participants are automatically assigned to the other group until the block of six is completed. This means that in a study of 30 participants exactly 15 will be assigned to each group, and in a study of 33 participants, the disproportion could be no greater than 18:15. Blocked randomization with a fixed block size is less suitable for nonblinded studies because the treatment assignment of the participants at the end of each block could be predicted and manipulated. This problem can be minimized by varying the size of the blocks randomly (ranging, for example, from four to eight) according to a schedule that is not known to the investigator.

Stratified blocked randomization ensures that an important predictor of the outcome is more evenly distributed between the study groups than chance alone would dictate. In a trial of the effect of a drug to prevent fractures, having a prior vertebral fracture is such a strong predictor of outcome and response to treatment that it may be best to ensure that similar numbers of people who have vertebral fractures are assigned to each group. This can be achieved by dividing participants into two groups—those with and those without vertebral fractures—as they enroll in the trial and then carrying out blocked randomization separately in each of these two "strata." Stratified blocked randomization can slightly enhance the power of a small trial by reducing the variation in outcome due to chance disproportions in important baseline variables. It is of little benefit in large trials (more than 1,000 participants) because chance assignment ensures nearly even distribution of baseline variables. An important limitation of stratified blocked randomization is the small number of baseline variables, not more than two or three, that can be balanced by this technique.

Randomizing equal numbers of participants to each group maximizes study power, but **unequal allocation of participants to treatment and control groups** may sometimes be appropriate (13). Occasionally, investigators increase the ratio of active to placebo treatment to make the trial more attractive to potential subjects who would like a greater chance of receiving active treatment if they enroll, or decrease the ratio (as in the Women's Health Initiative low-fat diet trial (14)) to save money if the intervention is expensive. A trial comparing multiple active treatments to one control group may increase the power of those comparisons by enlarging the control group (as in the Coronary Drug Project trial (15)). In this case there is no clear way to pick the best proportions to use, and disproportionate randomization might complicate the process of obtaining informed consent. Because the advantages are marginal (the effect of even a 2:1 disproportion on power is surprisingly modest (16)), the best decision is usually to assign equal numbers to each group.

Randomization of matched pairs is a strategy for balancing baseline confounding variables that requires selecting pairs of subjects who are matched on important factors like age and sex, then randomly assigning one member of each pair to each study group. A drawback of randomizing matched pairs is that it complicates recruitment and randomization, requiring that an eligible participant wait for randomization until a suitable match has been identified. In addition, matching is generally not necessary in large trials in which random assignment prevents confounding. However, a particularly attractive version of this design can be used when the circumstances permit a contrast of treatment and control effects in two parts of the same individual. In the Diabetic Retinopathy Study, for example, each participant had one eye randomly assigned to photocoagulation treatment while the other served as a control (17).

Blinding

Whenever possible, the investigator should design the interventions in such a fashion that the study participants, staff who have contact with them, persons making laboratory measurements, and those adjudicating outcomes have no knowledge of the study group assignment. When it is not possible to blind all of these individuals, it is

TABLE 10.2	In a Randomized Blinded Trial, Randomization Eliminates Confounding by Baseline Variables and Blinding Eliminates Confounding by Cointerventions
Explanation for Association	**Strategy to Rule Out Rival Explanation**
1. Chance	Same as in observational studies
2. Bias	Same as in observational studies
3. Effect—Cause	(Not a possible explanation in a trial)
4. Confounding → Prerandomization confounding variables	**Randomization**
→ Postrandomization confounding variables (cointerventions)	**Blinding**
5. Cause—Effect	

highly desirable to blind as many as possible (always, for example, blinding laboratory personnel). In a randomized trial, **blinding is as important as randomization**: it prevents bias due to use of cointerventions and biased ascertainment of outcomes.

Randomization only eliminates the influence of confounding variables that are present at the time of randomization; it does not eliminate differences that develop between the groups during follow-up (Table 10.2). In an unblinded study the investigator or study staff may give extra attention or treatment to participants he knows are receiving the active drug, and this "**cointervention**" may be the actual cause of any difference in outcome that is observed between the groups. For example, in an unblinded trial of the effect of exercise to prevent myocardial infarction, the investigator's eagerness to find a benefit might lead him to suggest that participants in the exercise group stop smoking. Cointerventions can also affect the control group if, for example, participants who know that they are receiving placebo seek out other treatments that affect the outcome. Concern by a participant's family or private physician might also lead to effective cointerventions if the study group is not blinded. Cointerventions that are delivered similarly in both groups may decrease the power of the study by decreasing outcome rates, but cointerventions that affect one group more than the other can cause bias in either direction.

The other important value of blinding is to prevent **biased ascertainment and adjudication of outcome.** In an unblinded trial, the investigator may be tempted to look more carefully for outcomes in the untreated group or to diagnose the outcome more frequently. For example, in an unblinded trial of estrogen therapy, the investigators may be more likely to ask women in the active treatment group about pain or swelling in the calf and to order ultrasound or other tests to make the diagnosis of deep vein thrombosis.

After a possible outcome event has been ascertained, it is important that personnel who will adjudicate the outcome are blinded. Results of the Canadian Cooperative Multiple Sclerosis trial nicely illustrate the importance of blinding in unbiased outcome adjudication (18). Persons with multiple sclerosis were randomly assigned to combined plasma exchange, cyclophosphamide and prednisone, or to sham plasma exchange and placebo medications. At the end of the trial, the severity of multiple sclerosis was assessed using a structured examination by neurologists blinded to treatment assignment and again by neurologists who were unblinded. Therapy was not effective based on the assessment of the blinded neurologists, but was statistically significantly effective based on the assessment of the unblinded neurologists.

Blinded assessment of outcome may not be important if the outcome of the trial is a "hard" outcome such as death, about which there is no uncertainty or opportunity for biased assessment. Most other outcomes, such as cause-specific death, disease diagnosis, physical measurements, questionnaire scales, and self-reported conditions, are susceptible to biased ascertainment.

After the study is over, it is a good idea to assess whether the participants and investigators were unblinded by asking them to guess which treatment the participant was assigned to; if a higher than expected proportion guesses correctly, the published discussion of the findings should include an assessment of the potential biases that partial unblinding may have caused.

What to do When Blinding is Difficult or Impossible. In some cases blinding is difficult or impossible, either for technical or ethical reasons. For example, it is difficult to blind participants if they are assigned to an educational, dietary or exercise intervention. However, the control group in such studies might receive a different form of education, diet or exercise of a type and intensity unlikely to be effective. Surgical interventions often cannot be blinded because it may be unethical to perform sham surgery in the control group. However, surgery is always associated with some risk, so it is very important to determine if the procedure is truly effective. For example, a recent randomized trial found that arthroscopic debridement of the cartilage of the knee was no more effective than sham arthroscopy for relieving osteoarthritic knee pain (19). In this case, the risk to participants in the control group may have been outweighed if thousands of patients were prevented from undergoing an ineffective procedure.

If the interventions cannot be blinded, the investigator should limit and standardize other potential cointerventions as much as possible and blind study staff who ascertain and adjudicate the outcomes. For example, an investigator testing the effect of yoga for relief of hot flashes could specify a precise regimen of yoga sessions in the treatment group and general relaxation sessions of equal duration in the control group. To minimize other differences between the groups, he could instruct both yoga and control participants to refrain from starting new recreational, exercise or relaxation activities or other treatments for hot flushes until the trial has ended. Also, study staff who collect information on the severity of hot flushes could be different from those who provide yoga training.

SUMMARY

1. The **choice and dose of intervention** is a difficult decision that balances **effectiveness** and **safety;** other considerations include **relevance** to clinical practice, **simplicity,** suitability for **blinding,** and feasibility of **enrolling subjects.**

2. The best **comparison group** is a **placebo control** that allows participants, investigators and study staff to be **blinded.**

3. **Clinically relevant outcome measures** such as pain, quality of life, occurrence of cancer, and death are the most meaningful outcomes of trials. **Intermediary**

markers, such as HIV viral load, are valid **surrogate markers** for clinical outcomes to the degree that treatment-induced changes in the marker consistently predict changes in the clinical outcome.

4. All clinical trials should include measures of potential **adverse effects** of the intervention.

5. The criteria for **selecting study participants** should identify those who are likely to **benefit and not be harmed** by treatment, easy to recruit, and likely to **adhere to treatment** and **follow-up** protocols. Choosing participants at **high risk** of an uncommon outcome can decrease sample size and cost, but may make recruitment more difficult and decrease generalizability of the findings.

6. **Baseline variables** should be measured parsimoniously to **track** the participants, **describe** their characteristics, **measure risk factors** for and baseline values of the outcome, and enable later examination of disparate intervention effects in various subgroups **(interactions);** serum, genetic material, and so on should be stored for later analysis.

7. **Randomization,** which eliminates bias due to baseline **confounding** variables, should be tamperproof; **matched pair** randomization is an excellent design when feasible, and in small trials **stratified blocked randomization** can reduce chance maldistributions of key predictors.

8. **Blinding** the intervention is **as important as randomization** and serves to control **cointerventions** and biased outcome **ascertainment** and **adjudication.**

◼ REFERENCES

1. Ettinger B, Black DM, Mitlak BH, et al. Reduction of vertebral fracture risk in post-menopausal women with osteoporosis treated with raloxifene: results from a 3-year randomized clinical trial. Multiple Outcomes of Raloxifene Evaluation (MORE) investigators. *JAMA* 1999;282:637–645.
2. The Women's Health Initiative Study Group. Design of the women's health initiative clinical trial and observational study. *Control Clin Trials* 1998;19:61–109.
3. Prentice RL. Surrogate endpoints in clinical trials: definition and operational criteria. *Stat Med* 1989;8:431–440.
4. Cummings SR, Karpf DB, Harris F, et al. Improvement in spine bone density and reduction in risk of vertebral fractures during treatment with antiresorptive drugs. *Am J Med* 2002;112:281–289.
5. Hulley S, Grady D, Bush T, et al. Randomized trial of estrogen plus progestin for secondary prevention of coronary heart disease in postmenopausal women. *JAMA* 1998;280:605–613.
6. Mosca L, Barrett-Connor E, Wenger NK, et al. Design and methods of the Raloxifene Use for The Heart (RUTH) Study. *Am J Cardiol* 2001;88:392–395.
7. Rossouw JE, Anderson GL, Prentice RL, et al. Risks and benefits of estrogen plus progestin in healthy postmenopausal women: principal results from the women's health initiative randomized controlled trial. *JAMA* 2002;288:321–333.
8. Fisher B, Costantins J, Wickerham D, et al. Tamoxifen for prevention of breast cancer: report of the National Surgical Adjuvant Breast and Bowel Project P-1 Study. *JNCI* 1998;90:1371–1388.

9. Fries R, Shariat K, von Wilmowsky H, et al. Sildenafil in the treatment of Raynaud's phenomenon resistant to vasodilatory therapy. *Circulation* 2005;112:2980–2985.
10. Freiman JA, Chalmers TC, Smith H Jr, et al. The importance of beta, the type II error and sample size in the design and interpretation of the randomized control trial. Survey of 71 "negative" trials. *N Engl J Med* 1978;299:690–694.
11. Cummings SR, Black DM, Thompson DE, et al. Effect of alendronate on risk of fracture in women with low bone density but without vertebral fractures: results from the fracture intervention trial. *JAMA* 1998;280:2077–2082.
12. Yusuf S, Collins R, Peto R. Why do we need some large, simple randomized trials? *Stat Med* 1984;3:409–420.
13. Avins AL. Can unequal be more fair? Ethics, subject allocation, and randomised clinical trials. *J Med Ethics* 1998;24:401–408.
14. Prentice RL, Caan B, Chlebowski RT, et al. Low-fat dietary pattern and risk of invasive breast cancer: the women's health initiative randomized controlled dietary modification trial. *JAMA* 2006;295:629–642.
15. CDP Research Group. The coronary drug project. Initial findings leading to modifications of its research protocol. *JAMA* 1970;214:1303–1313.
16. Friedman LM, Furberg C, DeMets DL. *Fundamentals of clinical trials*, 3rd ed. St. Louis, MO: Mosby Year Book, 1996.
17. Diabetic Retinopathy Study Research Group. Preliminary report on effects of photocoagulation therapy. *Am J Ophthalmol* 1976;81:383–396.
18. Noseworthy JH, O'Brien P, Erickson BJ, et al. The Mayo-Clinic Canadian cooperative trial of sulfasalazine in active multiple sclerosis. *Neurology* 1998;51:1342–1352.
19. Moseley JB, O'Malley K, Petersen NJ, et al. A controlled trial of arthroscopic surgery for osteoarthritis of the knee. *N Engl J Med* 2002;347:81–88.

11 Alternative Trial Designs and Implementation Issues

Deborah Grady, Steven R. Cummings, and Stephen B. Hulley

In the last chapter, we discussed the classic randomized, blinded, parallel group trial: how to select the intervention, choose outcomes, select participants, measure baseline variables, randomize, and blind. In this chapter, we describe **alternative clinical trial designs** and address the **conduct of clinical trials,** including **interim monitoring** during the trial.

ALTERNATIVE CLINICAL TRIAL DESIGNS

Other Randomized Designs

There are a number of variations on the classic parallel group randomized trial that may be useful when the circumstances are right.

The **factorial design** aims to answer two (or more) separate research questions in a single cohort of participants (Fig. 11.1). A good example is the Women's Health Study, which was designed to test the effect of low-dose aspirin and vitamin E on risk for cardiovascular events among healthy women (1). The participants were randomly assigned to four groups, and two hypotheses were tested by comparing two halves of the study cohort. First, the rate of cardiovascular events in women on aspirin is compared with women on aspirin placebo (disregarding the fact that half of each of these groups received vitamin E); then the rate of cardiovascular events in those on vitamin E is compared with all those on vitamin E placebo (now disregarding the fact that half of each of these groups received aspirin). The investigators have two complete trials for the price of one.

The factorial design can be very **efficient.** For example, the Women's Health Initiative randomized trial was able to test the effect of three interventions (hormone therapy, low-fat diet and calcium plus vitamin D) on a number of outcomes in one cohort (2). A limitation is the possibility of interactions between the effects of the treatments on the outcomes. For example, if the effect of aspirin on risk for cardiovascular disease is different in women treated with vitamin E compared to those

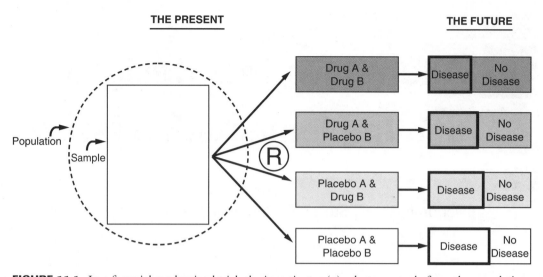

FIGURE 11.1. In a factorial randomized trial, the investigator (a) selects a sample from the population, (b) measures baseline variables, (c) randomly assigns two active interventions and their controls to four groups as shown, (d) applies interventions, (e) measures outcome variables during follow-up, (f) analyzes the results, first combining the two drug A groups to be compared with the two placebo A groups and then combining the two drug B groups to be compared with the two placebo B groups.

not treated with vitamin E, an interaction exists and the effect of aspirin would have to be calculated separately in these two groups. This would reduce the power of these comparisons, because only half of the participants would be included in each analysis. Factorial designs can actually be used to study such interactions, but trials designed to test interactions are more complicated and difficult to implement, larger sample sizes are required, and the results can be hard to interpret. Other limitations of the factorial design are that the same study population must be appropriate for each intervention and multiple treatments may interfere with recruitment and adherence.

Group or cluster randomization requires that the investigator randomly assign naturally occurring groups or clusters of participants to the intervention groups rather than assign individuals. A good example is a trial that enrolled players on 120 college baseball teams, randomly allocated half of the teams to an intervention to encourage cessation of spit-tobacco use, and observed a significantly lower rate of spit-tobacco use among players on the teams that received the intervention compared to control teams (3). Applying the intervention to groups of people may be more feasible and cost effective than treating individuals one at a time, and it may better address research questions about the effects of public health programs in the population. Some interventions, such as a low-fat diet, are difficult to implement in only one member of a family. Similarly, when participants in a natural group are randomized individually, those who receive the intervention are likely to discuss or share the intervention with family members, colleagues or acquaintances who have been assigned to the control group. For example, a clinician in a group practice who is randomly assigned to an educational intervention is very likely to discuss this intervention with his colleagues. In the cluster randomization design, the units of randomization and analysis are groups, not individuals. Therefore, the effective sample size is smaller than the number of individual participants and power is diminished. In fact, the effective sample size depends on the correlation of the effect of the intervention among participants in the clusters and is somewhere between the number of clusters and the number of participants (4). Another drawback is that sample size estimation and data analysis are more complicated in cluster randomization designs than for individual randomization (4).

In **equivalence trials,** an intervention is compared to an active control. Equivalence trials may be necessary when there is a known effective treatment for a condition, or an accepted "standard of care." In this situation, it may be unethical to assign participants to placebo treatment. For example, because bisphosphonates effectively prevent osteoporotic fractures in women at high risk, new drugs should be compared against or added to this standard of care. In general, there should be strong evidence that the active comparison treatment is effective for the types of participants who will be enrolled in the trial.

The objective of equivalence trials is to prove that the new intervention is at least as effective as the established one. It is impossible to prove that two treatments are *exactly* equivalent because the sample size would be infinite. Therefore, the investigator sets out to prove that the difference between the new treatment and the established treatment is no more than a defined amount. If the acceptable difference between the new and the established treatment is small, the sample size for an equivalence trial can be large—much larger than for a placebo-controlled trial. However, there is little clinical reason to test a new therapy if it does not have significant advantages over an established treatment, such as less toxicity or cost, or greater ease of use. Depending on how much advantage the new treatment is judged to have, the allowable difference between the efficacy of the new treatment and the established treatment may be substantial. In this case, the sample size estimate for an equivalence trial may be similar to that for a placebo-controlled trial.

An important problem with equivalence trials is that the traditional roles of the null and alternative hypotheses are reversed. The null hypothesis for equivalence trials is that the effects of the two treatments are not more different than a prespecified amount; the alternative hypothesis is that the difference does exceed this amount. In this case, failure to reject the null hypothesis results in accepting the hypothesis that the two treatments are equal. Inadequate sample size, poor adherence to the study treatments and large loss to follow-up all reduce the power of the study to reject the null hypothesis in favor of the alternative. Therefore, an inferior new treatment may appear to be equivalent to the standard when in reality the findings just represent an underpowered and poorly done study.

Nonrandomized Between-Group Designs

Trials that compare groups that have not been randomized are far less effective than randomized trials in controlling for the influence of confounding variables. Analytic methods can adjust for baseline factors that are unequal in the two study groups, but this strategy does not deal with the problem of unmeasured confounding. When the findings of randomized and nonrandomized studies of the same research question are compared, the apparent benefits of intervention are much greater in the nonrandomized studies, even after adjusting statistically for differences in baseline variables (5). The problem of confounding in nonrandomized clinical studies can be serious and not fully removed by statistical adjustment (6).

Sometimes participants are allocated to study groups by a **pseudorandom** mechanism. For example, every other subject (or every subject with an even hospital record number) may be assigned to the treatment group. Such designs sometimes offer logistic advantages, but the predictability of the study group assignment permits the investigator to tamper with it by manipulating the sequence or eligibility of new subjects.

Participants are sometimes assigned to study groups by the investigator according to certain specific criteria. For example, patients with diabetes may be allocated to receive either insulin four times a day or long-acting insulin once a day according to their willingness to accept four daily injections. The problem with this design is that those willing to take four injections per day might be more compliant with other health advice, and this might be the cause of any observed difference in the outcomes of the two treatment programs.

Nonrandomized designs are sometimes chosen in the mistaken belief that they are more ethical than randomization because they allow the participant or clinician to choose the intervention. In fact, studies are only ethical if they have a reasonable likelihood of producing the correct answer to the research question, and randomized studies are more likely to lead to a conclusive and correct result than nonrandomized designs. Moreover, the ethical basis for any trial is the uncertainty as to whether the intervention will be beneficial or harmful. This uncertainty, termed **equipoise,** means that an evidence-based choice of interventions is not possible and justifies random assignment.

Within-Group Designs

Designs that do not include randomization can be useful options for some types of questions. In a **time-series design,** measurements are made before and after each participant receives the intervention (Fig. 11.2). Therefore, each participant serves as his own control to evaluate the effect of treatment. This means that innate characteristics such as age, sex, and genetic factors are not merely balanced (as they are in between-group studies) but actually eliminated as confounding variables.

The major disadvantage of within-group designs is the lack of a concurrent control group. The apparent efficacy of the intervention might be due to **learning effects** (participants do better on follow-up cognitive function tests because they learned from the baseline test), **regression to the mean** (participants who were selected for the trial because they had high blood pressure at baseline are found to have lower

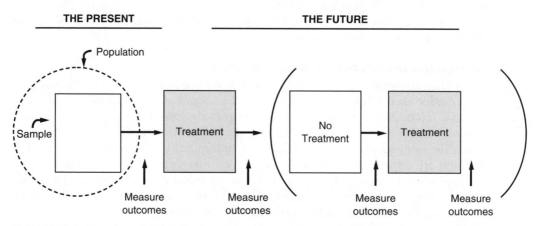

THE PRESENT **THE FUTURE**

FIGURE 11.2. In a time-series trial, the investigator (a) selects a sample from the population, (b) measures baseline and outcome variables, (c) applies the intervention to the whole cohort, (d) follows up the cohort and measures outcome variables again, (e) (optional) removes the intervention and measures outcome variables again, and so on.

blood pressure at follow-up simply due to random variation in blood pressure), or **secular trends** (upper respiratory infections are less frequent at follow-up because the trial started during flu season). Within-group designs sometimes use a strategy of repeatedly starting and stopping the treatment. If repeated onset and offset of the intervention produces similar patterns in the outcome, this provides strong support that these changes are due to the treatment. This approach is only useful when the outcome variable responds rapidly and reversibly to the intervention (e.g., the effect of a statin on LDL-cholesterol level). The design has a clinical application in the so-called "N-of-one" study in which an individual patient can alternate between active and inactive versions of a drug (using identical-appearing placebo prepared by the local pharmacy) to detect his particular response to the treatment (7).

The **crossover design** has features of both within- and between-group designs (Fig. 11.3). Half of the participants are randomly assigned to start with the control period and then switch to active treatment; the other half begin with the active treatment and then switch to control. This approach (or the Latin square for more than two treatment groups) permits between-group, as well as within-group analyses. The advantages of this design are substantial: it minimizes the potential for confounding because each participant serves as his own control and the paired analysis substantially increases the statistical power of the trial so that it needs fewer participants. However, the disadvantages are also substantial: a doubling of the duration of the study, and the added complexity of analysis and interpretation created by the problem of potential **carryover effects.** A carryover effect is the residual influence of the intervention on the outcome during the period after it has been stopped—blood pressure not returning to baseline levels for months after a course of diuretic treatment, for example. To reduce the carryover effect, the investigator can introduce an untreated "**washout**"

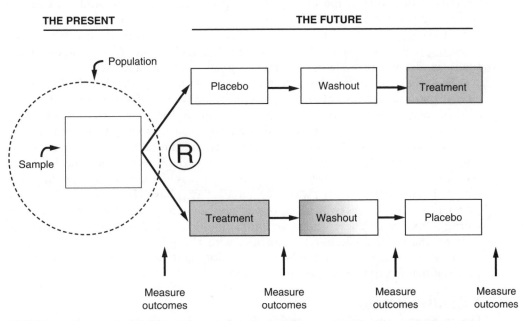

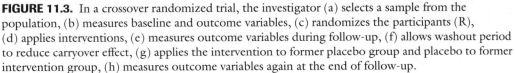

FIGURE 11.3. In a crossover randomized trial, the investigator (a) selects a sample from the population, (b) measures baseline and outcome variables, (c) randomizes the participants (R), (d) applies interventions, (e) measures outcome variables during follow-up, (f) allows washout period to reduce carryover effect, (g) applies the intervention to former placebo group and placebo to former intervention group, (h) measures outcome variables again at the end of follow-up.

period between treatments with the hope that the outcome variable will return to normal before starting the next intervention, but it is difficult to know whether all carryover effects have been eliminated. In general, crossover studies are chiefly a good choice when the number of study subjects is limited and the outcome responds rapidly and reversibly to an intervention.

A variation on the crossover design may be appropriate when participants are randomly assigned to usual care or to a very appealing intervention (such as weight loss, yoga or elective surgery). Participants assigned to usual care may be provided the active intervention at the end of the parallel, two-group period, making enrollment much more attractive. The outcome can be measured at the end of the intervention period in this group, providing within group crossover data on the participants who receive the **delayed intervention**.

Trials for Regulatory Approval of New Interventions

Many trials are done to test the effectiveness and safety of new treatments that might be considered for approval for marketing by the U.S. Food and Drug Administration (FDA) or another international regulatory body. Trials are also done to determine whether drugs that have FDA approval for one condition might be approved for the treatment or prevention of other conditions. The design and conduct of these trials is generally the same as for other trials, but regulatory requirements must be considered.

The FDA publishes general and specific guidelines on how such trials should be conducted (search for "FDA" on the web). It would be wise for investigators and staff conducting trials with the goal of obtaining FDA approval of a new medication or device to seek specific training on these general guidelines, called **"Good Clinical Practice."** In addition, the FDA provides specific guidelines for studies of certain outcomes. For example, studies designed to obtain FDA approval of treatments for hot flashes in menopausal women must currently include participants with at least seven hot flashes per day or 50 per week. FDA guidelines are regularly updated and similar guidelines are available from international regulatory agencies.

Trials for regulatory approval of new treatments are generally described by phase. This system refers to an orderly progression in the testing of a new treatment, from experiments in animals (**preclinical**) and initial unblinded, uncontrolled treatment of a few human volunteers to test safety (**phase I**), to small randomized blinded trials that test the effect of a range of doses on side effects and clinical outcomes (or surrogate outcomes) (**phase II**), to randomized trials large enough to test the hypothesis that the treatment improves the targeted condition (such as blood pressure) or reduces the risk of disease (such as stroke) with acceptable safety (**phase III**) (Table 11.1). **Phase IV** refers to large studies (which may or may not be randomized trials) conducted after a drug is approved. These studies are often conducted (and financed) by marketing departments of pharmaceutical companies with the goals of assessing the rate of serious side effects when used in large populations and identifying additional uses of the drug that might be approved by the FDA.

Pilot Clinical Trials

Designing and conducting a successful clinical trial requires extensive information on the type, dose and duration of the intervention, the likely effect of the intervention on the outcome, potential adverse effects and the feasibility of recruiting, randomizing

TABLE 11.1	Stages in Testing New Therapies
Preclinical	Studies in cell cultures and animals
Phase I	Unblinded, uncontrolled studies in a few volunteers to test safety
Phase II	Relatively small randomized blinded trials to test tolerability and different intensity or dose of the intervention on surrogate or clinical outcomes
Phase III	Relatively large randomized blinded trials to test the effect of the therapy on clinical outcomes
Phase IV	Large trials or observational studies conducted after the therapy has been approved by the FDA to assess the rate of serious side effects and evaluate additional therapeutic uses

and maintaining participants in the trial. Often, the only way to obtain some of this information is to conduct a good pilot study.

Pilot studies vary from a brief test of the feasibility of recruitment to a full-scale pilot in hundreds of participants. Pilot studies should be as carefully planned as the main trial, with clear objectives and methods. Many pilot studies are focused primarily on determining the **feasibility, time required** and **cost** of recruiting adequate numbers of eligible participants, and discovering if they are willing to accept randomization and can comply with the intervention. Pilot studies may also be designed to demonstrate that planned measurements, data collection instruments and data management systems are feasible and efficient. For pilot trials focused primarily on feasibility, a control group is generally not included.

An important goal of many pilot studies is to define the optimal intervention—the frequency, intensity and duration of the intervention that will result in minimal toxicity and maximal effectiveness. Phase I and II studies can be viewed as pilot studies with these goals.

Another important goal of pilot studies is to provide parameters to allow more accurate estimation of sample size. Sound estimates of the rate of the outcome or mean outcome measure in the placebo group, the effect of the intervention on the main outcome (**effect size**), and the statistical **variability** of this outcome are crucial to planning the sample size. In some situations, an estimate of the effect size and its variability can be achieved by delivering the intervention to all pilot subjects. For example, if it is known that a surgical procedure results in a certain volume of blood loss, evaluating the amount of blood loss in a small group of pilot study participants who undergo a new procedure might provide a good estimate of the effect size. However, if there is likely to be a placebo effect, it may be better to randomize pilot participants to receive the new intervention or placebo. For example, to obtain an estimate of the effect of a new treatment for pain related to dental extractions, the fact that pain responds markedly to placebo treatment would result in a biased estimate of effect if no placebo group is included.

Many trials fall short of estimated power not because the effect of the intervention is less than anticipated, but because the rate of outcome events in the placebo group is much lower than expected. This "**screening bias**" likely occurs because persons who fit the enrollment criteria for a clinical trial and agree to be randomized are healthier than the general population with the condition of interest. Therefore, in some trials, it is crucial to determine the rate of the outcome in the placebo group, which can only be done by randomizing participants to placebo in a pilot study.

A pilot study should have a short but complete protocol (approved by the Institutional Review Board), data collection forms and analysis plans. Variables should include the typical baseline measures, predictors and outcomes included in a clinical trial, but also estimates of the number of subjects available or accessible for recruitment, the number who are contacted or respond using different sources or recruitment techniques, the number and proportion eligible for the trial, those who are eligible but refuse (or say they would refuse) randomization, the time and cost of recruitment and randomization, and estimates of adherence to the intervention and other aspects of the protocol, including study visits. It may be very helpful to "debrief" both subjects and staff after the pilot study to obtain their views on how the trial methods could be improved.

A good pilot study requires substantial time and can be costly, but markedly improves the chance of funding for major clinical trials and the likelihood that the trial will be successfully completed.

■ CONDUCTING A CLINICAL TRIAL

Follow-up and Adherence to the Protocol

If a substantial number of study participants do not receive the study intervention, do not adhere to the protocol, or are lost to follow-up, the results of the trial are likely to be underpowered or biased. Strategies for **maximizing follow-up and adherence** are outlined in Table 11.2.

The effect of the intervention (and the power of the trial) is reduced to the degree that participants do not receive it. The investigator should try to choose a study drug or intervention that is easy to apply or take and is well tolerated. Adherence is likely to be poor if a behavioral intervention requires hours of practice by participants. Drugs that can be taken in a single daily dose are the easiest to remember and therefore preferable. The protocol should include provisions that will enhance adherence, such as instructing participants to take the pill at a standard point in the morning routine and giving them pill containers labeled with the day of the week.

There is also a need to consider how best to **measure adherence** to the intervention, using such approaches as self-report, pill counts, pill containers with computer chips that record when the container is opened, and serum or urinary metabolite levels. This information can identify participants who are not complying, so that approaches to improving adherence can be instituted and the investigator can interpret the findings of the study appropriately.

Adherence to study visits and measurements can be enhanced by discussing what is involved in the study before consent is obtained, by scheduling the visits at a time that is convenient and with enough staff to prevent waiting, by calling the participant the day before each visit, and by reimbursing travel expenses and other out-of-pocket costs.

Failure to follow trial participants and measure the outcome of interest can result in biased results, diminished credibility of the findings, and decreased statistical

TABLE 11.2	Maximizing Follow-up and Adherence to the Protocol
Principle	**Example**
Choose subjects who are likely to be adherent to the intervention and protocol	Require completion of two or more comprehensive visits before randomization
	Exclude those who are nonadherent in a prerandomization run-in period
	Exclude those who are likely to move or be noncompliant
Make the intervention easy	Use a single tablet once a day if possible
Make study visits convenient and enjoyable	Schedule visits often enough to maintain close contact but not frequently enough to be tiresome
	Schedule visits at night or on weekends, or collect information by phone or e-mail
	Have adequate and well-organized staff to prevent waiting
	Provide reimbursement for travel
	Establish inter-personal relationships with subjects
Make study measurements painless, useful and interesting	Choose noninvasive, informative tests that are otherwise costly or unavailable
	Provide test results of interest to participants and appropriate counseling or referrals
Encourage subjects to continue in the trial	Never discontinue subjects from follow-up for protocol violations, adverse events, or side effects
	Send participants birthday and holiday cards
	Send newsletters and e-mail messages
	Emphasize the scientific importance of adherence and follow-up
Find subjects who are lost to follow-up	Pursue contacts of subjects
	Use a tracking service

power. For example, a trial of nasal calcitonin spray to reduce the risk of osteoporotic fractures reported that treatment reduced fracture risk by 36% (8). However, about 60% of those randomized were lost to follow-up, and it was not known if fractures had occurred in these participants. Because the overall number of fractures was small, even a few fractures in the participants lost to follow-up could have altered the findings of the trial. This uncertainty diminished the credibility of the study findings (9).

Even if participants violate the protocol or discontinue the trial intervention, they should be followed so that their outcomes can be used in intention-to-treat analyses. In many trials, participants who violate the protocol by enrolling in another trial, missing study visits, or discontinuing the study intervention are discontinued from follow-up; this can result in biased or uninterpretable results. Consider, for example, a drug that causes a symptomatic side effect that results in more frequent discontinuation of the study medication in those on active treatment compared to those on placebo. If participants who discontinue study medication are not continued in follow-up, this can bias the findings if the side effect is associated with the main outcome.

Some strategies for achieving complete **follow-up** are similar to those discussed for cohort studies (Chapter 7). At the outset of the study, participants should be informed of the importance of follow-up and investigators should record the name, address, and telephone number of one or two close acquaintances who will always know where the participant is. In addition to enhancing the investigator's ability to assess vital status, the ability to contact participants by phone or e-mail may give him access to proxy outcome measures from those who refuse to come for a visit at the end. The Heart and Estrogen/Progestin Replacement Study (HERS) trial used all of these strategies: 89% of the women returned for the final clinic visit after an average of 4 years of follow-up, another 8% had a final telephone contact for outcome ascertainment, and information on vital status was determined for every participant by using phone contact, registered letters, contacts with close relatives, and a tracking service (10).

The design of the trial should make it as easy as possible for participants to adhere to the intervention and complete all follow-up visits and measurements. Long and stressful visits can deter some participants from attending. Participants are more likely to return for visits that involve noninvasive tests, such as electron beam computed tomography, than for invasive tests such as coronary angiography. Collecting follow-up information by phone or electronic means may improve adherence for participants who find visits difficult. On the other hand, participants may lose interest in a trial if there are not some social or interpersonal rewards for participation. Participants may tire of study visits that are scheduled monthly, and they may lose interest if visits only occur annually. Follow-up is improved by making the trial experience positive and enjoyable for study participants: designing trial measurements and procedures to be painless and interesting; performing tests that would not otherwise be available; providing results of tests to participants (if the result will not influence outcomes); sending newsletters, e-mail notes of appreciation, holiday, and birthday cards; giving inexpensive gifts; and developing strong interpersonal relationships with an enthusiastic and friendly study staff.

Two design aspects that are specific to trials may improve adherence and follow-up: screening visits before randomization and a run-in period. Asking participants to attend one or two **screening visits** before randomization may exclude participants who find that they cannot complete such visits. The trick here is to set the hurdles for entry into the trial high enough to exclude those who will later be nonadherent, but not high enough to exclude participants who will turn out to have satisfactory adherence.

A **run-in period** may be useful for increasing the proportion of study participants who adhere to the intervention and follow-up procedures (Fig. 11.4). During the baseline period, all participants are placed on placebo. A specified time later (usually a few weeks), only those who have complied with the intervention (e.g., taken at least 80% of the assigned study medication) are randomized. Excluding nonadherent participants before randomization in this fashion may increase the power of the study and permit a better estimate of the full effects of intervention. However, a run-in period delays entry into the trial, the proportion of participants excluded

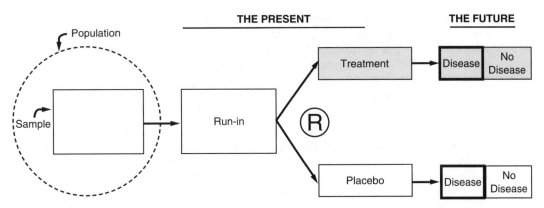

FIGURE 11.4. In a randomized trial preceded by a run-in period to test compliance, the investigator (a) selects a sample from the population, (b) measures baseline variables, (c) conducts the run-in (d) randomizes adherent participants (R), (e) applies interventions, (f) measures outcome variables during follow-up.

is generally small, and participants randomized to the active drug may notice a change in their medication following randomization, contributing to unblinding. It is also not clear that a placebo run-in is more effective in increasing adherence than the requirement that participants complete one or more screening visits before randomization. In the absence of a specific reason to suspect that adherence in the study will be poor, it is probably not necessary to include a run-in period in the trial design.

A variant of the **placebo run-in** design is the use of the active drug rather than the placebo for the run-in period. In addition to increasing adherence among those who enroll, an **active drug run-in** is designed to select participants who tolerate and respond to the intervention. The effect of treatment on an intermediary variable (i.e., a biomarker associated with the outcome) is used as the criterion for randomization. In a trial of the effect of an antiarrhythmic drug on mortality, for example, the investigators randomized only those participants whose arrhythmias were satisfactorily suppressed without undue side effects (11). This design maximized power by increasing the proportion of the intervention group that is responsive to the intervention. It also improved generalizability by mimicking the clinician's tendency to continue using a drug only when he sees evidence that it is working. However, the findings of trials using this strategy may not be generalizable to those excluded.

Using an active run-in may also result in underestimation of the rate of adverse effects. A trial of the effect of carvedilol on mortality in patients with congestive heart failure used a 2-week active run-in period. During the run-in, 17 people had worsening congestive heart failure and 7 died (12). These people were not randomized in the trial, and these adverse effects of drug treatment were not included as outcomes.

Adjudicating Outcomes

Most self-reported outcomes, such as history of stroke or a participant report of quitting smoking, are not 100% accurate. Self-reported outcomes that are important to the trial should be confirmed if possible. Occurrence of disease, such as a stroke, is generally adjudicated by (a) creating clear criteria for the outcome (e.g., a new, persistent neurologic deficit with corresponding lesion on computed tomography or magnetic resonance imaging scan), (b) collecting the clinical documents needed to make the assessment (e.g., discharge summaries and radiology reports), and (c) having experts review each potential case and judge whether the criteria for the diagnosis have been met. The adjudication is often done by two experts working independently, then resolving discordant cases by discussion between the two or with a third expert. Those who collect the information and adjudicate the cases must be blinded to the treatment assignment.

Monitoring Clinical Trials

Investigators must assure that participants not be exposed to a harmful intervention, denied a beneficial intervention, or continued in a trial if the research question is unlikely to be answered.

The most pressing reason to monitor clinical trials is to make sure that the intervention does not turn out unexpectedly to be harmful. If **harm** is judged to be clearly present and to outweigh any benefits, the trial should be stopped. Second, if an intervention is more effective than was estimated when the trial was designed, then **benefit** can be observed early in the trial. When clear benefit has been proved, it may be unethical to continue the trial and delay offering the intervention to participants on placebo and to others who could benefit. Third, if there is a very low probability of answering the research question, it may be unethical to continue participants in a trial that requires time and effort and that may cause some discomfort or risk. If a clinical trial is scheduled to continue for 5 years, for example, but after 4 years there is little difference in the rate of outcome events in the intervention and control groups, then the "conditional power" (the likelihood of answering the research question given the results thus far) becomes very small and consideration should be given to stopping the trial. Sometimes trials are stopped early on, if investigators are unable to recruit or retain enough participants to provide adequate power to answer the research question, or adherence to the intervention is very poor.

The research question might be answered by other trials before a given trial is finished. It is desirable to have more than one trial that provides evidence concerning a given research question, but if definitive evidence becomes available during a trial, the investigator should consider stopping.

Most clinical trials should include an interim monitoring plan. Trials funded by the National Institutes of Health (NIH) generally require interim monitoring, even if the intervention is considered safe (such as a behavioral intervention for weight loss). How interim monitoring will occur should be considered in the planning of any clinical trial. In small trials with interventions likely to be safe, the trial investigators might monitor safety or appoint a single independent data and safety monitor. In large trials and trials in which adverse effects of the intervention are unknown or potentially dangerous, interim monitoring is generally performed by a committee (usually known as the Data and Safety Monitoring Board [DSMB] or Data Monitoring Committee) consisting of experts in the disease or condition under study, biostatisticians, clinical trialists, ethicists and occasionally a representative of the patient group being studied. These experts are not involved in the trial, and should have no personal or financial interest in its continuation. DSMB guidelines and procedures should be detailed in writing before the trial begins. Guidance for developing DSMB procedures is provided by the FDA and the NIH. Items to include in these guidelines are outlined in Table 11.3.

TABLE 11.3	Monitoring a Clinical Trial

Elements to monitor
    Recruitment
    Randomization
    Adherence to intervention, and blinding
    Follow-up completeness
    Important variables
        Outcomes
        Adverse effects
        Potential co-interventions

Who will monitor
    Trial investigator or a single monitor if small trial with minor hazards
    Independent DSMB otherwise

Methods for interim monitoring
    Specify statistical approach and frequency of monitoring in advance
    Importance of judgment and context in addition to statistical stopping rules

Changes in the protocol that can result from monitoring
    Terminate the trial
    Modify the trial
        Stop one arm of the trial
        Add new measurements necessary for safety monitoring
        Discontinue high-risk participants
    Extend the trial in time
    Enlarge the trial sample

Stopping a trial should always be a careful decision that balances ethical responsibility to the participants and the advancement of scientific knowledge. Whenever a trial is stopped early, the chance to provide more conclusive results will be lost. The decision is often complex, and potential risks to participants must be weighed against possible benefits. Statistical tests of significance provide important but not conclusive information for stopping a trial. Trends over time and effects on related outcomes should be evaluated for consistency, and the impact of stopping the study early on the credibility of the findings should be carefully considered (Example 11.1).

There are many statistical methods for monitoring the interim results of a trial. Analyzing the results of a trial repeatedly is a form of multiple hypothesis testing and thereby increases the probability of a type I error. For example, if $\alpha = 0.05$ is used for each interim test and the results of a trial are analyzed four times during the trial and again at the end, the probability of making a type I error is increased from 5% to about 14% (13). To address this problem, statistical methods for interim monitoring generally decrease the α for each test so that the overall α is close to 0.05. There are multiple approaches to deciding how to "spend α" (Appendix 11.1).

Example 11.1 Trials That Have Been Stopped Early

Canadian Atrial Fibrillation Anticoagulation Study (CAFA) (14): *Atrial fibrillation is a risk factor for stroke and embolic events. The CAFA study was a blinded, randomized, placebo-controlled trial to evaluate the efficacy of warfarin in decreasing the rate of stroke, systemic embolism, or intracerebral or fatal bleeding in patients with nonrheumatic atrial fibrillation. The trial was designed to enroll 660 subjects and follow them on therapy for 3.5 years. During the trial (after 383 patients had been randomized and followed for a mean of 1.2 years), the results of two other randomized trials were reported showing a significant decrease in stroke risk and a low rate of major bleeding in those treated with warfarin. The Steering Committee decided that the evidence of benefit with warfarin was sufficiently compelling to stop the trial.*

Cardiac Arrhythmia Suppression Trial (CAST) (11): *The occurrence of ventricular premature depolarizations in survivors of myocardial infarction (MI) is a risk factor for sudden death. The CAST evaluated the effect of antiarrhythmic therapy (encainide, flecainide, or moricizine) in patients with asymptomatic or mildly symptomatic ventricular arrhythmia after MI on risk for sudden death. During an average of 10 months of follow-up, the participants treated with active drug had a higher total mortality (7.7% vs. 3.0%) and a higher rate of death from arrhythmia (4.5% vs. 1.5%) than those assigned to placebo. The trial was planned to continue for 5 years but this large and highly statistically significant difference led to the trial being stopped after 18 months.*

Coronary Drug Project (CDP) (15,16): *The CDP was a randomized, blinded trial to determine if five different cholesterol-lowering interventions (conjugated estrogen 5.0 mg/day; estrogen 2.5 mg/day; clofibrate 1.8 g/day; dextrothyroxine 6.0 mg/day; niacin 3.0 g/day) reduced the 5-year mortality rate. The CDP enrolled 8,341 men with MI who were followed for at least 5 years. With an average of 18 months of follow-up, the high-dose estrogen arm was stopped due to an excess of nonfatal MI (6.2% compared with 3.2%) and venous thromboembolic events (3.5% compared with 1.5%), as well as testicular atrophy, gynecomastia, breast tenderness, and decreased libido. At the same time, dextrothyroxine was stopped in the subgroup of men who had frequent premature ventricular beats on their baseline electrocardiogram because the death rate in this subgroup was 38.5% compared with 11.5% in the same subgroup receiving placebo. Dextrothyroxine therapy was stopped in all subjects shortly thereafter due to an excess mortality rate in the overall treated group. Two years before the planned end of the study, the 2.5-mg-dose estrogen arm was also stopped because there was no evidence of any beneficial effect and an increased risk of venous thromboembolic events.*

Physicians Health Study (17): *The Physicians Health Study was a randomized trial of the effect of aspirin (325 mg every other day) on cardiovascular mortality. The trial was stopped after 4.8 years of the planned 8-year follow-up. There was a statistically significant reduction in risk of MI in the treated group (relative risk for nonfatal MI = 0.56), but the number of cardiovascular disease deaths in each group was equal. The rate of cardiovascular disease deaths observed in the study was far lower than expected (88 after 4.8 years of follow-up vs. 733 expected), and the trial was stopped because of the beneficial effect of aspirin on risk for nonfatal MI coupled with the very low conditional power to detect a favorable impact of aspirin therapy on cardiovascular mortality.*

Adaptive Design

Clinical trials are generally conducted according to a protocol that does not change during the conduct of the study. However, for some types of treatments and conditions, it is possible to monitor results from the trial as it progresses and change the design of the trial based on interim analyses of the results (18). For example, consider a trial of several doses of a new treatment for menopausal hot flashes. The initial design may plan to enroll 40 women to a placebo group and 40 to each of three doses for 12 weeks of treatment over an enrollment period lasting 1 year. Review of the results after the first 10 women in each group have completed the first 4 weeks of treatment might reveal that there is a trend toward an effect only in the highest dose. It may be more efficient to stop assigning participants to the two lower doses and continue randomizing only to the highest dose. In this case, the design of the trial can be adapted to the interim results by changing the design in midstream to use only one dose versus the placebo. Other facets of a trial that could be changed based on interim results include increasing or decreasing the sample size or duration of the trial if interim results indicate that the effect size or rate of outcomes differ from the original assumptions.

These adaptive designs are feasible only for treatments that produce outcomes that are measured and analyzed early enough in the course of the trial that changes can be made in the design. To prevent bias in the ascertainment of outcomes, the interim analyses and consideration of change in design must be done by an independent group such as a DSMB that reviews unblinded data. Furthermore, multiple interim analyses will increase the probability of finding a result that is due to chance variations in the early results from the trial; the increased chance of a 'Type 1' error must be considered in the design and analysis of the results. Adaptive designs are also more complex to conduct and analyze, informed consent must include the range of possible changes in the study design or be repeated, and it is difficult to estimate the cost of an adaptive trial and the specific resources necessary to complete it.

With these precautions and limitations, adaptive designs are efficient and may be valuable, especially during the development of a new treatment, allowing earlier identification of the best dose and duration and ensuring that a high proportion of participants receive the optimal treatment.

Analyzing the Results

Statistical analysis of the primary hypothesis of a clinical trial is generally straightforward. If the outcome is dichotomous, the simplest approach is to compare the proportions in the study groups using a chi-squared test. When the outcome is continuous, a t test may be used, or a nonparametric alternative if the outcome is not normally distributed. In most clinical trials, the duration of follow-up is different for each participant, necessitating the use of survival time methods. More sophisticated statistical models such as Cox proportional hazards analysis can accomplish this and at the same time adjust for chance maldistributions of baseline confounding variables. The technical details of when and how to use these methods are described elsewhere (19).

Two important issues that should be considered in the analysis of clinical trial results are the primacy of the intention-to-treat analytic approach and the ancillary role for subgroup analyses. The investigator must decide what to do with nonadherence or **"cross-overs,"** participants assigned to the active treatment group who do not get treatment or discontinue it and those assigned to the control group who end up getting active treatment. An analysis done by **intention-to-treat** compares outcomes between the study groups with every participant analyzed according to his randomized group assignment, regardless of whether he adhered to the assigned intervention. Intention-to-treat analyses may underestimate the full effect of the treatment, but they guard against the more important problem of biased results.

An alternative to the intention-to-treat approach is to analyze only those who comply with the intervention. It is common, for example, to perform "**per protocol**" analyses that include only participants who were fully adherent to the protocol. This is defined in various ways, but often includes only participants in both groups who were adherent to the assigned study medication, completed a certain proportion of visits or measurements and had no other protocol violations. A subset of the per protocol analysis is an "**as-treated**" analysis in which only participants who were adherent to the intervention are included. These analyses *seem* reasonable because participants can only be affected by an intervention they actually receive. The problem arises, however, that participants who adhere to the study treatment and protocol may be different from those who drop out in ways that are related to the outcome. In the Postmenopausal Estrogen-Progestin Interventions Trial (PEPI), 875 postmenopausal women were randomly assigned to four different estrogen or estrogen plus progestin regimens and placebo (20). Among women assigned to the unopposed estrogen arm, 30% had discontinued treatment after 3 years because of endometrial hyperplasia, which is a precursor of endometrial cancer. If these women are eliminated in a per protocol analysis, the association of estrogen therapy and endometrial cancer will be missed.

The major disadvantage of the intention-to-treat approach is that participants who choose not to take the assigned intervention will, nevertheless, be included in the estimate of the effects of that intervention. Therefore, substantial discontinuation or crossover between treatments will cause intention-to-treat analyses to underestimate the magnitude of the effect of treatment. For this reason, results of trials are often evaluated with both intention-to-treat and per protocol analyses. For example, in the Women's Health Initiative randomized trial of the effect of estrogen plus progestin treatment on breast cancer risk, the hazard ratio was 1.24 ($P = 0.003$) from the intention-to-treat analysis and 1.49 in the as-treated analysis ($P < 0.001$) (21). If the results of intention-to-treat and per protocol analyses differ, the intention-to-treat results generally predominate for estimates of efficacy because they preserve the value of randomization and, unlike per protocol analyses, can only bias the estimated effect in the conservative direction (favoring the null hypothesis). However, for estimates of harm (e.g., the breast cancer findings noted above), as-treated or per protocol analyses provide the most conservative estimates, as interventions can only be expected to cause harm in exposed persons. Results can only be analyzed both by intention-to-treat and per protocol if follow-up measures are completed regardless of whether participants adhere to treatment, which should always be a goal.

Subgroup analyses are defined as comparisons between randomized groups in a subset of the trial cohort. These analyses have a mixed reputation because they are easy to misuse and can lead to wrong conclusions. With proper care, however, they can provide useful ancillary information and expand the inferences that can be drawn from a clinical trial. To preserve the value of randomization, subgroups should be defined by measurements that were made before randomization. For example, a trial of alendronate to prevent osteoporotic fractures found that the drug decreased risk of fracture by 14% among women with low bone density. Preplanned analyses by subgroups of bone density measured at baseline revealed that the treatment was effective (36% reduction in fracture risk; $P < 0.01$) among women whose bone density was more than 2.5 standard deviations below normal. In contrast, treatment was ineffective in women with higher bone density at baseline ($P = 0.02$ for the interaction) (22). It is important to note that the value of randomization is preserved: the fracture rate among women randomized to alendronate is compared with the rate among women randomized to placebo in each subgroup.

Subgroup analyses are prone, however, to producing misleading results for several reasons. Subgroups are, by definition, smaller than the entire trial population, and there may not be sufficient power to find important differences; investigators should avoid claiming that a drug "was ineffective" in a subgroup when the finding might reflect insufficient power to find an effect. Investigators often examine results in a large number of subgroups, increasing the likelihood of finding a different effect of the intervention in one subgroup by chance. For example, if 20 subgroups are examined, differences in one subgroup at $P < 0.05$ would be expected by chance. Optimally, planned subgroup analyses should be defined before the trial begins and the number of subgroups analyzed should be reported with the results of the study. A conservative approach is to require that claims about different responses in subgroups be supported by statistical evidence that there is an interaction between the effect of treatment and the subgroup characteristic, as in the alendronate trial noted above; if several subgroups are examined, a significance level of 0.01 should be used.

Subgroup analyses based on postrandomization factors do not preserve the value of randomization and often produce misleading results. Per protocol analyses limited to subjects who adhere to the randomized treatment are examples of this type of postrandomization subgroup analysis.

SUMMARY

1. There are several variations on the randomized trial design that can substantially increase efficiency under the right circumstances:
   a. The **factorial design** allows two independent trials to be carried out for the price of one.
   b. **Cluster randomization** permits efficient studies of naturally occurring groups.
   c. **Equivalence trials** compare a new intervention to an existing "standard of care;" this design may be the most ethical and clinically meaningful, but often requires a larger sample size than placebo-controlled trials.
   d. **Time-series designs** have a single (nonrandomized) group with outcomes compared within each subject during periods on and off the intervention.
   e. **Crossover designs** combine randomized and time-series designs to enhance control over confounding and minimize the required sample size if carryover effects are not a problem.

2. If a substantial number of study participants **do not adhere** to the study intervention or are **lost to follow-up,** the results of the trial are likely to be underpowered, biased, or uninterpretable.

3. An important difference between clinical trials and observational studies is that in a clinical trial, *something is being done to the participants.* During a trial, **interim monitoring** by an independent **DSMB,** is needed to assure that participants are not exposed to a harmful intervention, denied a beneficial intervention, or continued in a trial if the research question is unlikely to be answered.

4. **Intention-to-treat** analysis takes advantage of the control of confounding provided by randomization and should be the primary analysis approach. **Per protocol** analyses, a secondary approach that provides an estimate of the effect size in adherent subjects, should be interpreted with caution.

5. With proper care, **subgroup analyses** can expand the inferences that can be drawn from a clinical trial. To preserve the value of randomization, analyses should compare outcomes between subsets of randomly assigned study groups classified by **prerandomization** variables. To minimize misinterpretations, the investigator should specify the subgroups in advance, test **interactions** for statistical significance, and report the number of subgroups examined.

APPENDIX 11.1

Interim Monitoring of Trial Outcomes

Interim monitoring of trial results is a form of multiple testing, and thereby increases the probability of a type I error. To address this problem, α for each test (α_i) is generally decreased so that the overall α approximately $= 0.05$. There are multiple statistical methods for decreasing α_i.

One of the easiest to understand is the Bonferroni method, where $\alpha_i = \alpha/N$ if N is the total number of tests performed. For example, if the overall α is 0.05 and five tests will be performed, α_i for each test is 0.01. This method has several disadvantages, however. It requires using an equal threshold for stopping the trial at any interim analysis and results in a very low α for the final analysis. Most investigators would rather use a lower threshold for stopping a trial earlier rather than later in the trial and use an α close to 0.05 for the final analysis. In addition, this approach is too conservative because it assumes that each test is independent. Interim analyses are not independent, because each successive analysis is based on cumulative data, some of which were included in prior analyses. For these reasons, Bonferroni is not generally used.

A commonly used method suggested by O'Brien and Fleming (23) uses a very small initial α_i, then gradually increases it such that α_i for the final test is close to the overall α. O'Brien–Fleming provide methods for calculating α_i if the investigator chooses the number of tests to be done and the overall α. At each test, $Z_i = Z^*(N_i)^{1/2}$, where $Z_i = Z$ value for the ith test; Z^* is determined so as to achieve the overall significance level; N is the total number of tests planned and i is the ith test. For example, for five tests and overall $\alpha = 0.05$, $Z^* = 2.04$; the initial $\alpha = 0.00001$ and the final $\alpha_5 = 0.046$. This method is unlikely to lead to stopping a trial very early unless there is a striking difference in outcome between randomized groups. In addition, this method avoids the awkward situation of getting to the end of a trial and accepting the null hypothesis although the P value is substantially less than 0.05.

A major drawback to the preceding methods is that the number of tests and the proportion of data to be tested must be decided before the trial starts. In some trials, additional interim tests become necessary when important trends occur. DeMets and Lan (24) developed a method using a specified α-spending function that provides continuous stopping boundaries. The α_i at a particular time (or after a certain proportion of outcomes) is determined by the function and by the number of previous "looks." Using this method, neither the number of "looks" nor the proportion of data to be analyzed at each "look" must be specified before the trial. Of course, for each additional unplanned interim analysis conducted, the final overall α is a little smaller.

A different set of statistical methods based on curtailed sampling techniques suggests termination of a trial if future data are unlikely to change the conclusion. The multiple testing problem is irrelevant because the decision is based only on estimation of what the data will show at the end of the trial. A common approach is to compute the conditional probability of rejecting the null hypothesis at the end of the trial, based on the accumulated data. A range of conditional power is typically calculated, first assuming that H_0 is true (i.e., that any future outcomes in the treated and control groups will be equally distributed) and second assuming that H_a is true (i.e., that outcomes will be distributed unequally in the treatment and control groups as specified by H_a). Other estimates can also be used to provide a full range of reasonable effect sizes. If the conditional power to reject the null hypothesis across the range of assumptions is low, the null hypothesis is not likely to be rejected and the trial might be stopped.

REFERENCES

1. Ridker PM, Cook NR, Lee I, et al. A randomized trial of low-dose aspirin in the primary prevention of cardiovascular disease in women. *N Engl J Med* 2005;352:1293–1304.
2. The Women's Health Initiative Study Group. Design of the women's health initiative clinical trial and observational study. *Control Clin Trials* 1998;19:61–109.
3. Walsh M, Hilton J, Masouredis C, et al. Smokeless tobacco cessation intervention for college athletes: results after 1 year. *Am J Public Health* 1999;89:228–234.
4. Donner A, Birkett N, Buck C. Randomization by cluster: sample size requirements and analysis. *Am J Epidemiol* 1981;114:906–914.
5. Chalmers T, Celano P, Sacks H, et al. Bias in treatment assignment in controlled clinical trials. *N Engl J Med* 1983;309:1358–1361.
6. Pocock S. Current issues in the design and interpretation of clinical trials. *Br Med J* 1985;296:39–42.
7. Nickles CJ, Mitchall GK, Delmar CB et al. An n-of-1 trial service in clinical practice: testing the effectiveness of stimulants for attention-deficit/hyperactivity disorder. *Pediatrics* 2006;117:2040–2046.
8. Chestnut CH III, Silverman S, Andriano K, et al. A randomized trial of nasal spray salmon calcitonin in postmenopausal women with established osteoporosis: the prevent recurrence of osteoporotic fractures study. *Am J Med* 2000;109:267–276.
9. Cummings SR, Chapurlat R. What PROOF proves about calcitonin and clinical trials. *Am J Med* 2000;109:330–331.
10. Hulley S, Grady D, Bush T, et al. Randomized trial of estrogen plus progestin for secondary prevention of coronary heart disease in postmenopausal women. *JAMA* 1998;280:605–613.
11. Cardiac Arrhythmia Suppression Trial (CAST) Investigators. Preliminary report: effect of encainide and flecainide on mortality in a randomized trial of arrhythmia suppression after myocardial infarction. *N Engl J Med* 1989;321:406–412.
12. Pfeffer M, Stevenson L. Beta-adrenergic blockers and survival in heart failure. *N Engl J Med* 1996;334:1396–1397.
13. Armitage P, McPherson C, Rowe B. Repeated significance tests on accumulating data. *J R Stat Soc* 1969;132A:235–244.
14. Laupacis A, Connolly SJ, Gent M, et al. How should results from completed studies influence ongoing clinical trials? The CAFA Study experience. *Ann Intern Med* 1991;115:818–822.

15. Coronary Drug Project Research Group. The Coronary Drug Project. Initial findings leading to modifications of its research protocol. *JAMA* 1970;214:1303–1313.
16. Coronary Drug Project Research Group. The Coronary Drug Project. Findings leading to discontinuation of the 2.5-mg day estrogen group. *JAMA* 1973;226:652–657.
17. PHS Investigations. Findings from the aspirin component of the ongoing Physicians' Health Study. *N Engl J Med* 1988;318:262–264.
18. Chang M, Chow S, Pong A. Adaptive design in clinical research: issues, opportunities, and recommendations. *J Biopharm Stat* 2006;16:299–309.
19. Friedman LM, Furberg C, DeMets DL. *Fundamentals of clinical trials*, 3rd edn. St. Louis, MO: Mosby Year Book, 1996.
20. Writing Group for the PEPI Trial. Effects of estrogen or estrogen/progestin regimens on heart disease risk factors in postmenopausal women. *JAMA* 1995;273:199–208.
21. Chlebowski RT, Hendrix SL, Langer RD, et al. Influence of estrogen plus progestin on breast cancer and mammography in healthy postmenopausal women. The Women's Health Initiative Randomized Trial. *JAMA* 2003;289:3243–3253.
22. Cummings SR, Black D, Thompson D, et al. Effect of alendronate on risk of fracture in women with low bone density but without vertebral fractures: results from the fracture intervention trial. *JAMA* 1998;280:2077–2082.
23. O'Brien P, Fleming T. A multiple testing procedure for clinical trials. *Biometrics* 1979;35:549–556.
24. DeMets D, Lan G. The alpha spending function approach to interim data analyses. *Cancer Treat Res* 1995;75:1–27.

12 Designing Studies of Medical Tests

Thomas B. Newman, Warren S. Browner, Steven R. Cummings, and Stephen B. Hulley

Medical tests, such as those performed to screen for a risk factor, diagnose a disease, or estimate a patient's prognosis, are an important topic for clinical research. The study designs discussed in this chapter can be used when **studying whether, and in whom, a particular test should be done**.

Although clinical trials of medical tests are occasionally feasible and sometimes necessary, most designs for studies of medical tests are descriptive and resemble the observational designs in Chapters 7 and 8. There are, however, some important differences. The goal of most observational studies is to identify causal relationships (e.g., *whether estrogen use causes breast cancer*). Causality is generally irrelevant in studies of diagnostic tests. In addition, knowing that a test result is more closely associated with a condition or outcome than would be expected by chance alone is not nearly enough to determine its clinical usefulness. Instead, parameters that describe the performance of a medical test, such as **sensitivity, specificity**, and **likelihood ratios** are commonly estimated, with their associated confidence intervals. In this chapter we review studies of medical tests focusing not just on studies of test performance, but also on determining whether or under what circumstances a test is **clinically useful**.

DETERMINING WHETHER A TEST IS USEFUL

For a test to be useful it must pass muster on a series of increasingly difficult questions that address its **reproducibility, accuracy, feasibility**, and **effects on clinical decisions** and **outcomes** (Table 12.1). Favorable answers to each of these questions are necessary but insufficient criteria for a test to be worth doing. For example, if a test does not give consistent results when performed by different people or in different places, it can hardly be useful. If the test seldom supplies new information and hence seldom affects clinical decisions, it may not be worth doing. Even if it affects decisions, if these decisions do not improve the clinical outcome of patients who were tested, the test still may not be useful.

| TABLE 12.1 | Questions to Determine Usefulness of a Medical Test, Possible Designs to Answer Them, and Statistics for Reporting Results |

Question	Possible Designs	Statistics for Results*
How reproducible is the test?	Studies of intra- and interobserver and laboratory variability	Proportion agreement, kappa, coefficient of variation, mean and distribution of differences (avoid correlation coefficient)
How accurate is the test?	Cross-sectional, case–control, or cohort-type designs in which a test result is compared with a gold standard	Sensitivity, specificity, positive and negative predictive value, receiver operating characteristic curves, and likelihood ratios
How often do test results affect clinical decisions?	Diagnostic yield studies, studies of pre- and posttest clinical decision making	Proportion abnormal, proportion with discordant results, proportion of tests leading to changes in clinical decisions; cost per abnormal result or per decision change
What are the costs, risks, and acceptability of the test?	Prospective or retrospective studies	Mean costs, proportions experiencing adverse effects, proportions willing to undergo the test
Does doing the test improve clinical outcome or have adverse effects?	Randomized trials, cohort or case–control studies in which the predictor variable is receiving the test and the outcome includes morbidity, mortality, or costs related either to the disease or to its treatment	Risk ratios, odds ratios, hazard ratios, number needed to treat, rates and ratios of desirable and undesirable outcomes

* Most statistics in this table should be presented with confidence intervals.

Of course, if using a test improves outcome, favorable answers to the other questions can be inferred. However, demonstrating that doing a test improves outcome is impractical for most diagnostic tests. Instead, the potential effects of a test on clinical outcomes are usually assessed indirectly, by demonstrating that the test increases the likelihood of making the correct diagnosis or is safer or less costly than existing tests. When developing a new diagnostic or prognostic test, it may be worthwhile to consider what aspects of current practice are most in need of improvement. Are current tests unreliable, expensive, dangerous, or difficult to perform?

General Issues for Studies of Medical Tests

- *Gold standard for diagnosis.* Some diseases have a gold standard, such as the results of a tissue biopsy, that is generally accepted to indicate the presence (or absence) of that disease. Other diseases have "definitional" gold standards, such as defining coronary artery disease as a 50% obstruction of at least one major coronary artery as seen with coronary angiography. Still others, such as rheumatologic diseases, require that a patient have a minimum number of signs, symptoms, or specific laboratory abnormalities to meet the criteria for having the disease. Of course the accuracy of any signs, symptoms, or laboratory tests used to diagnose a disease cannot be studied if those same signs and symptoms are used as part of the gold standard for the diagnosis. Furthermore, if the gold standard is imperfect it can make a test either look worse than it really is (if in reality the test outperforms the gold standard), or better than it really is (if the gold standard is an imperfect measure of the condition of interest and the test has the same deficiencies).

- *Spectrum of disease severity and of test results.* Because the goal of most studies of medical tests is to draw inferences about populations by making measurements on samples, the way the sample is selected has a major effect on the validity of the inferences. **Spectrum bias** occurs when the spectrum of disease (or nondisease) in the sample differs from that in the population to which the investigator wishes to generalize. This can occur if the sample of subjects with disease is sicker, or the subjects without the disease are healthier, than those to whom the test will be applied in practice. Almost any test will perform well if the task is to distinguish between the very sick and the healthy, such as those with symptomatic pancreatic cancer and healthy controls. It is more difficult to distinguish between one disease and another that can cause similar symptoms, or between the healthy and those with early, presymptomatic disease. The subjects in a study of a diagnostic test should have spectra of disease and nondisease that resemble those of the population in which the test will be used. For example, a diagnostic test for pancreatic cancer might be studied in patients with abdominal pain and weight loss.

    Spectrum bias can occur from an inappropriate spectrum of test results as well as an inappropriate spectrum of disease. For example, consider a study of interobserver agreement among radiologists reading mammograms. If they are asked to classify the films as normal or abnormal, their agreement will be much higher if the "positive" films they examine are a set selected because they are clearly abnormal, and the "negative" films are a set selected as free of suspicious abnormalities.

- *Sources of variation, generalizability, and the sampling scheme.* For some research questions the main source of variation in test results is between patients. For example, some infants with bacteremia will have an elevated white blood cell count, whereas others will not. The proportion of bacteremic infants with high white blood cell counts is not expected to vary much according to who draws the blood or what laboratory measures it.

    On the other hand, for many tests the results may depend on the person doing or interpreting them, or the setting in which they are done. For example, sensitivity, specificity, and interrater reliability for interpreting mammograms depend on the readers' skill and experience as well as the quality of the equipment. Sampling those who perform and interpret the test can enhance the generalizability of studies of tests that require technical or interpretive skill. When accuracy may vary from institution to institution, the investigators will need to sample several different institutions to be able to assess the generalizability of the results.

- *Importance of blinding.* Many studies of diagnostic tests involve judgments, such as whether to consider a test result positive, or whether a person has a particular disease. Whenever possible, investigators should blind those interpreting test results from information about the patient being tested that is related to the gold standard. In a study of the contribution of ultrasonography to the diagnosis of appendicitis, for example, those reading the sonograms should not know the results of the history and physical examination. Similarly, the pathologists making the final determination of who does and does not have appendicitis (the gold standard to which sonogram results will be compared) should not know the results of the ultrasound examination. Blinding prevents biases, preconceptions, and information from sources other than the test from affecting these judgments.

- *Costs versus charges*. Investigators wishing to focus on test expense may be tempted to report charges rather than costs because charges are more readily available and are generally much higher than costs. However, test charges vary greatly among institutions and may have little relation to what is actually paid for the test or to its actual costs. In many cases, test charges resemble the rack rate on the inside door of a hotel room—a charge much higher than most customers actually pay. On the other hand, estimating how much an institution or society must spend per test is difficult, because many of the expenses, such as laboratory space and equipment, are fixed. One approach is to use the average amount actually paid for the test; another is to multiply charges by the institution's average cost-to-charge ratio.

STUDIES OF TEST REPRODUCIBILITY

Sometimes the results of tests vary according to when or where they were done or who did them. **Intraobserver variability** describes the lack of reproducibility in results when the same observer or laboratory performs the test at different times. For example, if a radiologist is shown the same chest radiograph on two occasions, what proportion of the time will he agree with himself on the interpretation? **Interobserver variability** describes the lack of reproducibility among two or more observers: if another radiologist is shown the same film, how likely is he to agree with the first radiologist?

Studies of reproducibility may be done when the level of reproducibility (or lack thereof) is the main research question. In addition, reproducibility is often studied with a goal of quality improvement, either for those making measurements as part of a research study of a different question, or as a part of clinical care. When reproducibility is poor—because either intra- or interobserver variability is large—a measurement is unlikely to be useful, and it may need to be either improved or abandoned.

Studies of reproducibility do not require a gold standard, so they can be done for tests or diseases where none exists. Of course, both (or all) observers can agree with one another and still be wrong: intra- and interobserver reproducibility address precision, not accuracy (Chapter 4).

Designs
The basic design to assess test reproducibility involves comparing tests done to results from more than one observer or on more than one occasion from a sample of patients or specimens. For tests that involve several steps in many locations, differences in any one of which might affect reproducibility, the investigator will need to decide on the breadth of the study's focus. For example, measuring interobserver agreement of pathologists about the interpretation of a set of cervical cytology slides in a single hospital may overestimate the overall reproducibility of Pap smears because the variability in how the sample was obtained and how the slide was prepared would not be assessed.

The extent to which an investigator needs to isolate the steps that might lead to interobserver disagreement depends partly on the goals of his study. Most studies should estimate the reproducibility of the entire testing process, because this is what determines whether the test is worth using. On the other hand, an investigator who is developing or improving a test may want to focus on the specific steps at which variability occurs, to improve the process. In either case, the investigator should lay out the exact process for obtaining the test result in the operations manual (Chapters 4 and 17) and then describe it in the methods section when reporting the study results.

Analysis

- *Categorical variables*. The simplest measure of interobserver agreement is the proportion of observations on which the observers agree exactly, sometimes called the **concordance rate**. However, when there are more than two categories or the observations are not evenly distributed among the categories (e.g., when the proportion "abnormal" on a dichotomous test is much different from 50%), the concordance rate can be hard to interpret, because it does not account for agreement that could result simply from both observers having some knowledge about the prevalence of abnormality. For example, if 95% of subjects are normal, two observers who randomly choose which 5% of tests to call "abnormal" will agree that results are "normal" about 90% of the time. A better measure of interobserver agreement, called **kappa** (Appendix 12A), measures the extent of agreement beyond what would be expected by chance alone. Kappa ranges from -1 (perfect disagreement) to 1 (perfect agreement). A kappa of 0 indicates that the amount of agreement was exactly that expected by chance. Kappa values above 0.8 are generally considered very good; levels of 0.6 to 0.8 are good.

- *Continuous variables*. Measures of interobserver variability for continuous variables depend on the design of the study. Some studies measure the agreement between just two machines or methods (e.g., temperatures obtained from two different thermometers). The best way to describe the data from such a study is to report the mean difference between the paired measurements and the distribution of the differences, perhaps indicating the proportion of time that the difference is clinically important. For example, if a clinically important difference in temperature is thought to be 0.3°C, a study comparing temperatures from tympanic and rectal thermometers could estimate the mean difference between the two and how often the two measurements differed by more than 0.3°C.[1]

   Other studies examine interobserver or interinstrument variability of a large group of different technicians, laboratories, or machines. These results are commonly summarized using the **coefficient of variation**, which is the standard deviation of the results on a single specimen divided by their mean, expressed as a percentage. If the results are normally distributed (i.e., if a histogram with results on the same specimen would be bell shaped), then about 95% of the results on different machines will be within two standard deviations of the mean. For example, given a coefficient of variation of a serum cholesterol measurement of 2% (2), the standard deviation of multiple measurements with a mean of 200 mg/dL would be about 4 mg/dL and about 95% of laboratories would be expected to report a value between 192 and 208 mg/dL.

---

[1] Although commonly used, the correlation coefficient is best avoided in studies of the reliability of laboratory tests because it is highly influenced by outlying values and does not allow readers to determine how frequently differences between the two measurements are clinically important. Confidence intervals for the mean difference should also be avoided because their dependence on sample size makes them potentially misleading. A narrow confidence interval for the mean difference between the two measurements does not imply that they generally closely agree—only that the mean difference between them is being measured precisely. For more extensive reading on this issue, see Bland and Altman (1).

STUDIES OF THE ACCURACY OF TESTS

Studies in this section address the question, "To what extent does the test give the right answer?" To be able to answer this question, a gold standard must be available in order to tell what the right answer is.

Designs

- *Sampling*. Studies of diagnostic tests can have designs analogous to case–control or cross-sectional studies, whereas studies of prognostic tests usually resemble cohort studies. In the case–control design, those with and without the disease are sampled separately and the test results in the two groups are compared. Unfortunately, it is often hard to reproduce a clinically realistic spectrum of the disease and absence of the disease in the two samples. Those with the disease should not have progressed to severe stages that are relatively easy to diagnose. Those without the target disease should be patients who had symptoms consistent with a particular disease and who turned out not to have it. Studies of tests that sample those with and without the target disease separately are also subject to a bias in the measurement of the test result if that measurement is made knowing whether the sample came from a case or control. Finally, studies with this sampling scheme cannot be used (without other information) to estimate **predictive value** or **posterior probability** (discussed below). Therefore, "case–control" sampling for diagnostic tests should be reserved for rare diseases for which no other sampling scheme is feasible.

  A single **cross-sectional** sample of patients being evaluated for a particular diagnosis generally will yield more valid and interpretable results. For example, Tokuda et al. (3) found that the severity of chills was a strong predictor of bacteremia in a series of 526 consecutive febrile adult emergency department patients. Because the subjects were enrolled before it was known whether they were bacteremic, the spectrum of patients in this study should be reasonably representative of patients who present to emergency rooms with fever.

  A variant of the cross-sectional sampling scheme that we call **tandem testing** is sometimes used to compare two (presumably imperfect) tests with one another. Both tests are done on a representative sample of patients who may or may not have the disease and the gold standard is selectively applied to the patients with positive results on either or both tests. Because subjects with negative results may be false-negatives, the gold standard should also be applied to a random sample of patients with concordant negative results. This design, which allows the investigator to determine which test is more accurate without the expense of measuring a gold standard in all the subjects with negative test results, has been used in studies comparing different cervical cytology methods (4).

  Prognostic test studies require either prospective or retrospective **cohort designs**. In prospective cohort studies, the test is done at baseline, and the subjects are then followed to see who develops the outcome of interest. A retrospective cohort study may be possible if a new test becomes available, such as viral load in HIV-positive patients, and a previously defined cohort with banked blood samples is available. Then the viral load can be measured in the stored blood, to see whether it predicts prognosis. The nested case–control design (Chapter 7) is particularly attractive if the outcome of interest is rare and the test is expensive.

- *Predictor variable: the test result*. Although it is simplest to think of the results of a diagnostic test as being either positive or negative, many tests have categorical, ordinal or continuous results. Whenever possible, investigators should use ordinal or continuous results to take advantage of all available information in the test. Most tests are more indicative of a disease if they are very abnormal than if they are slightly abnormal, and most also have a borderline range in which they do not provide much information.

- *Outcome variable: the disease (or its outcome)*. The outcome variable in a diagnostic test study is often the presence or absence of the disease, best determined with a gold standard. Wherever possible, the assessment of outcome should not be influenced by the results of the diagnostic test being studied. This is best accomplished by blinding those measuring the gold standard so that they do not know the results of the test. Sometimes uniform application of the gold standard is not ethical or feasible for studies of diagnostic tests, particularly screening tests. For example, Smith-Bindman et al. studied the accuracy of mammography according to characteristics of the interpreting radiologist (5). Women with positive mammograms were referred for further tests, eventually with pathologic evaluation as the gold standard. However, it is not reasonable to do biopsies in women whose mammograms are negative. Therefore, to determine whether these women had falsely negative mammograms the authors linked their mammography results with local tumor registries and used whether or not breast cancer was diagnosed in the year following mammography as the gold standard. This solution, although reasonable, assumes that all breast cancers that exist at the time of mammography will be diagnosed within 1 year, and that all cancers diagnosed within 1 year existed at the time of the mammogram. Measuring the gold standard differently depending on the result of the test in this fashion creates a potential for bias, discussed in more detail at the end of the chapter. **Prognostic tests** are studied in patients who already have the disease. The outcome is what happens to them, such as how long they live, what complications they develop, or what additional treatments they require. Again, blinding is important, especially if clinicians caring for the patients may make decisions based upon the prognostic factors being studied. For example, Rocker et al. (6) found that the attending physicians' estimates of prognosis, but not those of bedside nurses, were independently associated with intensive care unit mortality. This could be because the attending physicians were more skilled at estimating severity of illness, but it could also be because attending physician prognostic estimates had a greater effect than those of the nurses on decisions to withdraw support. To distinguish between these possibilities, it would be helpful to obtain estimates of prognosis from attending physicians other than those involved in making or framing decisions about withdrawal of support.

Analysis

- *Sensitivity, specificity, and positive and negative predictive values*. When results of a dichotomous test are compared with a dichotomous gold standard, the results can be summarized in a 2 × 2 table (Table 12.2). The sensitivity is defined as the proportion of subjects with the disease in whom the test gives the right answer (i.e., is positive), whereas the specificity is the proportion of subjects without the disease in whom the test gives the right answer (i.e., is negative). Positive and negative predictive values are the proportions of subjects with positive and negative tests in whom the test gives the right answer.
- *Receiver operating characteristic curves*. Many diagnostic tests yield ordinal or continuous results. With such tests, several values of sensitivity and specificity are

TABLE 12.2   Summarizing Results of a Study of a Dichotomous Tests in a 2 × 2 Table

		Gold Standard				
		Disease	No Disease	Total		
Test	Positive	a True-positive	b False-positive	a + b		Positive predictive value* a/(a + b)
	Negative	c False-negative	d True-negative	c + d		Negative predictive value* d/(c + d)
	Total	a + c	b + d			
		Sensitivity a/(a + c)	Specificity d/(b + d)			

* Positive and negative predictive values can be calculated from a 2×2 table like this only when the prevalence of disease is (a + c)/(a + b + c + d). This will not be the case if subjects with and without disease are sampled separately (e.g., 100 of each).

possible, depending on the cutoff point chosen to define a positive test. This trade-off between sensitivity and specificity can be displayed using a graphic technique originally developed in electronics: receiver operating characteristic (ROC) curves. The investigator selects several cutoff points and determines the sensitivity and specificity at each point. He then graphs the sensitivity (or true-positive rate) on the Y-axis as a function of $1-$ specificity (the false-positive rate) on the X-axis. An ideal test is one that reaches the upper left corner of the graph (100% true-positives and no false-positives). A worthless test follows the diagonal from the lower left to the upper right corners: at any cutoff the true-positive rate is the same as the false-positive rate (Fig. 12.1). The area under the ROC curve, which thus ranges from 0.5 for a useless test to 1.0 for a perfect test, is a useful summary of the overall accuracy of a test and can be used to compare the accuracy of two or more tests.

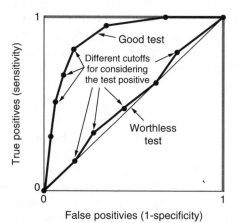

FIGURE 12.1. Receiver operating characteristic curves for good and worthless tests.

- *Likelihood ratios.* Although the information in a diagnostic test with continuous or ordinal results can be summarized using sensitivity and specificity or ROC curves, there is a better way. Likelihood ratios allow the investigator to take advantage of all information in a test. For each test result, the likelihood ratio is the ratio of the likelihood of that result in someone with the disease to the likelihood of that result in someone without the disease.[2]

$$\text{Likelihood ratio} = \frac{P(\text{Result}|\text{Disease})}{P(\text{Result}|\text{No Disease})}$$

The P is read as "probability of" and the "|" is read as "given." Thus $P(\text{Result}|\text{Disease})$ is the probability of result given disease, and $P(\text{Result}|\text{No Disease})$ is the probability of that result given no disease. The likelihood ratio is a ratio of these two probabilities.

The higher the likelihood ratio, the better the test result for ruling in a diagnosis; a likelihood ratio greater than 100 is very high (and very unusual among tests). On the other hand, the lower a likelihood ratio (the closer it is to 0), the better the test result is for ruling out the disease. A likelihood ratio of 1 means that the test result provides no information at all about the likelihood of disease.

An example of how to calculate likelihood ratios is shown in Table 12.3, which presents results from the Pediatric Research in Office Settings Febrile Infant study (10) on how well the white blood cell count predicted bacteremia or bacterial meningitis in young, febrile infants. A white blood cell count that is either less than 5,000 cells/mm^3 or at least 15,000 cells/mm^3 was more common among infants with bacteremia or meningitis than among other infants. The calculation of likelihood ratios simply quantifies this: 8% of the infants with bacteremia or bacterial meningitis had less than 5,000 cells/mm^3, whereas only 4% of those without bacteremia or meningitis did. Therefore the likelihood ratio is 8%/4% = 2.

- *Relative risks and risk differences.* The analysis of studies of prognostic tests or risk factors for disease is similar to that of other cohort studies. If everyone in a prognostic test study is followed for a set period of time (say 3 years) with few losses to follow-up, then the results can be summarized with absolute risks, relative risks and risk differences. Especially when follow-up is complete and of short duration, results of prognostic tests are sometimes summarized like diagnostic tests, using sensitivity, specificity, predictive value, likelihood ratios and ROC curves. On the other hand, when the study subjects are followed for varying lengths of

[2]For dichotomous tests the likelihood ratio for a positive test is

$$\frac{\text{sensitivity}}{(1 - \text{specificity})}$$

and the likelihood ratio for a negative test is

$$\frac{(1 - \text{sensitivity})}{\text{specificity}}.$$

Detailed discussions of how to use likelihood ratios and prior information (the prior probability of disease) to estimate a patient's probability of disease after knowing the test result (the posterior probability) are available in standard clinical epidemiology texts (7–9). The formula is

$$\text{Prior odds} \times \text{Likelihood Ratio} = \text{Posterior odds},$$

where prior and posterior odds are related to their respective probabilities by

$$\text{odds} = \frac{P}{1 - P}.$$

TABLE 12.3	Example of Calculation of Likelihood Ratios from a Study of Predictors of Bacterial Meningitis or Bacteremia Among Young Febrile Infants

White Blood Cell Count (per mm^3)	Meningitis or Bacteremia		Likelihood Ratio
	Yes	No	
<5,000	5	96	
	8%	4%	2.0
5,000–9,999	18	854	
	29%	39%	0.7
10,000–14,999	8	790	
	12%	36%	0.3
15,000–19,999	17	286	
	27%	13%	2.1
≥20,000	15	151	
	24%	7%	3.4
Total	63	2,177	
	100%	100%	

time, a survival-analysis technique that accounts for the length of follow-up time is preferable (11).

STUDIES OF THE EFFECT OF TEST RESULTS ON CLINICAL DECISIONS

A test may be accurate, but if the disease is very rare, the test may be so seldom positive that it is not worth doing in most situations. Another diagnostic test may be positive more often but not affect clinical decisions because it does not provide new information beyond what was already known from the medical history, physical examination, or other tests. The study designs in this section address the yield of diagnostic tests and their effects on clinical decisions.

Types of Studies
- *Diagnostic yield studies*. Diagnostic yield studies address such questions as the following:
  - When a test is ordered for a particular indication, how often is it abnormal?
  - Can a test result be predicted from other information available at the time of testing?
  - What happens to patients with abnormal results? Do they appear to benefit?
  Diagnostic yield studies estimate the proportion of positive tests among patients with a particular indication for the test. Of course, showing that a test is often positive is not sufficient to indicate the test should be done. However, a diagnostic yield study showing a test is almost always negative may be sufficient to question its use for that indication,

For example, Siegel et al. (12) studied the yield of stool cultures in hospitalized patients with diarrhea. Although not all patients with diarrhea receive stool cultures, it seems reasonable to assume that those who do are, if anything, more likely to have a positive culture than those who do not. Overall, only 40 (2%) of 1,964 stool cultures were positive. Moreover, none of the positive results were in the 997 patients who had been in the hospital for more than 3 days. Because a negative stool culture is unlikely to affect management in these patients with a low likelihood of bacterial diarrhea, it is of little value in that setting. Therefore, the authors were able to conclude that stool cultures are unlikely to be useful in patients with diarrhea who have been in the hospital for more than 3 days.

- *Before/after studies of clinical decision making*. These designs directly address the effect of a test result on clinical decisions. The design generally involves a comparison between what clinicians do (or say they would do) before and after obtaining results of a diagnostic test. For example, Carrico et al. (13) prospectively studied the value of abdominal ultrasound in 94 children with acute lower abdominal pain. They asked the clinicians requesting the sonograms to record their diagnostic impression and what their treatment would be if a sonogram were not available. After doing the sonograms and providing the clinicians with the results, they asked again. They found that sonographic information changed the initial treatment plan in 46% of patients.

Of course (as discussed later), altering a clinical decision does not guarantee that a patient will benefit. Therefore, if a study with this design shows effects on decisions, it is most useful when the natural history of the disease and the efficacy of treatment are clear. In the preceding example, there is very likely a benefit from changing the decision from "discharge from hospital" to "laparotomy" in children with appendicitis, or from "laparotomy" to "observe" in children with nonspecific abdominal pain.

STUDIES OF FEASIBILITY, COSTS, AND RISKS OF TESTS

An important area for clinical research relates to the practicalities of diagnostic testing. What proportion of patients will return a postcard with tuberculosis skin test results? What proportion of colonoscopies are complicated by hypotension? What are the medical and psychological effects of false-positive screening tests in newborns?

Design Issues

Studies of the feasibility, costs, and risks of tests are generally descriptive. The sampling scheme is important because tests often vary among the people or institutions doing them, as well as the patients receiving them.

Among studies that sample individual patients, several sampling schemes are possible. A straightforward choice is to study everyone who receives the test, as in a study of the return rate of postcards after tuberculosis skin testing. Alternatively, for some questions, the subjects in the study may be only those with results that were positive or falsely positive. For example, Bodegard et al. (14) studied families of infants who had tested falsely positive on a newborn screening test for hypothyroidism and found that fears about the baby's health persisted for at least 6 months in almost 20% of the families.

Adverse effects can occur not just from false-positive results, but also from tests in which the measurement may be correct but a patient's reaction leads to a decrement in quality of life. Rubin and Cummings (15), for example, studied women who had undergone bone densitometry to test for osteoporosis. They found that women who had been told that their bone density was abnormal were much more likely to limit their activities because of fear of falling.

Analysis

Results of these studies can usually be summarized with simple descriptive statistics like means and standard deviations, medians, ranges, and frequency distributions. Dichotomous variables, such as the occurrence of adverse effects, can be summarized with proportions and their 95% CIs. For example, Waye et al. (16) reported that 3 of 2,097 ambulatory colonoscopies (0.14%; 95% CI, 0.030% to 0.042%) resulted in hypotension that required intravenous fluids.

There are generally no sharp lines that divide tests into those that are or are not feasible, or those that have or do not have an unacceptably high risk of adverse effects. For this reason it is helpful in the design stage of the study to specify criteria for deciding that the test is acceptable. What rate of follow-up would be insufficient? What rate of complications would be too high?

STUDIES OF THE EFFECT OF TESTING ON OUTCOMES

The best way to determine the value of a medical test is to see whether patients who are tested have a better outcome (e.g., live longer) than those who are not. Randomized trials are the ideal design for making this determination, but trials of diagnostic tests are often difficult to do. The value of tests is therefore usually estimated from observational studies. The key difference between the designs described in this section and the experimental and observational designs discussed elsewhere in this book is that the predictor variable for this section is *testing*, rather than a treatment, risk factor, or test result.

Designs

Testing itself is unlikely to have any direct benefit on the patient's health. It is only when a test result leads directly to the use of effective preventive or therapeutic interventions that the patient may benefit. Therefore, one important caveat about outcome studies of testing is that the predictor variable actually being studied is not just a test (e.g., a fecal occult blood test), but everything that follows (e.g., procedures for following up abnormal results, colonoscopy, etc.).

The outcome variable of these studies must be a measure of morbidity or mortality, not simply a diagnosis or stage of disease. For example, showing that men who are screened for prostate cancer have a greater proportion of cancers diagnosed at an early stage does not by itself establish the value of screening. It is possible that some of those cancers would not have caused any problem if they had not been detected or that treatment of the detected cancers is ineffective.

The outcome should be broad enough to include plausible adverse effects of testing and treatment, and may include psychological as well as medical effects of testing. Therefore, a study of the value of prostate-specific antigen screening for prostate cancer should include treatment-related morbidity (e.g., impotence or incontinence, perioperative myocardial infarction) and mortality. When many more people are tested than are expected to benefit (as is usually the case), less severe adverse outcomes among those without the disease may be important, because they will occur much more frequently. While negative test results may be reassuring and relieving to some patients, in others the psychological effects of labeling or false-positive results, loss of insurance, and troublesome (but nonfatal) side effects of preventive medications may outweigh infrequent benefits.

- *Observational studies*. Observational studies are generally quicker, easier, and less costly than experimental studies. However, they have important disadvantages as well, especially because patients who are tested tend to differ from those who are not tested in important ways that may be related to the risk of a disease or its prognosis. For example, those getting the test may be at *lower* risk of an adverse health outcome, because people who volunteer for medical tests and treatments tend to be healthier than average, an example of **volunteer bias**. On the other hand, those tested may be at *higher* risk, because patients are more likely to be tested when they or their clinicians are concerned about a disease or its sequelae, an example of **confounding by indication** for the test (Chapter 9).

    An additional common problem with observational studies of testing is the lack of standardization and documentation of any interventions or changes in management that follow positive results. If a test does not improve outcome in a particular setting, it could be because follow-up of abnormal results was poor, because patients were not compliant with the planned intervention, or because the particular intervention used in the study was not ideal.

Example 12.1 An Elegant Observational Study of a Screening Test

Selby et al. (17) did a nested case–control study in the Kaiser Permanente Medical Care Program to determine whether screening sigmoidoscopy reduces the risk of death from colon cancer. They compared the rates of previous sigmoidoscopy among patients who had died of colon cancer with controls who had not. They found an adjusted odds ratio of 0.41 (95% CI, 0.25 to 0.69), suggesting that sigmoidoscopy resulted in a 60% decrease in the death rate from cancer of the rectum and distal colon.

A potential problem is that patients who undergo sigmoidoscopy may differ in important ways from those who do not, and that those differences might be associated with a difference in the expected death rate from colon cancer. To address this possible confounding, Selby et al. examined the apparent efficacy of sigmoidoscopy at preventing death from cancers of the proximal colon, above the reach of the sigmoidoscope. If patients who underwent sigmoidoscopy were less likely to die of colon cancer for other reasons, then sigmoidoscopy would appear to be protective against these cancers as well. However, sigmoidoscopy had no effect on mortality from cancer of the proximal colon (adjusted odds ratio = 0.96; 95% CI, 0.61 to 1.50), suggesting that confounding was not the reason for the apparent benefit in distal colon cancer mortality.

- *Clinical trials*. The most rigorous design for assessing the benefit of a diagnostic test is a clinical trial, in which subjects are randomly assigned to receive or not to receive the test. Presumably the result of the test is then used to guide clinical management. A variety of outcomes can be measured and compared in the two groups. Randomized trials minimize or eliminate confounding and selection bias and allow measurement of all relevant outcomes such as mortality, morbidity, cost, and satisfaction. Standardizing the testing and intervention process enables others to reproduce the results.

Unfortunately, randomized trials of diagnostic tests are often not practical, especially for diagnostic tests already in use in the care of sick patients. Randomized trials are generally more feasible and important for tests that might be used in large numbers of apparently healthy people, such as new screening tests.

Randomized trials, however, may bring up ethical issues about withholding potentially valuable tests. Rather than randomly assigning subjects to undergo a test or not, one approach to minimizing this ethical concern is to randomly assign some subjects to receive an intervention that increases the use of the test, such as frequent postcard reminders and assistance in scheduling. The primary analysis must still follow the "intention-to-treat" rule—that is, the entire group that was randomized to receive the intervention must be compared with the entire comparison group. However, this rule will tend to create a conservative bias; the observed efficacy of the intervention will underestimate the actual efficacy of the test, because some subjects in the control group will get the test and some subjects in the intervention group will not. This problem can be addressed in secondary analyses that assume all the difference between the two groups is due to different rates of testing. The actual benefits of testing in the subjects as a result of the intervention can then be estimated algebraically (18).

Analysis

Analysis of studies of the effect of testing on outcome are those appropriate to the specific design used—odds ratios for case–control studies, and risk ratios or hazard ratios for cohort studies or experiments. A convenient way to express the results is to project the results of the testing procedure to a large cohort (e.g., 100,000), listing the number of initial tests, follow-up tests, people treated, side effects of treatment, costs, and lives saved.

■ PITFALLS IN THE DESIGN OR ANALYSIS OF DIAGNOSTIC TEST STUDIES

As with other types of clinical research, errors in the design or analysis of studies of diagnostic tests are common. Some of the most common and serious of these, along with steps to avoid them, are outlined below.

Verification Bias 1: Selective Application of a Single Gold Standard

A common sampling strategy for studies of medical tests is to study (either prospectively or retrospectively) patients at risk for disease who receive the gold standard for diagnosis. However, this causes a problem if the findings being studied are also used to decide who gets the gold standard. For example, consider a study of predictors of fracture in children presenting to the emergency department with ankle injuries, in which only children who had x-rays for ankle injuries were included. If those without a particular finding, for example, ankle swelling, were less likely to get an x-ray, both false-negatives and true-negatives (c and d in the 2×2 table in Table 12.4) would be reduced, thereby increasing sensitivity ($a/(a + c)$) and decreasing specificity ($d/(d + b)$), as shown in Table 12.4. This bias, called **verification bias, work-up bias**, or **referral bias**, is illustrated numerically in Appendix 12B.

TABLE 12.4	How Verification Bias Leads to Overestimation of Sensitivity and Underestimation of Specificity, by Decreasing the Number of Subjects in the Study with No Swelling, and Hence Both Cells c and d

	Fracture	**No Fracture**
Swelling	a	b
No swelling	c ↓	d ↓

This type of verification bias can be avoided by using strict criteria for application of the gold standard that do not include the test being studied. Another strategy is to use a different gold standard for those in whom the usual gold standard is not indicated. However, this can cause other problems as discussed below.

Verification Bias 2: Different Gold Standards for Those Testing Positive and Negative

A different type of verification bias, which might be called **double gold standard bias**, occurs when different gold standards are used for those with positive and negative test results. An example is the previously mentioned study of mammography (5) in which the gold standard for those with positive mammograms was a biopsy, whereas for those with negative mammograms it was a period of follow-up to see if a cancer became evident. Having two different gold standards for the disease is a problem if the gold standards might not agree with one another.

Another example is a study of ultrasonography to diagnose intussusception in young children (19). All children with a positive ultrasound scan for intussusception received the gold standard, a contrast enema. In contrast, the majority of children with a negative ultrasound were observed in the emergency room and intussusception was ruled out clinically. For cases of intussusception that resolve spontaneously, the two gold standards would give different results: the contrast enema would be positive, and clinical follow-up would be negative. If these cases have a negative ultrasound, the double gold standard can turn what would appear to be a false-negative result (when the ultrasound is negative and the contrast enema is positive) into a true negative (when the ultrasound is negative and clinical follow-up reveals no intussusception). This increases both sensitivity and specificity (Table 12.5). A numerical example of this double gold standard type of verification bias is provided in Appendix 12.C.

Because sometimes using an invasive gold standard for everyone is not feasible, investigators considering a study with two gold standards should make every effort to use other data sources (e.g., autopsy studies examining the prevalence of asymptomatic cancers among patients who died from other causes in a study of a cancer screening test) to assess the degree to which double gold standard bias might threaten the validity of the study.

TABLE 12.5	How Using Clinical Follow-up as the Gold Standard for Children with a Negative Ultrasound Moves Self-resolving Cases of Intussusception From Cell c to Cell d and Changes False-Negatives into True-Negatives	
	Intussusception	No Intussusception
Ultrasound +	a	b
Ultrasound −	c ———————→ d	

Inadequate Sample Size

A basic principle is that if there are plenty of instances of what the investigator is trying to measure, the sample size is likely to be adequate. However, if the disease or outcome being tested for is rare, this may require testing a very large number of people. Many laboratory tests, for example, are not expensive, and a yield of 1% or less might justify doing them, especially if they can diagnose a serious treatable illness. Therefore, to conclude that a test is not useful, the upper confidence interval for the yield should be low enough to exclude a clinically significant yield.

For example, Sheline and Kehr (20) retrospectively reviewed routine admission laboratory tests, including the Venereal Disease Research Laboratory (VDRL) test for syphilis among 252 psychiatric patients and found that the laboratory tests identified 1 patient with previously unsuspected syphilis. If this patient's psychiatric symptoms were indeed due to syphilis, it would be hard to argue that it was not worth the $3,186 spent on VDRLs to make this diagnosis. But if the true rate of unsuspected syphilis were close to the 0.4% seen in this study, a study of this sample size could easily have found no cases. In that situation, the upper limit of the 95% CI would have been 1.2%. This confidence limit would not be low enough to exclude a clinically significant yield of the VDRL in such psychiatric patients.

Inappropriate Exclusion

When calculating proportions, such as the proportion of subjects with a positive test result in a diagnostic yield study, excluding subjects from the numerator without excluding similar subjects from the denominator is a common error. The basic rule is that if any subjects who test positive are excluded from the numerator, similar subjects must also be excluded from the denominator. In a study of routine laboratory tests in emergency department patients with new seizures (21), for example, 11 of 136 patients (8%) had a correctable laboratory abnormality (hypoglycemia, hypocalcemia, etc.) as a sole or contributory cause for their seizure. In 9 of the 11 patients, however, the abnormality was suspected on the basis of the history or physical examination. The authors therefore reported that only 2 of 136 patients (1.5%) had abnormalities not suspected on the basis of the history or physical examination. But if all patients with suspected abnormalities are excluded from the numerator, then similar patients must be excluded from the denominator as well. The correct denominator for this proportion is therefore not all 136 patients tested, but only those who were not suspected of having any laboratory abnormalities on the basis of their medical history or physical examination.

Institution-Specific Results

Generalizability is especially important for tests that require skill or training to do or interpret. For example, just because pathologists in a particular institution cannot agree on what constitutes an abnormal Pap smear does not mean that pathologists elsewhere would have the same problem. In some cases, investigators are motivated to study questions that seem particularly problematic in their own institution. The results obtained may be internally valid but of little interest elsewhere.

Nongeneralizable findings can also occur in institutions that do exceptionally well. For example, it is possible that the value of abdominal ultrasonography in children with belly pain reported by Carrico et al. (13) is greater than would be found elsewhere, because of the particular skill of their ultrasonographers.

Dropping Borderline or Uninterpretable Results

Sometimes a test may fail to give any answer at all, such as if the assay failed, the test specimen deteriorated, or the test result fell into a gray zone of being neither positive nor negative. It is not usually legitimate to ignore these problems, but how to handle them depends on the specific research question and study design. In studies dealing with the expense or inconvenience of tests, failed attempts to do the test are clearly important results. On the other hand, for most other studies of diagnostic tests, instances of failure of the test to provide a result should be divided into those that likely are and are not related to characteristics of the patient. Thus patients whose specimens were lost or in whom the assays failed for reasons unrelated to the patient can generally be excluded without distorting results.

Patients with "nondiagnostic" imaging studies or a borderline result on a test need to be counted as having had that specific result on the test. In effect, this may change a dichotomous test to an ordinal one—positive, negative, and indeterminate. ROC curves can then be drawn and likelihood ratios can be calculated for the "indeterminate" as well as positive and negative results.

SUMMARY

1. The usefulness of **medical tests** can be assessed using designs that address a series of increasingly stringent questions (Table 12.1). For the most part, standard **observational designs** provide **descriptive statistics** of test characteristics with confidence intervals.

2. The **subjects** for a study of a diagnostic test should be chosen from patients who have a **spectrum** of disease and nondisease that reflects the anticipated use of the test in clinical practice.

3. If possible, the investigator should **blind** those interpreting the test results from other information about the patients being tested.

4. Measuring the **reproducibility** of a test, including the **intra-** and **interobserver variability**, is often a good first step in evaluating a test.

5. Studies of the **accuracy of tests** require a **gold standard** for determining if a patient has, or does not have, the disease or outcome being studied.

6. The results of studies of the accuracy of diagnostic tests can be summarized using **sensitivity, specificity, predictive value, ROC curves**, and **likelihood ratios**. Studies of the value of prognostic tests can be summarized with **risk ratios** or **hazard ratios**.

7. Because of the difficulty of demonstrating that doing a test improves outcome, studies of the effects of tests on **clinical decisions** and the **accuracy, feasibility, costs,** and **risks** of tests are often most useful when they suggest a test should not be done.

8. The most rigorous way to study a diagnostic test is to do a **clinical trial**, in which subjects are randomly assigned to receive or not to receive the test, and outcomes, such as mortality, morbidity, cost, and satisfaction, are compared. However, there may be practical and ethical impediments to such trials; with appropriate attention to possible biases and confounding, **observational studies** of these questions can be helpful.

◼ APPENDIX 12A

Calculation of Kappa to Measure Interobserver Agreement

When there are two observers or when the same observer repeats a measurement on two occasions, the agreement can be summarized in a "c by c" table, where c is the number of categories that the measurement can have. For example, consider two observers listening for an S4 gallop on cardiac examination (Table 12A.1). They record it as either present or absent. The simplest measure of interobserver agreement is the concordance rate—that is, the proportion of observations on which the two observers agree. The concordance rate can be obtained by summing the numbers along the diagonal from the upper left to the lower right and dividing it by the total number of observations. In this example, out of 100 patients there were 10 patients in whom both observers heard a gallop, and 75 in whom neither did, for a concordance rate of $(10 + 75)/100 = 85\%$.

When the observations are not evenly distributed among the categories (e.g., when the proportion "abnormal" on a dichotomous test is substantially different from 50%), the concordance rate can be misleading. For example, if the two observers each hear a gallop on five patients but do not agree on which patients have the gallop, their observed agreement will still be 90% (Table 12A.2). In fact, if two observers

TABLE 12A.1	Interobserver Agreement on Presence of an S4 Gallop		
	Gallop Heard by Observer 1	**No Gallop Heard by Observer 1**	**Total, Observer 2**
Gallop heard by observer 2	10	5	15
No gallop heard by observer 2	10	75	85
Total, observer 1	20	80	100

Note: The concordance rate is the percentage of the time two observers agree with one another. In this example, both observers either heard or did not hear the gallop in $(10 + 75)/100 = 85\%$ of cases.

TABLE 12A.2	High Agreement When Both Observers Know Gallops are Uncommon		
	Gallop Heard by Observer 1	**No Gallop Heard by Observer 1**	**Total, Observer 2**
Gallop heard by observer 2	0	5	5
No gallop heard by observer 2	5	90	95
Total, observer 1	5	95	100

Note: When both observers know that an abnormality is uncommon, they will have a high concordance rate, even if they do not agree on which subjects are abnormal. In this case the observers agree 90% of the time, although they do not agree at all on who has a gallop.

both know an abnormality is uncommon, they can have nearly perfect agreement just by never or rarely saying that it is present.

To get around this problem, another measure of interobserver agreement, called *kappa* (κ), is sometimes used. Kappa measures the extent of agreement beyond what would be expected from knowing the "*marginal values*" (i.e., the row and column totals). Kappa ranges from -1 (perfect disagreement) to 1 (perfect agreement). A kappa of 0 indicates that the amount of agreement was exactly that expected by chance. κ is estimated as:

$$\frac{\text{Observed agreement (\%)} - \text{Expected agreement (\%)}}{100\% - \text{Expected agreement (\%)}}$$

The "expected" proportion in each cell is simply the proportion in that cell's row (i.e., the row total divided by the sample size) times the proportion in that cell's column (i.e., the column total divided by the sample size). The expected agreement is obtained by adding the expected proportions in the cells along the diagonal of the table, in which the observers agreed.

For example, in Table 12A.1, the observers appear to have done quite well: they have agreed 85% of the time. But how well did they do compared with agreement by chance? By chance alone they will agree about 71% of the time: (20% $\times$ 15%) + (80% $\times$ 85%) = 71%. Because the observed agreement was 85%, kappa is (85% $-$ 71%)/(100% $-$ 71%) = 0.48—respectable, if somewhat less impressive than 85% agreement. But now consider Table 12A.2. Although the observed agreement was 90%, the expected agreement is (5% $\times$ 5%) + (95% $\times$ 95%) = 90.5%. Therefore, kappa is (90% $-$ 90.5%)/(100% $-$ 90.5%) = -0.05%—a tiny bit worse than chance alone.

When there are more than two categories of variables, it is important to distinguish between ordinal variables, which are intrinsically ordered, and nominal variables, which are not. For ordinal variables, kappa fails to capture all the information in the data, because it does not give partial credit for coming close. For example, if a radiograph can be classified as "normal," "questionable," and "abnormal," having one observer call it normal and the other call it questionable is better agreement than if one says it is normal and the other says it is abnormal. To give credit for partial agreement, a weighted kappa[3] should be used.

[3] The formula for weighted kappa is the same as that for regular kappa except that observed and expected agreement are summed not just along the diagonal, but for the whole table, with each cell first multiplied by a weight for that cell. Any weighting system can be used, but the most common are $w_{ij} = 1 - |i - j|/(c - 1)$ and $w_{ij} = 1 - [(i - j)/(c - 1)]^2$ where w_{ij} is the weight for the number in i^{th} row and the jth column and c is the number of categories.

APPENDIX 12B

Numerical Example of Verification Bias: 1

Consider two studies examining ankle swelling as a predictor of fractures in children with ankle injuries. The first study is a **consecutive sample** of 200 children. In this study, all children with ankle injuries are x-rayed, regardless of swelling. The sensitivity and specificity of ankle swelling are 80% and 75%, as shown in Table 12B.1:

TABLE 12B.1	Ankle Swelling as a Predictor of Fracture Using a Consecutive Sample	
	Fracture	**No Fracture**
Swelling	32	40
No swelling	8	120
Total	40	160

Sensitivity = 32/40 =80%

Specificity = 120/160 =75%

The second study is a **selected** sample, in which only half the children without ankle swelling are x-rayed. Therefore, the numbers in the "No swelling" row will be reduced by half. This raises the apparent sensitivity from 32/40 (80%) to 32/36 (89%) and lowers the apparent specificity from 120/160 (75%) to 60/100 (60%), as shown in Table 12B.2:

TABLE 12B.2	Verification Bias: Ankle Swelling as a Predictor of Fracture Using a Selected Sample	
	Fracture	**No Fracture**
Swelling	32	40
No swelling	4	60
Total	36	100

Sensitivity = 32/36 =89%

Specificity = 60/100 =60%

Note: If we knew that the children with no swelling who received an x-ray were otherwise similar to those who did not receive an x-ray, we could estimate the verification bias and correct for it algebraically. In practice, the children who receive an x-ray are probably more likely to have a fracture than those who do not, so the effect of verification bias on sensitivity in the example above is likely a worst-case scenario. (That is, if the clinicians were good at predicting who did not have a fracture, all those not x-rayed would not have had any fractures, and the sensitivity of the test would not have been biased upwards. Specificity, however, would still be underestimated.)

APPENDIX 12C

Numerical Example of Verification Bias: 2

Results of the study by Eshed et al. (19) of ultrasonography to diagnose intussusception are shown in Table 12C.1:

TABLE 12C.1	Results of a Study of Ultrasound Diagnosis of Intussusception	
	Intussusception	**No Intussusception**
Ultrasound +	37	7
Ultrasound −	3	104
Total	40	111

Sensitivity = 37/40 =93%

Specificity = 104/111 =94%

The 104 subjects with a negative ultrasound listed as having "No Intussusception" actually included 86 who were followed clinically and did not receive a contrast enema. If about 10% of these subjects (i.e., nine children) actually had an intussusception that resolved spontaneously, but that would still have been identified if they had a contrast enema, and all subjects had received a contrast enema, those nine children would have changed from true-negatives to false-negatives, as shown in Table 12C.2:

TABLE 12C.2	Effect on Sensitivity and Specificity if Nine Children with Spontaneously Resolving Intussusception had Received the Contrast Enema Gold Standard Instead of Clinical Follow-up	
	Intussusception	**No Intussusception**
Ultrasound +	37	7
Ultrasound −	3 + 9 = 12	104 − 9 = 95
Total	49	102

Sensitivity = 37/49 =76%

Specificity = 95/102 =93%

Now consider the 37 subjects with positive ultrasound scans, who had intussusception based on their contrast enema. Suppose about 10% of those intussusceptions would have resolved spontaneously, if given the chance. Then about four children would change from true-positives to false-positives, is shown in Table 12C.3:

TABLE 12C.3	Effect on Sensitivity and Specificity if Four Children with Spontaneously Resolving Intussusception had Received the Clinical Follow-up Gold Standard Instead of the Contrast Enema

	Intussusception	No Intussusception
Ultrasound +	$37 - 4 = 33$	$7 + 4 = 11$
Ultrasound −	3	104
Total	36	115

Sensitivity = 33/36 =92%

Specificity = 104/115 =90%

Therefore, for spontaneously resolving cases of intussusception, the ultrasound scan will appear to give the right answer whether it is positive or negative, increasing both sensitivity and specificity.

REFERENCES

1. Bland J, Altman D. Statistical methods for assessing agreement between two methods of clinical measurement. *Lancet* 1986;1: 307–310.
2. Watson JE, Evans RW, Germanowski J, et al. Quality of lipid and lipoprotein measurements in community laboratories. *Arch Pathol Lab Med* 1997;121(2): 105–109.
3. Tokuda Y, Miyasato H, Stein GH, et al. The degree of chills for risk of bacteremia in acute febrile illness. *Am J Med* 2005;118(12): 1417.
4. Sawaya GF, Washington AE. Cervical cancer screening: which techniques should be used and why? *Clin Obstet Gynecol* 1999;42(4): 922–938.
5. Smith-Bindman R, Chu P, Miglioretti DL, et al. Physician predictors of mammographic accuracy. *J Natl Cancer Inst* 2005;97(5): 358–367.
6. Rocker G, Cook D, Sjokvist P, et al. Clinician predictions of intensive care unit mortality. *Crit Care Med* 2004;32(5): 1149–1154.
7. Guyatt G, Rennie D. *Users' guides to the medical literature. A manual for evidence-based practice*. Chicago, IL: AMA Press, 2002.
8. Fletcher R, Fletcher S. *Clinical epidemiology, the essentials*, 4th ed. Baltimore, MD: Lippincott Williams & Wilkins, 2005.
9. Straus S, Richardson W, Glasziou P, et al. *Evidence-based medicine: how to practice and teach EBM*. New York: Elsevier/Churchill Livingstone, 2005.
10. Pantell RH, Newman TB, Bernzweig J, et al. Management and outcomes of care of fever in early infancy. *JAMA* 2004;291(10): 1203–1212.
11. Vittinghoff E, Glidden D, Shiboski S, et al. *Regression methods in biostatistics: linear, logistic, survival, and repeated measures models*. New York: Springer-Verlag, 2005.
12. Siegel DL, Edelstein PH, Nachamkin I. Inappropriate testing for diarrheal diseases in the hospital. *JAMA* 1990;263(7): 979–982.

13. Carrico CW, Fenton LZ, Taylor GA, et al. Impact of sonography on the diagnosis and treatment of acute lower abdominal pain in children and young adults. *AJR Am J Roentgenol* 1999;172(2): 513–516.

14. Bodegard G, Fyro K, Larsson A. Psychological reactions in 102 families with a newborn who has a falsely positive screening test for congenital hypothyroidism. *Acta Paediatr Scand Suppl* 1983;304: 1–21.

15. Rubin SM, Cummings SR. Results of bone densitometry affect women's decisions about taking measures to prevent fractures. *Ann Intern Med* 1992;116(12 Pt 1): 990–995.

16. Waye JD, Lewis BS, Yessayan S. Colonoscopy: a prospective report of complications. *J Clin Gastroenterol* 1992;15(4): 347–351.

17. Selby JV, Friedman GD, Quesenberry CJ, et al. A case-control study of screening sigmoidoscopy and mortality from colorectal cancer. *N Engl J Med* 1992;326(10): 653–657.

18. Sheiner LB, Rubin DB. Intention-to-treat analysis and the goals of clinical trials. *Clin Pharmacol Ther* 1995;57(1): 6–15.

19. Eshed I, Gorenstein A, Serour F, et al. Intussusception in children: can we rely on screening sonography performed by junior residents? *Pediatr Radiol* 2004;34(2): 134–137.

20. Sheline Y, Kehr C. Cost and utility of routine admission laboratory testing for psychiatric inpatients. *Gen Hosp Psychiatry* 1990;12(5): 329–334.

21. Turnbull TL, Vanden Hoek TL, Howes DS, et al. Utility of laboratory studies in the emergency department patient with a new-onset seizure. *Ann Emerg Med* 1990;19(4): 373–377.

13 Utilizing Existing Databases

Deborah Grady and Norman Hearst

Many research questions can be answered quickly and efficiently using data that have already been collected. There are three general approaches to using existing data. **Secondary data analysis** is the use of existing data to investigate research questions other than the main ones for which the data were originally gathered. **Ancillary studies** add one or more measurements to a study, often in a subset of the participants, to answer a separate research question. **Systematic reviews** combine the results of multiple previous studies of a given research question, often including calculation of a summary estimate of effect that has greater precision than the individual study estimates. Making creative use of existing data is a fast and effective way for new investigators with limited resources to begin to answer important research questions.

ADVANTAGES AND DISADVANTAGES

The main **advantages** of using existing data are speed and economy. A research question that might otherwise require much time and money to investigate can sometimes be answered **rapidly** and **inexpensively.** For example, in the Multiple Risk Factor Intervention Trial (MRFIT), a large heart disease prevention trial in men, information about the smoking habits of the wives of the study subjects was recorded to examine whether this influenced the men's ability to quit smoking. After the study was over, one of the investigators realized that the data provided an opportunity to investigate the health effects of passive smoking—a new finding at the time. A twofold excess in the incidence of heart disease was found in nonsmoking men married to smoking wives when compared with similar nonsmoking men married to nonsmoking wives (1).

Existing data sets also have **disadvantages.** The selection of the population to study, which data to collect, the quality of data gathered, and how variables were measured and recorded are all predetermined. The existing data may have been collected from a population that is not ideal (*men only rather than men and women*), the measurement approach may not be what the investigator would prefer (*history of* *hypertension, a dichotomous historical variable, in place of actual blood pressure*) and the quality of the data may be poor (*frequent missing or incorrect values*). Important confounders and outcomes may not have been measured or recorded. All these factors contribute to the main disadvantage of using existing data: the investigator has little or **no control** over what data have been collected, and how.

SECONDARY DATA ANALYSIS

Secondary data sets may come from previous research studies, medical records, health care billing files, death certificates, and many other sources. **Previous research studies,** often conducted at the investigator's institution, may provide a rich source of secondary data. Many studies collect more data than the investigators analyze and contain interesting findings that have gone unnoticed. Access to such data is controlled by the study's **principal investigator**; the new researcher should therefore seek out information about the work of senior investigators at his institution. One of the most important ways a good mentor can be helpful to a new investigator is by providing knowledge of and access to relevant data both from his own and other institutions. Most large **NIH-funded studies** are now required to make their data publicly available after a certain period of time. These data sets are usually available through the Internet and can provide extensive data addressing related research questions.

Other sources of secondary data are large regional and **national data sets** that are publicly available and do not have a principal investigator. Computerized databases of this sort are as varied as the reasons people have for collecting information. We will give several examples that deserve special mention, and readers can locate others in their own areas of interest.

Tumor registries are government-supported agencies that collect complete statistics on cancer incidence, treatment, and outcome in defined geographic areas. These registries currently include about one quarter of the US population, and the area of coverage is expected to increase during the coming years. One of the purposes of these registries is to provide data to outside investigators. Combined data for all the registries are available from the Surveillance, Epidemiology, and End Results (SEER) Program. For example, investigators used the SEER registry of breast cancer diagnoses to determine the specificity of screening mammography in a large cohort of women in the San Francisco Bay Area. Women with negative mammograms in whom cancer was not diagnosed within 13 months were considered to have had true negative mammography (2).

Death certificate registries can be used to follow the mortality of any cohort. The **National Death Index** includes all deaths in the United States since 1978. This can be used to ascertain the vital status of subjects of an earlier study or of those who are part of another data set that includes important predictor variables. An example is the follow-up of men with coronary disease who were treated with high-dose nicotinic acid (or placebo) to lower serum cholesterol in the Coronary Drug Project. Although there was no difference in death rates at the end of the 5 years of randomized treatment, a mortality follow-up 9 years later using the National Death Index revealed a significant difference (3). Whether an individual is alive or dead is public information, so follow-up was available even for men who had dropped out of the study.

The National Death Index can be used when any two of three basic individual identifiers (name, birth date, and social security number) are known. Ascertainment of the fact of death is 99% complete with this system, and additional information from the death certificates (notably cause of death) can then be obtained from state records. On the state and local level, many jurisdictions now have computerized vital statistics systems, in which individual data (such as information from birth or death certificates) are entered as they are received.

Secondary data can be especially useful for studies to evaluate patterns of utilization and clinical outcomes of medical treatment. This approach can complement the information available from randomized trials and examine questions that trials cannot answer. These types of existing data include **administrative and clinical databases** such as those developed by Medicare, the Department of Veterans Affairs, Kaiser Permanente Medical Group, the Duke Cardiovascular Disease Databank, and **registries** such as the San Francisco Mammography Registry and the National Registry of Myocardial Infarction (NRMI). Information from these sources (many of which can be found on the Web) can be very useful for studying rare adverse events and for assessing real-world utilization and effectiveness of an intervention that has been shown to work in a clinical trial setting. For example, the NRMI was used to examine risk factors for intracranial hemorrhage after treatment with recombinant tissue-type plasminogen activator (tPA) for acute myocardial infarction (MI). The registry included 71,073 patients who received tPA; among these, 673 had intracranial hemorrhage confirmed by computed tomography or magnetic resonance imaging. A multivariate analysis showed that a tPA dose exceeding 1.5 mg/kg was significantly associated with developing an intracranial hemorrhage when compared with lower doses (4). Given that the overall risk of developing an intracranial hemorrhage was less than 1%, a clinical trial collecting primary data to examine this outcome would have been prohibitively large and expensive.

Another valuable contribution from this type of secondary data analysis is a better understanding of the difference between efficacy and effectiveness. The randomized clinical trial is the gold standard for determining the **efficacy** of a therapy under highly controlled circumstances in selected clinical settings. In the "real world," however, patients and treatments are often different. The choice of drugs and dosage by the treating physician and the adherence to medications by the patient are much more variable. These factors often act to make the new therapy less effective than demonstrated in trials. Assessing the **effectiveness** of treatments in actual practice can sometimes be accomplished through studies using secondary data. For example, primary angioplasty has been demonstrated to be superior to thrombolytic therapy in clinical trials of treating patients with acute MI (5). But this may only be true when success rates for angioplasty are as good as those achieved in the clinical trial setting. Secondary analyses of community data sets have not found a benefit of primary angioplasty over thrombolytic therapy (6,7).

Secondary data analysis is often the best approach for studying the utilization of accepted therapies. Although clinical trials can demonstrate efficacy of a new therapy, this benefit can only occur if the therapy is adopted by practicing physicians. Understanding **utilization rates,** addressing regional variation and use in specific populations (such as the elderly, ethnic minorities, the economically disadvantaged, and women), can have major public health implications. For example, despite convincing data that angiotensin converting enzyme inhibitors decrease mortality in patients with MI, a secondary analysis of community data has shown that many patients with clear indications for such therapy do not receive it (8).

Two data sets may also be linked to answer a research question. Investigators who were interested in how military service effects health used the 1970 to 1972 draft lottery involving 5.2 million 20-year-old men who were assigned eligibility for military service randomly by date of birth (the first data set) linked to later mortality based on state **death certificate registries** (the second source of data). The predictor variable (*date of birth*) was a randomly assigned proxy for military service during the Vietnam era. Men who had been randomly assigned to be eligible for the draft had significantly greater mortality from suicide and motor vehicle accidents in the ensuing 10 years (9). The study was done for less than $2,000 (not including the investigators' time), yet it was a more unbiased approach to examining the effect of military service on specific causes of subsequent death than other studies of this topic with much larger budgets.

When individual data are not available, aggregate data sets can sometimes be useful. The term **aggregate data** means that information is available only for groups of subjects (e.g., *death rates from cervical cancer in each of the 50 states*). With such data, associations can only be measured among these groups by comparing group information on a risk factor (such as *tobacco sales*) with the rate of an outcome. Studies using aggregate data are called **ecologic studies**.

The advantage of aggregate data is its availability. Its major drawback is the fact that associations are especially susceptible to confounding: groups tend to differ from each other in many ways, not all of which are causally related. Furthermore, associations observed in the aggregate do not necessarily hold for the individual. For example, sales of cigarettes may be greater in states with high suicide rates, but the individuals who commit suicide may not be the ones doing most of the smoking. This situation is referred to as the **ecologic fallacy.** Aggregate data are most appropriately used to test the plausibility of a new hypothesis or to generate new hypotheses. Interesting results can then be pursued in another study that uses individual data.

Getting Started

After choosing a research topic and becoming familiar with the literature in that area (including a thorough literature search and advice from a senior mentor), the next step is to investigate whether the research question can be addressed with an existing database. The help of a **senior colleague** can be invaluable in finding an appropriate data set. An experienced researcher has defined areas of interest in which he stays current and is aware of important data sets and the investigators who control these data, both at his own institution and elsewhere. This person can help identify and gain access to the appropriate database. Often, the research question needs to be altered slightly (by modifying the definition of the predictor or outcome variables, for example) to fit the available data.

The best solution may be close at hand, a **database at the home institution.** For example, a University of California, San Francisco (UCSF) fellow who was interested in the role of lipoproteins in coronary disease noticed that one of the few interventions known to lower the level of lipoprotein(a) was estrogen. Knowing that the Heart and Estrogen/Progestin Replacement Study (HERS), a major clinical trial of hormone treatment to prevent coronary disease, was being managed at UCSF, the fellow approached the investigators with his interest. Because no one else had specifically planned to examine the relationship between this lipoprotein, hormone treatment and coronary heart disease events, the fellow designed an analysis and publication plan. After receiving permission from the HERS study leadership, he worked with coordinating center statisticians, epidemiologists, and programmers to carry out an analysis that he subsequently published in a leading journal (10).

Sometimes a research question can be addressed that has little to do with the original study. For example, another fellow from UCSF was interested in the value of repeated screening Pap tests in women over 65 years old. He realized that the mean age of participants in the HERS trial was 67 years, that participants were required to have a normal Pap test to enter and then received screening Pap tests annually during follow-up. By following up on Pap test outcomes, he was able to document that 110 Pap tests were abnormal among over 2500 women screened over a 2-year period, and only one woman was ultimately found to have abnormal follow-up histology. Therefore, all but one of the abnormal Pap tests were falsely positive (11). This study strongly influenced the US Preventive Services Task Force's current recommendation that Pap tests should not be performed in low-risk women over age 65 with previous normal tests.

Sometimes it is necessary to **venture further afield.** Working from a list of predictor and outcome variables whose relation might help to answer the research question, an investigator can seek to locate databases that include these variables. Phone calls or e-mail messages to the authors of previous studies or to government officials might result in access to files containing useful data. It is essential to conquer any anxiety that the investigator may feel about contacting strangers to ask for help. Most people are surprisingly cooperative, either by providing data themselves or by suggesting other places to try.

Once the data for answering the research question have been located, the next challenge is to obtain **permission** to use them. It is a good practice to use official letterhead on correspondence and to adopt any institutional titles that are appropriate. Young investigators should determine if their mentors are acquainted with the investigators who control the database, as an introduction may be more effective than a cold contact. It is generally most effective to work with an investigator who is interested in the research topic and involved in the study whose database you would like to examine. This investigator can facilitate access to the data, assure that you understand the study methods and how the variables were measured, and often becomes a valued colleague and collaborator. Databases that result from multicenter studies and clinical trials generally have clear mechanisms for obtaining access to the data that include the requirement for a written analysis proposal and approval by an analysis or publications committee.

The investigator should be very specific about **what information** is sought and confirm the request in writing. It is a good idea to keep the size of the request to a minimum and to offer to pay any cost of preparing the data. If the data set is controlled by another group of researchers, the investigator can suggest a collaborative relationship. In addition to providing an incentive to share the data, this can engage a coinvestigator who is familiar with the database. It is wise to clearly define such a relationship early on, including who will be first author of the planned publications. Important arrangements of this sort often benefit from a face-to-face meeting.

ANCILLARY STUDIES

Research with secondary data takes advantage of the fact that the data needed to answer a research question are already available. In an **ancillary study,** the investigator adds one or several measurements to an existing study to answer a different research question. For example, in the HERS trial of the effect of hormone therapy on risk for coronary events in 2,763 elderly women, an investigator added measurement of the frequency and severity of urinary incontinence. Adding a one-page questionnaire created a large trial of the effect of hormone therapy on urinary incontinence, with little additional time or expense (12).

Ancillary studies have many of the **advantages** of secondary data analysis with fewer constraints. They are both inexpensive and efficient, and the investigator can design a few key ancillary measurements specifically to answer the research question. Ancillary studies can be added to any type of study, including cross-sectional and case–control studies, but large prospective cohort studies and randomized trials are particularly well suited to such studies.

Ancillary studies in randomized trials have the problem that the measurements may be most informative when added before the trial begins, and it may be difficult for an outsider to identify trials in the planning phase. Even when a variable was not measured at baseline, however, a single measurement during or at the end of the trial can produce useful information. By adding cognitive function measures at the end of the HERS trial, the investigators were able to compare the cognitive function of elderly women treated with hormone therapy for 4 years with the cognitive function of those treated with placebo (13).

A good opportunity for ancillary studies is provided by the **banks of stored serum, DNA, images,** and so on, that are found in most large clinical trials and cohort studies. The opportunity to propose new measurements using these specimens can be an extremely cost-effective approach to answering a novel research question, especially if it is possible to make these measurements on a subset of specimens using a nested case–control or case–cohort design (Chapter 7). In HERS, for example, genetic analyses of fewer than 100 cases and controls showed that the excess number of thromboembolic events in the hormone-treated group was not due to an interaction with factor V Leiden (14).

Getting Started

Opportunities for ancillary studies should be actively pursued, especially by new investigators with limited time and resources. A good place to start is to identify studies with research questions that include either the predictor or the outcome variable of interest. For example, an investigator interested in the effect of weight loss on pain associated with osteoarthritis might start by identifying trials of interventions (such as *diet, exercise, behavior change,* or *drugs*) for weight loss. Such studies can be identified by searching lists of studies funded by the federal government, by contacting pharmaceutical companies that manufacture drugs for weight loss, and by talking with experts in weight loss who are familiar with ongoing studies. To create an ancillary study, the investigator would simply add a measure of arthritis symptoms among subjects enrolled in these studies. Alternatively, he might identify studies that have joint pain as an outcome, and add change in weight as an ancillary measure.

After identifying a study that provides a good opportunity for ancillary measures, the next step is to obtain the cooperation of the study investigators. Most researchers will consider adding brief ancillary measures to an established study if they address an important question and do not substantially interfere with the conduct of the main study. Investigators will be reluctant to add measures that require a lot of the participant's time (*cognitive function testing*) or are invasive and unpleasant (*colonoscopy*) or costly (*positron emission tomography scanning*).

Generally, formal permission from the principal investigator or the appropriate study committee is required to add an ancillary study. Most large, multicenter studies have established procedures requiring a written application. The proposed ancillary study is generally reviewed by a committee that can approve, reject, or revise the ancillary study. Many ancillary measures require funding, and the ancillary study investigator must find a way to pay these costs. Of course, the cost of an ancillary study is much less than the cost of conducting the same trial independently. Some large studies may have their own mechanisms for funding ancillary studies, especially if the research question is important and considered relevant by the funding agency. The NIH has recently issued several requests for proposals to add ancillary studies to large NIH-funded trials.

The **disadvantages** of ancillary studies are few. If the main study is already in progress, new variables can be added, but variables already being measured cannot be changed. In some cases there may be practical problems in obtaining permission from the investigators or sponsor to perform the ancillary study, training those who will make the measurements, or obtaining separate informed consent from participants. Because the ancillary study investigator may not have designed or conducted the main study, it may also be difficult to obtain access to the full database for analysis. These issues, including a clear understanding of authorship of scientific papers that result from the ancillary study and the rules governing their preparation and submission, need to be clarified before starting the study.

SYSTEMATIC REVIEWS

Systematic reviews identify completed studies that address a research question, and evaluate the results of these studies to arrive at conclusions about a body of research. In contrast to other approaches to reviewing the literature, systematic reviews use a well-defined and uniform approach to identify all relevant studies, display the results of eligible studies, and, when appropriate, calculate a summary estimate of the overall results. The statistical aspects of a systematic review (calculating summary effect estimates and variance, statistical tests of heterogeneity, and statistical estimates of publication bias) are called **meta-analysis.**

A systematic review can be a good **opportunity for a new investigator.** Although it takes a surprising amount of time and effort, a systematic review generally does not require substantial financial or other resources. Completing a good systematic review requires that the investigator become intimately familiar with the literature regarding the research question. For new investigators, this detailed knowledge of published studies is invaluable. Publication of a good systematic review can also establish a new investigator as an "expert" on the research question. Moreover, the findings, with power enhanced by the larger sample size available from the combined studies and peculiarities of individual study findings revealed by comparison with the others, often represent an important scientific contribution. Systematic review findings can be particularly useful for developing practice guidelines.

The elements of a good systematic review are listed in Table 13.1. Just as for other studies, the methods for completing each of these steps should be described in a written protocol before the systematic review begins.

The Research Question
As with any research, a good systematic review has a well-formulated, clear research question that meets the usual FINER criteria (Chapter 2). Feasibility depends largely on the existence of a set of studies of the question. The research question

TABLE 13.1	Elements of a Good Systematic Review

1. Clear research question
2. Comprehensive and unbiased identification of completed studies
3. Definition of inclusion and exclusion criteria
4. Uniform and unbiased abstraction of the characteristics and findings of each study
5. Clear and uniform presentation of data from individual studies
6. Calculation of a summary estimate of effect and confidence interval based on the findings of all eligible studies when appropriate
7. Assessment of the heterogeneity of the findings of the individual studies
8. Assessment of potential publication bias
9. Subgroup and sensitivity analyses

should describe the disease or condition of interest, the population and setting, the intervention and comparison treatment (for trials), and the outcomes of interest. For example, *''Among persons admitted to an intensive care unit with unstable angina, does treatment with aspirin plus intravenous heparin reduce the risk of myocardial infarction and death during the hospitalization more than treatment with aspirin alone (15)?''*

Identifying Completed Studies

Systematic reviews are based on a comprehensive and unbiased search for completed studies. The search should follow a well-defined strategy established before the results of the individual studies are known. The process of identifying studies for potential inclusion in the review and the sources for finding such articles should be explicitly documented before the study. Searches should not be limited to **MEDLINE,** which includes only about half of all published English-language clinical research studies and often does not list non-English-language references. Depending on the research question, other electronic databases such as AIDSLINE, CANCERLIT, and EMBASE can be included, as well as manual review of the bibliography of relevant published studies, previous reviews, evaluation of the **Cochran Collaboration** database, and consultation with experts. The search strategy should be clearly described so that other investigators can replicate the search.

Criteria for Including and Excluding Studies

The protocol for a systematic review should provide a good rationale for including and excluding studies, and these **criteria should be established** *a priori.* Criteria for including or excluding studies from meta-analyses typically designate the period during which studies were published, the population that is acceptable for study, the disease or condition of interest, the intervention to be studied, whether blinding is required, acceptable control groups, required outcomes, maximal acceptable loss to follow-up, and minimal acceptable length of follow-up. Once these criteria are established, each potentially eligible study should be reviewed for eligibility independently by two or more investigators, with disagreements resolved by another reviewer or by consensus. When determining eligibility, it may be best to blind reviewers to the date, journal, authors, and results of trials.

Published systematic reviews should **list studies that were considered** for inclusion and the specific reason for excluding a study. For example, if 30 potentially eligible trials are identified, these 30 trials should be fully referenced and a reason should be given for each exclusion.

Collecting Data from Eligible Studies

Data should be abstracted from each study in a uniform and unbiased fashion. Generally, this is done **independently by two or more abstractors** using predesigned forms that include variables that define eligibility criteria, design features, the population included in the study, the number of individuals in each group, the intervention (for trials), the main outcome, secondary outcomes, and outcomes in subgroups. The data abstraction forms should include any data that will subsequently appear in the text, tables or figures describing the studies included in the systematic review, or in tables or figures presenting the outcomes. When the two abstractors disagree, a third abstractor may settle the difference, or a consensus process may be used. The process for abstracting data from studies for the systematic review should be clearly described in the manuscript.

The published reports of some studies that might be eligible for inclusion in a systematic review may not include important information, such as design features, risk estimates, and standard deviations.. Often it is difficult to tell if design features such as blinding were not implemented or were just not described in the publication. The reviewer can sometimes calculate relative risks and confidence intervals from crude data presented from randomized trials, but it is generally unacceptable to calculate risk estimates and confidence intervals based on crude data from observational studies because there is not sufficient information to adjust for potential confounders. Every effort should be made to contact the authors to retrieve important information that is not included in the published description of a study. If this necessary information cannot be calculated or obtained, the study findings are generally excluded.

Presenting the Findings Clearly

Systematic reviews generally include three types of information. First, important characteristics of each study included in the systematic review are presented in tables. These often include the study sample size, number of outcomes, length of follow-up, characteristics of the population studied, and methods used in the study. Second, the review displays the results of the individual studies (risk estimates, confidence intervals or P values) in a table or figure. Finally, in the absence of significant heterogeneity (see below), the meta-analysis presents summary estimates and confidence intervals based on the findings of all the included studies as well as sensitivity and subgroup analyses.

The summary effect estimates represent a main outcome of the meta-analysis but should be presented in the context of all the information abstracted from the individual studies. The characteristics and findings of individual studies included in the systematic review should be displayed clearly in tables and figures so that the reader can form opinions that do not depend solely on the statistical summary estimates.

Meta-Analysis: Statistics for Systematic Reviews

- *Summary effect estimate and confidence interval.* Once all completed studies have been identified, those that meet the inclusion and exclusion criteria have been chosen, and data have been abstracted from each study, a summary estimate (summary relative risk, summary odds ratio, etc.) and confidence interval may be calculated. The summary effect is essentially an average effect weighted by the inverse of the variance of the outcome of each study. Methods for calculating the summary effect and confidence interval are discussed in Appendix 13.1. Those not interested in the details of calculating mean weighted estimates from multiple studies should at least be aware that different approaches can give different results. For example, recent meta-analyses of the effectiveness of condoms for preventing heterosexual transmission of HIV have given summary estimates ranging from 80% to 94% decrease in transmission rates, although they are based on the results of almost identical sets of studies (16,17).

- *Heterogeneity.* Combining the results of several studies is not appropriate if the studies differ in clinically important ways, such as the intervention, outcome, controls, blinding, and so on. It is also inappropriate to combine the findings if the results of the individual studies differ widely. Even if the methods used in the studies appear to be similar, the fact that the results vary markedly suggests that something important was different in the individual studies. This variability in the findings of the individual studies is called **heterogeneity** (and the study findings are said to be **heterogeneous**); if there is little variability, the study findings are said to be **homogeneous.**

  How can the investigator decide whether methods and findings are similar enough to combine into summary estimates? First, he can review the individual studies to determine if there are substantial differences in study design, study populations, intervention, or outcome. Then he can examine the results of the individual studies. If some trials report a substantial beneficial effect of an intervention and others report considerable harm, heterogeneity is clearly present. Sometimes, it is difficult to decide if heterogeneity is present. For example, if one trial reports a 50% risk reduction for a specific intervention but another reports only a 30% risk reduction, is heterogeneity present? Statistical approaches (tests of homogeneity) have been developed to help answer this question (Appendix 13.1), but ultimately, this requires judgment. Every reported systematic review should include some discussion of heterogeneity and its effect on the summary estimates.

Assessment of Publication Bias

Publication bias occurs when published studies are not representative of all studies that have been done, usually because positive results tend to be submitted and published more often than negative results. There are two main ways to deal with publication bias. **Unpublished studies can be identified** and the results included in the summary estimate. Unpublished results may be identified by querying investigators and reviewing abstracts, meeting presentations, and doctoral theses. The results of unpublished studies can be included with those of the published trials in the overall summary estimate, or sensitivity analyses can determine if adding these unpublished results substantially changes the summary estimate determined from published results. However, including unpublished results in a systematic review is problematic for several reasons. It is often difficult to identify unpublished studies and even more difficult to abstract the required data. Frequently, inadequate information is available to determine if the study meets inclusion criteria for the systematic review or to evaluate the quality of the methods. For these reasons, unpublished data are not often included in meta-analyses.

Alternatively, the extent of potential **publication bias can be estimated** and this information used to temper the conclusions of the systematic review. Publication bias exists when unpublished studies have different findings from published studies. Unpublished studies are more likely to be small (large studies usually get published, regardless of the findings) and to have found no association between the risk factor or intervention and the outcome (markedly positive studies usually get published, even if small). If there is no publication bias, there should be no association between a study's size (or the variance of the outcome estimate) and findings. The degree of this association is often measured using **Kendall's Tau,** a coefficient of correlation. A strong or statistically significant correlation between study outcome and sample size suggests publication bias. In the absence of publication bias, a plot of study sample size versus outcome (e.g., log relative risk) should have a bell or **funnel shape** with the apex near the summary effect estimate.

The funnel plot in Fig. 13.1A suggests that there is little publication bias because small studies with both negative and positive findings were published. The plot in Fig. 13.1B, on the other hand, suggests publication bias because the distribution appears truncated in the corner that should contain small, negative studies.

When substantial publication bias is likely, summary estimates should not be calculated or should be interpreted cautiously. Every reported systematic review should include some discussion of potential publication bias and its effect on the summary estimates.

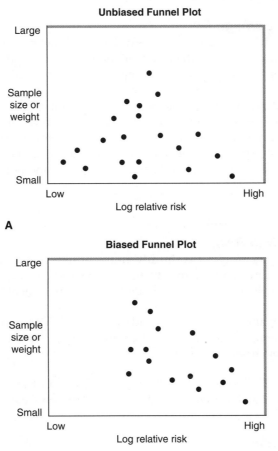

FIGURE 13.1. **A:** Funnel plot that does not suggest publication bias because there are studies with a range of large and small sample sizes, and low relative risks are reported by some smaller studies. **B:** Funnel plot suggestive of publication bias because the smaller studies primarily report high relative risks.

Subgroup and Sensitivity Analyses

Subgroup analyses may be possible using data from all or some subset of the studies included in the systematic review. For example, in a systematic review of the effect of postmenopausal estrogen therapy on endometrial cancer risk, some of the studies presented the results by duration of estrogen use. Subgroup analyses of the results of studies that provided such information demonstrated that longer duration of use was associated with higher risk for cancer (18).

Sensitivity analyses indicate how "sensitive" the findings of the meta-analysis are to certain decisions about the design of the systematic review or inclusion of certain studies. For example, if the authors decided to include studies with a slightly different design or methods in the systematic review, the findings are strengthened if the summary results are similar whether or not the questionable studies are included. Systematic reviews should generally include sensitivity analyses if any of the design decisions appear questionable or arbitrary.

Garbage In, Garbage Out

The biggest drawback to a systematic review is that it can produce a reliable-appearing summary estimate based on the results of individual studies that are of poor quality. The process of assessing quality is complex and problematic. We favor relying on relatively strict criteria for good study design when setting the inclusion criteria. If the individual studies that are summarized in a systematic review are of poor quality, no amount of careful analysis can prevent the summary estimate from being unreliable. A special instance of this problem is encountered in systematic reviews of observational data. If the results of these studies are not adjusted for potential confounding variables, the results of the meta-analysis will also be unadjusted and potentially confounded.

SUMMARY

Secondary Data Analysis

1. Secondary data analysis has the **advantage** of greatly reducing the time and cost of doing research and the **disadvantage** of providing the investigator little or no control over the study population, design, or measurements.

2. One good source of data for secondary analysis is a **completed research project** at the investigator's institution; others are the large number of **public databases** now available from many sources.

3. Large community-based data sets are useful for studying the **effectiveness** and **utilization** of an intervention in the community, and for discovering **rare adverse events.**

Ancillary Studies

1. A clever ancillary study can answer a new research question with **little cost and effort.** As with secondary data analyses, the investigator **cannot control the design,** but he is able to **specify a few key additional measurements.**

2. Good opportunities for ancillary studies may be found in **cohort studies** or **clinical trials** that include either the predictor or outcome variable for the research question of interest. **Stored banks of serum, DNA, images,** and so on, provide the opportunity for cost-effective nested case–control and case-cohort designs.

3. Most large studies have written **policies** that allow investigators (including outside scientists) to propose and carry out ancillary studies.

Systematic Reviews

1. A good systematic review, like any other study, requires a complete **written protocol** before the study begins. The protocol should include the **research question,** methods for **identifying all eligible studies,** methods for **abstracting data** from the studies, and **statistical methods.**

2. The statistical aspects of a systematic review, termed **meta-analysis,** include the **summary effect estimate and confidence interval,** tests for evaluating **heterogeneity** and **potential publication bias,** and planned **subgroup** and **sensitivity analyses.**

3. The **characteristics** and **findings** of individual studies should be displayed clearly in tables and figures so that the reader can form opinions that do not depend solely on the statistical summary estimates.

4. The biggest drawback to a systematic review is that the results can be no more reliable than the **quality of the studies** on which it is based.

APPENDIX 13.1

Statistical Methods for Meta-Analysis

SUMMARY EFFECTS AND CONFIDENCE INTERVALS

The primary goal of meta-analysis is to calculate a summary effect size and confidence interval. An intuitive way to do this is to multiply each trial relative risk (an effect estimate) by the sample size (a weight that reflects the accuracy of the relative risk), add these products, and divide by the sum of the weights. In actual practice, the inverse of the variance of the effect estimate from each individual study ($1/\text{variance}_i$) is used as the weight for each study. The inverse of the variance is a better estimate of the precision of the effect estimate than the sample size because it takes into account the number of outcomes and their distribution. The weighted mean effect estimate is calculated by multiplying each study weight ($1/\text{variance}_i$) by the log of the relative risk (or any other risk estimate, such as the log odds ratio, risk difference, etc.), adding these products, and dividing by the sum of the weights. Small studies generally result in a large variance (and a wide confidence interval around the risk estimate) and large studies result in a small variance (and a narrow confidence interval around the risk estimate). Therefore, in a meta-analysis, large studies get a lot of weight (1/small variance) and small studies get little weight (1/big variance).

To determine if the summary effect estimate is statistically significant, the variability of the estimate of the summary effect is calculated. There are various formulas for calculating the variance of summary risk estimates (19,20). Most use something that approximates the inverse of the sum of the weights of the individual studies ($1/\Sigma \text{ weight}_i$). The variance of the summary estimate is used to calculate the 95% confidence interval around the summary estimate ($\pm 1.96 \times \text{variance}^{1/2}$).

RANDOM- VERSUS FIXED-EFFECT MODELS

There are multiple statistical approaches available for calculating a summary estimate (20). The choice of statistical method is usually dependent on the type of outcome (relative risk, risk reduction, difference score, etc.). In addition to the statistical model, the investigator must also choose to use either a fixed-effect or random-effect model. The fixed-effect model simply calculates the variance of a summary estimate based on the inverse of the sum of the weights of each individual study. The random-effect model adds variance to the summary effect in proportion to the variability of the results of the individual studies. Summary effect estimates are generally similar using either the fixed- or random-effect model, but the variance of the summary effect is greater in the random-effect model to the degree that the results of the individual studies differ, and the confidence interval around the summary effect is correspondingly larger, so that summary results are less likely to be statistically significant. Many journals now require authors to use a random-effect model because it is considered "conservative." Meta-analyses should state clearly whether they used a fixed- or random-effect model.

Simply using a random-effect model does not obviate the problem of heterogeneity. If the studies identified by a systematic review are clearly heterogeneous, a summary estimate should not be calculated.

STATISTICAL TESTS OF HOMOGENEITY

Tests of homogeneity assume that the findings of the individual trials are the same (the null hypothesis) and use a statistical test (test of homogeneity) to determine if the data (the individual study findings) refute this hypothesis. A chi-square test is commonly used (19). If the data do support the null hypothesis (P value ≥ 0.10), the investigator accepts that the studies are homogeneous. If the data do not support the hypothesis (P value < 0.10), he rejects the null hypothesis and assumes that the study findings are heterogeneous. In other words, there are meaningful differences in the populations studied, the nature of the predictor or outcome variables, or the study results.

All meta-analyses should report tests of homogeneity with a P value. These tests are not very powerful and it is hard to reject the null hypothesis and prove heterogeneity when the sample size—the number of individual studies—is small. For this reason, a P value somewhat higher than the typical value of 0.05 is typically used as a cutoff. If substantial heterogeneity is present, it is inappropriate to combine the results of trials into a single summary estimate.

REFERENCES

1. Svendsen KH, Kuller LH, Martin MJ, et al. Effects of passive smoking in the multiple risk factor intervention trial (MRFIT). *Am J Epidemiol* 1987;126:783–795.
2. Kerlikowske K, Grady D, Barclay J, et al. Likelihood ratios for modern screening mammography. *JAMA* 1996;276:39–43.
3. Canner PL. Mortality in CDP patients during a nine-year post-treatment period. *J Am Coll Cardiol* 1986;8:1243–1255.

4. Gurwitz JH, Gore JM, Goldberg RJ, et al. Risk for intracranial hemorrhage after tissue plasminogen activator treatment for acute myocardial infarction. Participants in the National Registry of Myocardial Infarction 2. *Ann Intern Med* 1998;129:597–604.

5. Weaver WD, Simes RJ, Betriu A, et al. Comparison of primary coronary angioplasty and intravenous thrombolytic therapy for acute myocardial infarction: a quantitative review. *JAMA* 1997;278:2093–2098; published erratum appears in *JAMA* 1998;279:876.

6. Every NR, Parsons LS, Hlatky M, et al. A comparison of thrombolytic therapy with primary coronary angioplasty for acute myocardial infarction. Myocardial infarction triage and intervention investigators. *N Engl J Med* 1996;335:1253–1260.

7. Tiefenbrunn AJ, Chandra NC, French WJ, et al. Clinical experience with primary percutaneous transluminal coronary angioplasty compared with alteplase (recombinant tissue-type plasminogen activator) in patients with acute myocardial infarction: a report from the Second National Registry of Myocardial Infarction (NRMI-2). *J Am Coll Cardiol* 1998;31:1240–1245.

8. Barron HV, Michaels AD, Maynard C, et al. Use of angiotensin-converting enzyme inhibitors at discharge in patients with acute myocardial infarction in the United States: data from the National Registry of Myocardial Infarction 2. *J Am Coll Cardiol* 1998;32:360–367.

9. Hearst N, Newman TB, Hulley SB. Delayed effects of the military draft on mortality: a randomized natural experiment. *N Engl J Med* 1986;314:620–624.

10. Shlipak M, Simon J, Vittinghoff E, et al. Estrogen and progestin, lipoprotein (a), and the risk of recurrent coronary heart disease events after menopause. *JAMA* 2000;283:1845–1852.

11. Sawaya GF, Grady D, Kerlikowske K, et al. The positive predictive value of cervical smears in previously screened postmenopausal women: the Heart and Estrogen/progestin Replacement Study (HERS). *Ann Intern Med* 2000;133:942–950.

12. Grady D, Brown J, Vittinghoff E, et al. Postmenopausal hormones and incontinence: the Heart and Estrogen/Progestin Replacement Study. *Obstet Gynecol* 2001;97:116–120.

13. Grady D, Yaffe K, Kristof M, et al. Effect of postmenopausal hormone therapy on cognitive function: the Heart and Estrogen/progestin Replacement Study. *Am J Med* 2002;113:543–548.

14. Herrington DM, Vittinghoff E, Howard TD, et al. Factor V Leiden, hormone replacement therapy, and risk of venous thromboembolic events in women with coronary disease. *Arterioscler Thromb Vasc Biol* 2002;22:1012–1017.

15. Oler A, Whooley M, Oler J, et al. Heparin plus aspirin reduces the risk of myocardial infarction or death in patients with unstable angina. *JAMA* 1996;276:811–815.

16. Pinkerton SD, Abramson PR. Effectiveness of condoms in preventing HIV transmission. *Soc Sci Med* 1997;44:1303–1312.

17. Weller S, Davis K. Condom effectiveness in reducing heterosexual HIV transmission. *Cochrane Database Syst Rev* 2002;(1):CD003255.

18. Grady D, Gebretsadik T, Kerlikowske K, et al. Hormone replacement therapy and endometrial cancer risk: a meta-analysis. *Obstet Gynecol* 1995;85:304–313.

19. Petitti D. *Meta-analysis, decision analysis and cost effectiveness analysis*. New York: Oxford University Press, 1994.

20. Cooper H, Hedges LV. *The handbook of research synthesis*. New York: Russell Sage Foundation, 1994.

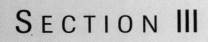

Implementation

14 Addressing Ethical Issues

Bernard Lo

Research with human participants raises ethical concerns because people accept risks and inconvenience primarily to advance scientific knowledge and to benefit others. For the public to be willing to participate in clinical research and to provide public funding, it needs to trust that such research is conducted according to strict ethical standards (1).

In this chapter we begin by reviewing ethical principles and the federal regulations about informed consent and institutional review boards (IRBs) in the United States. We then turn to a number of ethical considerations including scientific misconduct, conflict of interest, authorship, and confidentiality.

ETHICAL PRINCIPLES

Three ethical principles guide research with human participants (2). The principle of **respect for persons** requires investigators to obtain informed consent from research participants, to protect participants with impaired decision-making capacity, and to maintain confidentiality. Research participants are not passive sources of data, but individuals whose rights and welfare must be respected.

The principle of **beneficence** requires that the research design be scientifically sound and that the risks of the research be acceptable in relation to the likely benefits. Risks to participants include both physical harm from research interventions and also psychosocial harm, such as breaches of confidentiality, stigma, and discrimination. The risks of participating in the study can be reduced, for example, by screening potential participants to exclude those likely to suffer adverse effects and monitoring participants for adverse effects.

The principle of **justice** requires that the benefits and burdens of research be distributed fairly. Vulnerable populations, such as people with poor access to health care, those with impaired decision-making capacity, and institutionalized persons, may lack the capacity to make informed and free choices about participating in research.

225

Such populations may seem attractive to study if access and follow-up are convenient, but vulnerable populations should not be targeted for research if other populations would also be suitable participants.

Justice also requires equitable access to the benefits of research. Traditionally, clinical research has been regarded as risky, and potential subjects have been thought of as guinea pigs who needed protection from dangerous interventions that would confer little or no personal benefit. Increasingly, however, clinical research is regarded as providing access to new therapies for such conditions as HIV infection, cancer, and organ transplantation. Patients who seek promising new drugs for fatal conditions want increased access to clinical research, not greater protection (3). In addition, groups that are underrepresented on clinical research have suboptimal clinical care because of a weak evidence base. Children, women, and members of ethnic minorities historically have been underrepresented in clinical research. NIH-funded clinical researchers must have adequate representation of children, women, and members of ethnic minorities in studies, or else justify why they are underrepresented.

FEDERAL REGULATIONS FOR RESEARCH ON HUMAN SUBJECTS

Federal regulations are intended to assure that human subjects research is conducted in an ethically acceptable manner (4). (Although the regulations refer to human "subjects," the term "participants" is generally preferred today.) These regulations apply to all federally funded research and to research that will be submitted to the U.S. Food and Drug Administration (FDA) in support of a new drug or device application. In addition, most universities require that all research on human subjects conducted by affiliated faculty and staff comply with these regulations, including research funded privately or conducted off-site.

These federal regulations define **research** as "systematic investigation designed to develop or contribute to generalizable knowledge (4)." Research is therefore distinguished from unproven clinical care that is directed toward benefiting the individual patient and not toward publication. **Human subjects** are living individuals about whom an investigator obtains either "data through intervention or interaction with the individual" or "identifiable private information." **Private information** comprises (1) information that a person can reasonably expect is not being observed or recorded and (2) information that has been provided for specific purposes and that "the individual can reasonably expect will not be made public (e.g., a medical record)." Information is identifiable if "the identity of the subject is or may be readily ascertained by the investigator or associated with the information." Research data that is identified by a code is not considered individually **identifiable** if the key that links data to participants is destroyed before the research begins or if the investigators have no access to the key.

Researchers who have questions about these federal regulations should consult their IRB or read the full text of federal regulations, which are available on the website of the Office for Human Research Protections (OHRP) of the Department of Health and Human Services.

The federal regulations provide two main protections for human subjects, IRB approval and informed consent.

Institutional Review Board Approval

Federal regulations require that research with human subjects be approved by an **IRB**. The IRB mission is to ensure that the research is ethically acceptable and that the welfare and rights of research participants are protected. Although most IRB members are researchers, IRBs must also include community members and persons knowledgeable about legal and ethical issues concerning research.

When approving a research study, the IRB must determine that:

- risks to participants are minimized,
- risks are reasonable in relation to anticipated benefits and the importance of the knowledge that is expected to result,
- selection of participants is equitable,
- informed consent will be sought from participants or their legally authorized representatives, and
- confidentiality is adequately maintained (4).

The IRB system is decentralized. Each local IRB implements federal regulations using its own forms, procedures, and guidelines, and there is no appeal to a higher body. As a result, protocol for a multicenter study may be approved by the IRB of one institution but not by the IRB of another institution. Usually these differences can be resolved through discussions or protocol modifications.

IRBs have been criticized for several reasons (5,6). They may place undue emphasis on consent forms and fail to scrutinize the research design. Review of the scientific merit of the research is usually beyond the expertise of the IRB and is left to the funding agency. Although IRBs need to review any protocol revisions and monitor adverse events, typically they do not check whether research was actually carried out in accordance with the approved protocols. Many IRBs lack the resources and expertise to adequately fulfill their mission of protecting research participants. For these reasons, federal regulations and IRB approval should be regarded only as a minimal ethical standard for research. Ultimately, the **judgment and character of the investigator** are the most essential element for assuring that research is ethically acceptable.

Exceptions to Institutional Review Board Review.   Certain research may be exempted from IRB review or may receive expedited review.

IRBs may be **exempted** from review of certain types of research, most commonly surveys, interviews, and research with existing specimens, records, or data (Table 14.1). The ethical justification for such exemptions is that the research involves low risk, almost all people would consent to such research, and obtaining consent from each subject would make such studies prohibitively expensive or difficult.

An IRB may allow certain research to undergo **expedited review** by a single reviewer rather than the full committee (Table 14.2). The Department of Health and Human Services publishes a list of types of research that are eligible for expedited review (7), which can be obtained at its website.

The concept of **minimal risk to participants** plays a key role in federal regulations, as indicated in Tables 14.1 and 14.2. Minimal risk is defined as that "ordinarily encountered in daily life or during the performance of routine physical or psychological tests." Both the magnitude and probability of risk must be considered. The IRB must judge whether a specific project may be considered minimal risk.

TABLE 14.1	What Research is Exempt from Institutional Review Board Review?

1. Surveys, interviews, or observations of public behavior unless:
   - subjects can be identified, either directly or through identifiers and
   - disclosure of subjects' responses could place them at risk for legal liability or damage their reputation, financial standing, or employability.

2. Studies of existing records, data, or specimens, provided that:
   - samples exist and are publicly available (e.g., data tapes released by state and federal agencies) or
   - information is recorded by the investigator in such a manner that subjects cannot be identified, either directly or through identifiers. Coded data is considered identifiable if the codes could be broken with the cooperation of others.

3. Research on normal educational practices

The HIPAA Health Privacy Regulations. The federal Health Privacy Regulations (commonly known as HIPAA, after the Health Insurance Portability and Accountability Act) require researchers to obtain permission from patients to use protected health information in research (8–10). The Privacy Rule protects individually identifiable health information, which is termed **protected health information**. Under the Privacy Rule, individuals must sign an authorization to allow the health care provider to use or disclose protected health information in a research project. The regulations specify information that must be included in the authorization form. This HIPAA authorization form is in addition to the informed consent form required by the IRB. Researchers must obtain authorization for each use of protected information for research. Furthermore, under the Privacy Rule research participants may have the right to access health information and to obtain a record of disclosures of their protected health information.

Informed and Voluntary Consent

Investigators must obtain informed and voluntary consent from research participants.

Disclosure of Information to Participants. Investigators must disclose information that is relevant to the potential participant's decision whether or not to participate in the research. Specifically, investigators must discuss with potential participants:

TABLE 14.2	What Research May Undergo Expedited Institutional Review Board (IRB) Review?

1. Research that involves no more than minimal risk and is one of the categories of research listed by the Department of Health and Human Services as eligible for expedited review. Examples include:
   - collection of specimens through venipuncture
   - collection of specimens through noninvasive procedures routinely employed in clinical practice, such as electrocardiograms and magnetic resonance imaging. However, procedures using x-rays must be reviewed by the full IRB.
   - research involving data, records, or specimens that have been collected or will be collected for clinical purposes and research using surveys or interviews that is not exempt from IRB review.

2. Minor changes in previously approved research

The nature of the research project. The prospective subject should be told explicitly that research is being conducted, what the purpose of the research is, and how participants are being recruited. The actual study hypothesis need not be stated.

The Procedures of the Study. Participants need to know what they will be asked to do in the research project. On a practical level, they should be told how much time will be required and how often. Procedures that are not standard clinical care should be identified as such. Alternative procedures or treatments that may be available outside the study should be discussed. If the study involves blinding or randomization, these concepts should be explained in terms the participant can understand. In interview or questionnaire research, participants should be informed of the topics to be addressed.

The Risks and Potential Benefits of the Study and the Alternatives to Participating in the Study. Medical, psychosocial, and economic harms and benefits should be described in lay terms. Also, potential participants need to be told the alternatives to participation, for example, whether the intervention in a clinical trial is available outside the study. Concerns have been voiced that often the information provided to participants understates the risks and overstates the benefits (11,12). For example, research on new drugs is sometimes described as offering benefits to participants. However, most promising new interventions, despite encouraging preliminary results, show no significant advantages over standard therapy. Often participants have a "therapeutic misconception" that the research intervention is designed to provide them a personal benefit (13). Investigators should make clear that it is not known whether the study drug is more effective than standard therapy and that promising drugs can cause serious harms.

Consent Forms. Written consent forms are generally required to document that the process of informed consent—discussions between an investigator and the subject—has occurred. The consent form needs to contain all the information that must be disclosed under the provisions of 45 CFR § 46.116 . Alternatively, a short form may be used, which states that the required elements of informed consent have been presented orally. If the short form is used, there must be a witness to the oral presentation, and the witness must sign the short consent form as well as the participant.

IRBs usually have sample consent language and forms that they prefer investigators to use. IRBs may require more information to be disclosed than the Common Rule requires. Investigators should be familiar with the templates and suggestions from their IRBs.

Participants' Understanding of Disclosed Information. Ethically, the crucial issue regarding consent is not what information the researcher discloses but whether participants understand the risks and benefits of the research project. Research participants commonly have serious misunderstandings about the goals of research and the procedures and risks of the specific protocol (1,14). In discussions and consent forms, researchers should avoid technical jargon and complicated sentences. IRBs have been criticized for excessive focus on consent forms rather than on whether potential participants have understood pertinent information (1). Strategies to increase comprehension by participants include having a study team member or a neutral educator spend more time talking one-on-one with study participants, simplifying consent forms, using a question and answer format, providing information over several visits, and using audiotapes or videotapes (15). In research that involves substantial risk or is controversial, investigators should consider assessing whether participants have appreciated the disclosed information (16).

The Voluntary Nature of Consent. Ethically valid consent must be voluntary as well as informed. Researchers must minimize the possibility of coercion or undue influence. Examples of undue influence are excessive payments to participants or asking staff members or students to volunteer for research. An undue influence is ethically problematical because participants might discount the risks of a research project or find it too difficult to decline to participate. Participants must understand that declining to participate in the study will not compromise their medical care and that they may withdraw from the project at any time.

Exceptions to consent. Table 14.3 explains how informed consent or written consent forms may not be needed in several situations. First, activities that do not obtain identifiable private information on living persons is not considered human subjects research. Second, the activity may qualify for an exemption from the Common Rule. These provisions permit exceptions to informed consent for many projects that carry out secondary analyses of existing data or biological materials. Under HIPAA, the exceptions to individual authorization for research differ somewhat from exceptions and waivers of informed consent under the Common Rule. HIPAA allows research to

---

TABLE 14.3   **Is Informed Consent Required Under the Common Rule?**

1. Is the activity human subjects research as defined in § 46.012(e) and (f)?
   - Is there an intervention or interaction with a living person?
   - Does the researcher obtain identifiable private information?
   If the answer to both questions is NO, then the Common Rule does not apply

2. Does the activity quality for an exemption from the Common Rule under 45 CFR § 46.101(b)
   - Existing data, documents, records, or specimens, provided that the investigator records data in a way that it cannot be linked to the subject OR that the data or specimens are publicly available.
   - Surveys, interviews, observation of public behavior, provided that subjects cannot be identified AND responses could not put participants at risk for legal, financial, or social risk.
   - Educational practices in educational settings.

3. Does the project qualify for a waiver or modification of informed consent under § 46.116(d)?
   - the research involves no more than minimal risk to the subjects; AND
   - the waiver or alteration will not adversely affect the rights and welfare of the subjects; AND
   - the research could not practicably be carried out without the waiver or alteration; AND
   - whenever appropriate, the subjects will be provided with additional pertinent information after participation.

4. Does the research project qualify for a waiver of signed consent forms under § 46.117(c)?
   - The only record linking the subject and the research would be the consent document and the principal risk is a breach of confidentiality OR
   - The research is minimal risk and involves no procedures for which written consent is normally required outside the research context.
   - The research presents no more than minimal risk to participants and
   - The waiver or alteration would not adversely affect the rights and welfare of participants and
   - The research otherwise could not practicably be carried out

be carried out without authorization if the data set does not contain certain specified participant identifiers.

Subjects Who Lack Decision-Making Capacity. When participants are not capable of giving informed consent, permission to participate in the study should be obtained from the subject's legally authorized representative. Also, the protocol should be subjected to additional scrutiny, to ensure that the research question could not be studied in a population that is capable of giving consent.

Risks and Benefits

Researchers need to maximize the benefits and minimize the risks of research projects. Researchers must anticipate risks that might occur in the study; and modify the protocol to reduce risks to an acceptable level. Measures might include identifying and excluding persons who are very susceptible to adverse events, appropriate monitoring for adverse events, and training staff in how to identify and respond to serious adverse events. An important aspect of minimizing risk is maintaining participants' confidentiality.

Confidentiality

Breaches of confidentiality may cause stigma or discrimination, particularly if the research addresses sensitive topics such as psychiatric illness, alcoholism, or sexual behaviors. Strategies for protecting confidentiality include coding research data, storing it in locked cabinets, protecting or destroying the key that identifies subjects, and limiting personnel who have access to identifiers. However, investigators should not make unqualified promises of confidentiality. Confidentiality may be breached if research records are audited or subpoenaed, or if conditions are identified that legally must be reported. Researchers have a moral and legal obligation to override confidentiality to prevent harm in such situations as child abuse, certain infectious diseases, and serious threats of violence by psychiatric patients. In projects where information about such situations can be foreseen, the protocol should specify how field staff should respond, and participants should be informed of these plans.

Investigators can forestall subpoenas in legal disputes by obtaining confidentiality certificates from the Public Health Service if the research project involves sensitive information, such as sexual attitudes or practices, use of alcohol or drugs, illegal conduct, or mental health, or any information that could reasonably lead to stigma or discrimination (17). These certificates allow the investigator to withhold names or identify characteristics of the participants from people not connected with the project, even if faced with a subpoena or court order. The research need not be federally funded. However, these certificates do not apply to audits by funding agencies or the FDA.

■ RESEARCH PARTICIPANTS WHO REQUIRE ADDITIONAL PROTECTIONS

Some participants might be "at greater risk for being used in ethically inappropriate ways in research" (18). Such vulnerable persons might have difficulty giving voluntary and informed consent or might be more susceptible to adverse events.

Types of Vulnerability

Identifying different types of vulnerability allows researchers to adopt safeguards tailored to the specific type of vulnerability.

Cognitive or Communicative Impairments. Persons with impaired cognitive function may have difficulty understanding information about a study and deliberating about the risks and benefits of the study.

Vulnerability because of Power Differences. Persons who reside in institutions, such as prisoners or nursing home residents, might feel pressure to participate in research. In these institutions, those in authority control the daily routine and life choices of the residents (19). Residents might not appreciate that they may decline to participate in research, without retaliation by authorities or jeopardy to other aspects of their everyday lives.

In addition, if the investigator in the research project is also a participant's treating physician, the participant might find it difficult to decline to participate in research. Participants might fear that if they decline, the physician will not be as interested in their care or that they might have difficult getting timely appointments. This might particularly be a concern for patients at a specialized clinic or hospital, who have few alternative sources of care.

Social and Economic Disadvantages. Persons with poor access to health care and low socioeconomic status may join a research study to obtain payment, a physical examination, or screening tests, although they would regard the risks as unacceptable if they had a higher income. Poor education or low health literacy may make it both difficult for participants to comprehend information about the study and also make them unduly influenced by other people.

Special Federal Regulations for Vulnerable Participants
Research on Children. Investigators must obtain both the permission of the parents and the assent of the child when developmentally appropriate. In addition, research with children involving more than minimal risk is circumscribed. Such research is permissible if it presents the prospect of direct benefit to the child. If the research offers no such prospect, it may still be approved by the IRB, provided that the increase over minimal risk is minor and the research is likely to yield generalizable knowledge of vital importance about the child's disorder or condition.

Research on Prisoners. Prisoners may not feel free to refuse to participate in research and may be unduly influenced by cash payments, living conditions, or parole considerations. Federal regulations limit the types of research that are permitted and require both stricter IRB review and approval by the Department of Health and Human Services.

Research on Pregnant Women, Fetuses, and Embryos. Extra protections and restrictions are required when research is carried out on fetuses and embryos or pregnant women.

■ RESPONSIBILITIES OF INVESTIGATORS

Scientific Misconduct
In several highly publicized cases, researchers made up or altered research data or enrolled ineligible participants in clinical trials (20–23). Such conduct gives incorrect answers to the research question, undermines public trust in research, and threatens public support of federally funded research (24).

The federal government defines research misconduct as fabrication, falsification, and plagiarism, as the website of the Office for Research Integrity explains. **Fabrication** is making up results and recording or reporting them. **Falsification** is manipulating research materials, equipment, or procedures or changing or omitting data or results, so that the research record misrepresents the actual findings. **Plagiarism** is appropriating another person's ideas, results, or words without giving appropriate credit.

The federal definition of misconduct requires perpetrators to act intentionally in the sense that they are aware that their conduct is wrong. Research misconduct does not include honest error or legitimate scientific differences of opinion, which are a normal part of the research process. The federal definition also excludes other wrong actions, such as double publication, failure to share research materials, and sexual harassment (25). Such inappropriate behavior should be dealt with by the principal investigator and institution.

When research misconduct is alleged, both the federal funding agency and the investigator's institution have the responsibility to carry out a fair and timely inquiry or investigation (26). During an investigation, both whistleblowers and accused scientists have rights that must be respected. Whistleblowers need to be protected from retaliation, and accused scientists need to be told the charges and given an opportunity to respond. Punishment for proven research misconduct may include suspension of a grant, debarment from future grants, and other administrative, criminal, or civil procedures.

Authorship

Authorship of scientific papers results in prestige, promotions, and grants for researchers. Therefore investigators are eager to receive credit for publications. Researchers also need to take responsibility for problems with published articles (27). In several cases of scientific misconduct, coauthors of manuscripts containing fabricated, falsified, or plagiarized data denied knowledge of the misconduct. The rise in multiple-authored papers has made it more difficult to assign accountability for published articles.

Problems with authorship include guest authorship and ghost authorship. Guest or honorary authors are persons who have made only trivial contributions to the paper, for example, by providing access to participants, reagents, laboratory assistance, or funding (28). Ghost authors are individuals who made substantial contributions to the paper but are not listed as authors; generally ghost authors are employees of pharmaceutical companies or public relations officers. In one study, 21% of articles had guest authors and 13% ghost authors (29).

Medical journals have set criteria for authorship (30). Authors must make substantial contributions to (a) the conception and design of the project, or the data analysis and interpretation, and (b) the drafting or revising of the article; they must also (c) give final approval of the manuscript. Mere acquisition of funding, data collection, or supervision of a research group does not justify authorship, instead warranting an acknowledgment. Because there is no agreement on criteria for first, middle, or last author, it has been suggested that the contributions of each author to the project be described in the published article (31).

Disagreements commonly arise among the research team regarding who should be an author or the order of authors. These issues are best discussed explicitly and decided at the beginning of a project. Collaborators subsequently might not carry out the tasks they agreed to, for example, failing to carry out data analyses or prepare a first draft. Changes in authorship should be negotiated when decisions are made to shift responsibilities for the work. Detailed suggestions have been made on how to carry out such negotiations diplomatically (32).

Conflicts of Interest

Researchers may have conflicting interests that might impair their objectivity and undermine public trust in research (33,34). Even the perception of a conflict of interest may be deleterious (35).

Types of Conflicts of Interests.

- *Dual roles for clinician-investigators.* An investigator may be the personal physician of an eligible research participant. Such participants might fear that their future care will be jeopardized if they decline to participate in the research, or they may not distinguish between research and treatment. Furthermore, what is best for a particular participant may differ from what is best for the research project. In this situation, the welfare of the participant should be paramount, and the physician must do what is best for the participant.
- *Financial conflicts of interests.* Studies of new drugs are commonly funded by pharmaceutical companies or biotechnology firms. The ethical concern is that certain financial ties may lead to bias in the design and conduct of the study, the overinterpretation of positive results, or failure to publish negative results (33,36, 37). If investigators hold stock or stock options in the company making the drug or device under study, they may reap large financial rewards if the treatment is shown to be effective, in addition to their compensation for conducting the study. Furthermore, investigators may lose well-paying consulting arrangements if the drug proves ineffective.

Responding to Conflicting Interests.
Researchers can respond to some conflicts of interests by substantially eliminating the potential for bias. Other situations, however, have such great potential for conflicts of interest that they should be avoided.

- *Minimize conflicting interests.* In well-designed clinical trials, several standard precautions help keep competing interests in check. Investigators can be **blinded** to the intervention a subject is receiving, to prevent bias in assessing outcomes. An independent **data safety monitoring board** (DSMB), whose members have no conflict of interest, can review interim data and terminate the study if the data provide convincing evidence of benefit or harm. The **peer review** process for grants, abstracts, and manuscripts also helps eliminate biased research.

    Physicians should separate the roles of investigator in a research project and clinician providing the research participant's medical care, whenever possible. A member of the research team who is not the treating physician should handle consent discussions and follow-up visits that are part of the study.

    If research is funded by a pharmaceutical company, academic-based investigators need to ensure that the contract gives them **control over the primary data and statistical analysis**, and the **freedom to publish findings**, whether or not the investigational drug is found to be effective (36,38). The investigator has an ethical obligation to take responsibility for all aspects of the research, ensuring that the work is done rigorously. The sponsor may review the manuscripts, make suggestions, and ensure that patent applications have been filed before the article is submitted to a journal. However, the sponsor must not have power to veto or censor publication (36).

- *Disclose conflicting interests.* Conflicts of interest should be disclosed to the IRB and research participants. In a landmark court case, the California Supreme Court declared that physicians need to "disclose personal interests unrelated to the patient's health, whether research or economic, that may affect the physician's professional judgment (39)." Medical journals commonly require authors to disclose such conflicts of interest when manuscripts are submitted or published (40,41). Although disclosure itself is a small step, it may deter investigators from ethically problematical practices.
- *Manage conflicts of interest.* If a particular study presents concerns about a conflict of interest, the research institution may require additional safeguards, such as closer monitoring of the informed consent process.
- *Prohibit certain situations.* To minimize conflicts of interest, researchers from academic institutions should not hold stock or stock options in a company that has a financial interest in the intervention being studied, nor be an officer in the company (42–44). Many universities, however, allow investigators to have de minibus holdings under $10,000.

ETHICAL ISSUES SPECIFIC TO CERTAIN TYPES OF RESEARCH

Randomized Clinical Trials

Although randomized controlled trials are the most rigorous design for evaluating interventions (see Chapter 10), they present special ethical concerns because the intervention is determined by chance. The ethical justification for assigning treatment by randomization is that the arms of the protocol are in equipoise. That is, current evidence does not prove that either arm is superior. Even if some experts believe that one arm offers more effective treatment, other experts believe the opposite (45). Furthermore, individual participants and their personal physicians must find randomization acceptable. If physicians believe strongly that one arm of the trial is superior and can provide the intervention in that arm outside the study, they cannot in good faith recommend that their patients enter the trial. Also, the participant might not consider the arms equivalent, for example, when the trade-offs between benefit and adverse effects differ markedly in a comparison of medical and surgical approaches to a disease (46).

Interventions for control groups also raises ethical concerns. According to the principle of "do no harm," it is problematic to withhold therapies that are known to be effective. Hence the control group should receive the current standard of care. However, placebo controls may still be justified in short-term studies that do not offer serious risks to participants, such as studies of mild hypertension and mild, self-limited pain. Participants need to be informed of effective interventions that are available outside the research study. Dilemmas about the control group are particularly difficult when the research participants have such poor access to care that the research project is the only practical way for them to receive adequate health care.

It is unethical to continue a clinical trial if there is compelling evidence that one arm is safer or more effective. Furthermore, it would be wrong to continue a trial that will not answer the research question because of low enrollment, few outcome events, or high drop out rates. The periodic analysis of interim data in a clinical trial by an independent DSMB can determine whether a trial should terminated prematurely (47). Such interim analyses should not be carried out by the researchers themselves, because unblinding investigators to interim findings can lead to bias if the study continues. Procedures for examining interim data and statistical stopping rules should be specified in the protocol (Chapter 11).

Clinical trials in developing countries present additional ethical dilemmas, as Chapter 18 discusses.

Research on Previously Collected Specimens and Data

Such research offers the potential for significant discoveries. For example, DNA testing on a large number of stored biological specimens that are linked to clinical data may identify genes that increase the likelihood of developing a disease or responding to a particular treatment. Large biobanks of blood and tissue samples allow future studies to be carried out without the collection of additional samples. Research on previously collected specimens and data offers no physical risks to participants. However, there are ethical concerns. Consent for future studies is problematic because no one can anticipate what kind of research might be carried out later. Furthermore, participants may object to the use of data and samples in certain ways (48). Breaches of confidentiality may occur and may lead to stigma and discrimination. Even if individual participants are not harmed, groups may be harmed. Historically, genetics research in the United States led to eugenics abuses, such as forced sterilization of persons with mental retardation or psychiatric illness (49).

When biological specimens are collected, consent forms should allow participants to agree to or refuse certain broad categories of future research using the specimens. For example, participants might agree to allow their specimens to be used in future research on related conditions or for any kind of future study that is approved by an IRB and scientific review panel. Participants should also know whether the code identifying individual participants will be retained or shared with other researchers. Furthermore, participants should understand that research discoveries from the biobank may be patented and developed into commercial products. Several national biobanks in Europe have required commercial users of the biobanks to make payments to the government, so that the population that contributed the samples will derive some financial benefit.

OTHER ISSUES

Payment to Research Participants

Participants in clinical research deserve payment for their time and effort and reimbursement for out-of-pocket expenses such as transportation and childcare. Practically speaking, compensation may be needed to enroll and retain participants. The widespread practice is to offer higher payment for studies that are very inconvenient or risky. However, such incentives also raise ethical concerns about undue inducement. If participants are paid more to participate in riskier research, poor persons may undertake risks against their better judgment. To avoid undue influence, it has been suggested that participants be compensated only for actual expenses and the time, at an hourly rate for unskilled labor (50).

SUMMARY

1. Investigators must assure that their projects observe the **ethical principles** of **respect for persons, beneficence**, and **justice**.

2. Investigators must assure that research meets the requirements of applicable **federal regulations. Informed consent** from participants and **IRB** review are the key features of these regulations. During the informed consent process, investigators must explain to potential participants the **nature of the project** and the **risks, potential benefits**, and **alternatives**.

3. **Vulnerable populations,** such as **children, prisoners, pregnant women,** and people with **cognitive deficiency** or **social disadvantage** require additional protections.

4. Researchers must have **ethical integrity**. They must not commit scientific misconduct, including **fabrication, falsification**, or **plagiarism**. They should deal with **conflicts of interest** appropriately and follow criteria for appropriate **authorship**.

5. In certain types of research, additional ethical issues must be addressed. In randomized clinical trials, the intervention arms must be in **equipoise**, control groups must receive **appropriate interventions**, and the trial must not be continued once it has been demonstrated that one intervention is safer or more effective. When research is carried out on previously collected specimens and data, special attention needs to be given to **confidentiality**.

REFERENCES

1. Institute of Medicine. *Responsible research: a systems approach to protecting research participants*. Washington, DC: National Academies Press, 2003.
2. National Commission for the Protection of Human Subjects of Biomedical and Behavioral Research. *The belmont report: ethical principles and guidelines for the protection of human subjects of biomedical and behavioral research*. Washington, DC: US Government Printing Office, 1979.
3. Levine C, Dubler NN, Levine RJ. Building a new consensus: ethical principles and policies for clinical research on HIV/AIDS. *IRB* 1991;13:1–17.
4. Department of Health and Human Services. *Protection of human subjects*. 45 CFR 56. Available at <http://www.hhs.gov/ohrp/humansubjects/guidance/45cfr46.htm>. 2005
5. US General Accounting Office. *Continued vigilance critical to protecting human subjects*. Washington, DC: Government Accounting Office, 1996.
6. Office of the Inspector General. *Institutional review boards: their role in reviewing approved research*. Washington, DC: Department of Health and Human Services, 1998.
7. Institutional Review Board (IRB). *Through an expedited review procedure*. 63 Federal Register 60364–60367. Available at: <http://www.hhs.gov/ohrp/humansubjects/guidance/expedited98.htm>. (1998)
8. Department of Health and Human Services. 45 CFR Parts 160 and 164. Standards for Privacy of Individually Identifiable Health Information. *Fed Regist* 2002;67:53182–53273.
9. National Institutes of Health. Protecting Personal Health Information in Research: Understanding the HIPAA Privacy Rule. http://privacyruleandresearch.nih.gov/. Accessed July 28, 2003.

10. Gunn PP, Fremont AM, Bottrell M, et al. The Health Insurance Portability and Accountability Act Privacy Rule: a practical guide for researchers. *Med Care* 2004;42(4):321–327.

11. Advisory Committee on Human Radiation Experiments. *Final report*. New York: Oxford University Press, 1998.

12. King NM. Defining and describing benefit appropriately in clinical trials. *J Law Med Ethics* 2000;28(4):332–343. Winter

13. Lidz CW, Appelbaum PS. The therapeutic misconception: problems and solutions. *Med Care* 2002;40(9 Suppl):V55–V63.

14. Wendler D, Emanuel EJ, Lie RK. The standard of care debate: can research in developing countries be both ethical and responsive to those countries' health needs? *Am J Public Health* 2004;94(6):923–928.

15. Flory J, Emanuel E. Interventions to improve research participants' understanding in informed consent for research: a systematic review. *JAMA* 2004;292(13):1593–1601.

16. Woodsong C, Karim QA. A model designed to enhance informed consent: experiences from the HIV prevention trials network. *Am J Public Health* 2005;95(3):412–419.

17. Wolf L, Lo B. Using the law to protect confidentiality of sensitive research data. *IRB* 1999;21:4–7.

18. National Bioethics Advisory Commission. *Ethical and policy issues in international research*. Rockville, MD: National Bioethics Advisory Commission, 2001.

19. Goffman E. *Asylums;~essays on the social situation of mental patients and other inmates*. Garden City, NY: Anchor Books, 1961.

20. Culliton B. Coping with fraud: the Darsee case. *Science* 1983;220:31–35.

21. Relman AS. Lessons from the Darsee affair. *N Engl J Med* 1983;308:1415–1417.

22. Engler RL, Covell JW, Friedman PJ, et al. Misrepresentation and responsibility in medical research. *N Engl J Med* 1987;317(22):1383–1389.

23. Kassirer JP, Angell M. The journal's policy on cost-effectiveness analyses. *N Engl J Med* 1994;331(10):669–670.

24. Dingell JD. Shattuck lecture—misconduct in medical research. *N Engl J Med* 1993;328:1610–1615.

25. Friedman PJ. Advice to individuals involved in misconduct accusations. *Acad Med* 1996;71(7):716–723.

26. Mello MM, Brennan TA. Due process in investigations of research misconduct. *N Engl J Med* 2003;349(13):1280–1286.

27. Rennie D, Flanagin A. Authorship! authorship! guests, ghosts, grafters, and the two-sided coin. *JAMA* 1994;271:469–471.

28. Shaprio DW, Wenger NS, Shapiro MS. The contributions of authors to multiauthored biomedical research papers. *JAMA* 1994;271:438–442.

29. Flanagin A, Carey LA, Fontranarosa PB, et al. Prevalence of articles with honorary authors and ghost authors in peer-reviewed medical journals. *JAMA* 1998;280:222–224.

30. Lundberg GD, Glass RM. What does authorship mean in a peer-reviewed medical journal? *JAMA* 1996;276:75.

31. Rennie D, Yank V, Emanuel L. When authorship fails: a proposal to make contributors accountable. *JAMA* 1997;278:579–585.

32. Browner WS. *Publishing and presenting clinical research*. Baltimore, MD: Lippincott Williams & Wilkins, 1999.

33. Relman AS. Economic incentives in clinical investigation. *N Engl J Med* 1989;320:933–934.

34. Bekelman JE, Li Y, Gross CP. Scope and impact of financial conflicts of interest in biomedical research: a systematic review. *JAMA* 2003;289(4):454–465.

35. Thompson DF. Understanding financial conflicts of interest. *N Engl J Med* 1993;329:573–576.

36. Rennie D, Flanagin A. Thyroid storm. *JAMA* 1997;277:1238–1243.

37. DeAngelis CA. Conflict of interest and the public trust. *JAMA* 2000;284:2237–2238.

38. Hillman AL, Eisenberg JM, Pauly MV, et al. Avoiding bias in the conduct and reporting of cost-effectiveness research sponsored by pharmaceutical companies. *N Engl J Med* 1991;324(19):1362–1365.

39. Moore v. Regents of University of California, 51 Cal.3d 120; Cal Rptr. 146, 793 P.2d 479 (1990).

40. Rennie D, Flanagin A. Conflicts of interest in the publication of science. *JAMA* 1991; 266:266–267.

41. Angell M, Kassirer JP. Editorials and conflicts of interest. *N Engl J Med* 1996;335(14): 1055–1056.

42. Healy B, Campeau L, Gray R, et al. Conflict-of-interest guidelines for a multicenter clinical trial of treatment after coronary-artery bypass-graft surgery. *N Engl J Med* 1989; 320(14):949–951.

43. Topol EJ, Armstrong P, Van de Werf F, et al. Confronting the issues of patient safety and investigator conflict of interest in an international trial of myocardial reperfusion. *J Am Coll Cardiol* 1992;19:1123–1128.

44. Association of American Medical Colleges. *Protecting subjects, preserving trust, promoting progress—policy and guidelines for the oversight of individual financial interests in human subjects research*. Washington, DC: Association of American Medical Colleges, 2001.

45. Freedman B. Equipoise and the ethics of clinical research. *N Engl J Med* 1987;317:141– 145.

46. Lilford RJ. Ethics of clinical trials from a bayesian and decision analytic perspective: whose equipoise is it anyway? *BMJ* 2003;326(7396):980–981.

47. Slutsky AS, Lavery JV. Data safety and monitoring boards. *N Engl J Med* 2004;350(11): 1143–1147.

48. National Bioethics Advisory Commission. *Research on human stored biologic materials*. Rockville, MD: National Bioethics Advisory Commission, 1999.

49. Kevles DJ. *In the name of eugenics: genetics and the uses of human heredity*. New York: Knopf, 1985.

50. Dickert N, Grady C. What's the price of a research subject? Approaches to payment for research participation. *N Engl J Med* 1999;341:198–203.

15 Designing Questionnaires and Interviews

Steven R. Cummings and Stephen B. Hulley

Much of the data in clinical research is gathered using **questionnaires** or **interviews**. For many studies, the validity of the results depends on the quality of these **instruments**. In this chapter we will describe the components of questionnaires and interviews and outline procedures for developing them.

DESIGNING GOOD INSTRUMENTS

Open-Ended and Closed-Ended Questions

There are two basic types of questions, open-ended and closed-ended, which serve somewhat different purposes. **Open-ended questions** are particularly useful when it is important to hear what respondents have to say in their own words. For example:

What habits do you believe increase a person's chance of having a stroke?

_____

_____

Open-ended questions leave the respondent **free** to answer with fewer limits imposed by the researcher. They allow participants to report more information than is possible with a discrete list of answers, but the responses may be less complete. A major **disadvantage** is that open-ended questions usually require qualitative methods or special systems (such as coding dictionaries for symptoms and health conditions) to code and analyze the responses, which takes more time than entering data from closed-ended responses, and may require subjective judgments. Open-ended questions are often used in exploratory phases of question design because they facilitate understanding a concept as respondents express it. Phrases and words used by respondents can form the basis for more structured items in a later phase.

Closed-ended questions are more common and form the basis for most standardized measures. These questions ask respondents to choose from two or more preselected answers:

Which of the following do you believe increases the chance of having a stroke?

(check all that apply)

☐ *Smoking*

☐ *Being overweight*

☐ *Stress*

☐ *Drinking alcohol*

Because closed-ended questions provide a list of possible alternatives from which the respondent may choose, they are quicker and **easier to answer** and the answers are **easier to tabulate** and analyze. In addition, the list of possible answers often helps clarify the meaning of the question. Finally, closed-ended questions are well suited for use in multi-item scales designed to produce a single score.

On the other hand closed-ended questions have several **disadvantages.** They lead respondents in certain directions and do not allow them to express their own, potentially more accurate, answers. The set of answers may not be **exhaustive** (i.e., not include all possible options, e.g., the list does not include *sexual activity* or *dietary salt*). One solution is to include an option such as "*Other (please specify)*" or "*None of the above.*" When a single response is desired, the respondent should be so instructed and the set of possible responses should also be **mutually exclusive** (i.e., the categories should not overlap) to ensure clarity and parsimony.

When the question allows more than one answer, instructing the respondent to mark "*all that apply*" is not ideal. This does not force the respondent to consider each possible response, and a missing item may represent either an answer that does not apply or an overlooked item. It is better to ask respondents to mark each possible response as either "*yes*" or "*no*" as in the example.

Which of the following do you believe increases the chance of having a stroke?

	Yes	No	Don't know
Smoking	☐	☐	☐
Being overweight	☐	☐	☐
Stress	☐	☐	☐
Drinking alcohol	☐	☐	☐

The visual analog scale (VAS) is another option for recording answers to closed-ended questions using lines or other drawings. The participant is asked to mark a line at a spot, along the continuum from one extreme to the other, that best represents his characteristic. It is important that the words that anchor each end describe the most extreme values for the item of interest. Here is a VAS for pain severity:

Please use an X to mark the place on this line that best describes the severity of your pain in general over the past week.

_____

None   *Unbearable*

For convenience of measurement, the lines are often 10-cm long and the score is the distance, in centimeters, from the lowest extreme (Example 15.1).

Example 15.1 Illustrated Use of a Visual Analog Scale for Rating the Severity of Pain

_____X_____
None   *Unbearable*

This is a 10-cm line, and the mark is 3.0 cm from the end (30% of the distance from none to unbearable) so the respondent's pain would be recorded as having a severity of 3.0, or 30%.

VASs are attractive because they rate characteristics on a continuous scale; they may be more sensitive to change than ratings based on categorical lists of adjectives. An alternative approach is to provide numbers to circle instead of a line. This may be easier to score, but some participants may find it difficult to understand, so it is important to explain and give examples of how to answer the question.

Formatting

On questionnaires, it is customary to describe the purpose of the study and how the data will be used in a brief statement on the cover. Similar information is usually presented at the beginning of an interview as part of obtaining consent. To ensure accurate and standardized responses, all instruments must have instructions specifying how they should be filled out. This is true not only in self-administered questionnaires, but also for the forms that interviewers use to record responses.

Sometimes it is helpful to provide an example of how to complete a question, using a simple question that is easily answered (Example 15.2).

Example 15.2 Instructions on How to Fill Out a Questionnaire that Assesses Dietary Intake

These questions are about your usual eating habits during the past 12 months. Please mark your usual serving size and write down how often you eat each food in the boxes next to the type of food.

For example, if you drink a medium (6 oz) glass of apple juice about three times a week, you would answer:

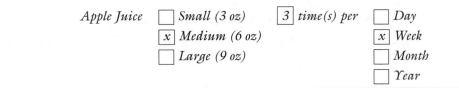

To improve the flow of the instrument, questions concerning major subject areas should be grouped together and introduced by headings or short descriptive statements. To warm up the respondent to the process of answering questions, it is helpful to begin with emotionally neutral questions such as name and contact information. More sensitive questions can then be placed in the middle, and questions about personal characteristics such as income or sexual function are often placed at the end of the instrument. For each question or set of questions, particularly if the format differs from that of other questions on the instrument, instructions must indicate clearly how to respond.

If the instructions include different time frames, it is sometimes useful to repeat the time frame at the top of each new set of questions. For example, questions such as

How often have you visited a doctor during the past year?

During the past year, how many times have you been a patient in an emergency department?

How many times were you admitted to the hospital during the past year?

can be shortened and tidied as follows:

During the past year, how many times have you

> *visited a doctor?*

> *been a patient in an emergency department?*

> *been admitted to a hospital?*

The **visual design** of the instruments should make it as easy as possible for respondents to complete all questions in the correct sequence. If the format is too complex, respondents or interviewers may skip questions, provide the wrong information, and even refuse to complete the instruments.

A **neat** format with **plenty of space** is more attractive and easier to use than one that is crowded or cluttered. Although investigators often assume that a questionnaire will appear shorter by having fewer pages, the task is more difficult when more questions are crowded onto a page. Response scales should be spaced widely enough so that it is easy to circle or check the correct number without the mark accidentally including the answer above or below. When an open-ended question is included, the space for responding should be big enough to allow respondents with large handwriting to write comfortably in the space. People with visual problems, including many elderly subjects, will appreciate large type (e.g., font size 14) and high contrast (black on white).

Possible answers to closed-ended questions should be lined up vertically and preceded by boxes or brackets to check, or by numbers to circle, rather than open blanks:

How many different medicines do you take everyday? (Check one)

☐ *None*

☐ *1–2*

☐ *3–4*

☐ *5–6*

☐ *7 or more*

(Note that these response options are exhaustive and mutually exclusive.)

Sometimes the investigator may wish to follow up certain answers with more detailed questions. This is best accomplished by a **branching question**. Respondents' answers to the initial question, often referred to as a "screener," determine whether they are directed to answer additional questions or skip ahead to later questions. For example:

Have you ever been told that you have high blood pressure?

☐ *Yes* ⟶ *How old were you when you were first told you had high blood pressure?*

         ☐☐ *years old*

☐ *No*

↓

Go to question 11

Branching questions save time and allow respondents to avoid irrelevant or redundant questions. Directing the respondent to the next appropriate question is done by using arrows to point from response to follow-up questions and including directions such as "*Go to question 11*" (see Appendix 15.1).

If questionnaires or data will be entered by **scanning** the forms, the format of the questions and the page may be dictated by the requirements of the software used for scanning. It is important to understand the requirements of the data entry program and use the appropriate software to develop the forms (Chapter 16).

Wording
Every word in a question can influence the validity and reproducibility of the responses. The objective should be to construct questions that are simple, are free of ambiguity, and encourage accurate and honest responses without embarrassing or offending the respondent.

- *Clarity.* Questions must be as clear and specific as possible. In general, concrete words are preferred over abstract words. For example, to measure the amount of exercise respondents get, asking, "*How much exercise do you usually get?*" is less clear than "*During a typical week, how many hours do you spend in vigorous walking?*"
- *Simplicity.* Questions should use simple, common words that convey the idea and avoid technical terms and jargon. For most people, for example, it is clearer to ask about "*drugs you can buy without a doctor's prescription*" than to ask about "*over-the-counter medications*": sentences should also be simple, using the fewest words and simplest grammatical structure that convey the meaning.

- *Neutrality.* Avoid "loaded" words and stereotypes that suggest that there is a most desirable answer. Asking, "*During the last month, how often did you drink too much alcohol?*" will discourage respondents from admitting that they drink a lot of alcohol. "*During the last month, how often did you drink more than five drinks in one day?*" is a more factual, less judgmental, and less ambiguous question.

Sometimes it is useful to set a tone that permits the respondent to admit to behaviors and attitudes that may be considered undesirable. For example, when asking about a patient's compliance with prescribed medications, an interviewer or a questionnaire may use an introduction: "*People sometimes forget to take medications their doctor prescribes. Does that ever happen to you?*" Wording of these introductions can be tricky. It is important to give respondents permission to admit certain behaviors without encouraging them to exaggerate.

Collecting information about potentially **sensitive** areas like sexual behavior or income is especially difficult. Some people feel more comfortable answering these types of questions in self-administered questionnaires than in interviews, but a skillful interviewer can sometimes reveal open and honest answers. In personal interviews, it may be useful to put potentially embarrassing responses on a card so that the respondent can answer by simply pointing to a response.

Setting the Time Frame

Many questions are designed to measure the frequency of certain habitual or recurrent behaviors, like drinking alcohol or taking medications. To measure the frequency of the behavior it is essential to have the respondent describe it in terms of some unit of time. If the behavior is usually the same day after day, such as taking one tablet of a diuretic every morning, the question can be very simple: "*How many tablets do you take a day?*"

Many behaviors change from day to day, season to season, or year to year. To measure these, the investigator must first decide what aspect of the behavior is most important to the study: the average or the extremes. For example, a study of the effect of chronic alcohol intake on the risk of cardiovascular disease may need a measurement of average consumption during a period of time. On the other hand, a study of the role of alcohol in the occurrence of falls may need to know how frequently the respondent drank enough alcohol to become intoxicated.

Questions about average behavior can be asked in two ways: asking about "usual" or "typical" behavior or counting actual behaviors during a period of time. For example, an investigator may determine average intake of beer by asking respondents to estimate their usual intake:

About how many beers do you have during a typical week (one beer is equal to one 12-oz can or bottle, or one large glass)?

☐☐ *beers per week*

This format is simple and brief. It assumes, however, that respondents can accurately average their behavior into a single estimate. Because drinking patterns often change markedly over even brief intervals, the respondent may have a difficult time deciding what is a typical week. Faced with questions that ask about usual or typical behavior, people often report the things they do most commonly and ignore the extremes. Asking about drinking on typical days, for example, will under-estimate alcohol consumption if the respondent drinks unusually large amounts on weekends.

An alternative approach is to quantify exposure during a certain period of time.

During the last 7 days, how many beers did you have (one beer is equal to one 12-oz can or bottle, or one large glass)?

☐☐ *beers in the last 7 days*

The goal is to ask about the shortest recent segment of time that accurately represents the characteristic over the whole period of interest for the research question. The best length of time depends on the characteristic. For example, patterns of sleep can vary considerably from day to day, but questions about sleep habits during the past week may adequately represent patterns of sleep during an entire year. On the other hand, the frequency of unprotected sex may vary greatly from week to week so questions about unprotected sex should cover longer intervals.

Using **diaries** may be a more accurate approach to keep track of events, behaviors, or symptoms that happen episodically (such as *falls*) or that vary from day to day (such as *pain following surgery* or *vaginal bleeding*). This may be valuable when the timing or duration of an event is important or the occurrence is easily forgotten. Participants can enter these data into electronic devices, and the approach allows the investigator to calculate an average daily score of the object or behavior being assessed. However, this approach can be time consuming for participants and can lead to more missing data than the more common retrospective questions. The use of diaries assumes that the time period assessed was typical, and the self-awareness involved in using diaries can alter the behavior being recorded.

Avoid Pitfalls
- *Double-barreled questions.* Each question should contain only one concept. Questions that use the words *or* or *and* sometimes lead to unsatisfactory responses. Consider this question designed to assess caffeine intake: "*How many cups of coffee or tea do you drink during a day?*" Coffee contains much more caffeine than tea and differs in other ways, so a response that combines the two beverages is not as precise as it could be. When a question attempts to assess two things at one time, it is better to break it into two separate questions. "(1) *How many cups of coffee do you drink during a typical day?*" and "(2) *How many cups of tea do you drink during a typical day?*"
- *Hidden assumptions.* Sometimes questions make assumptions that may not apply to all people who participate in the study. For example, a standard depression item asks how often respondents have felt this way in the past week: "*I felt that I could not shake off the blues even with help from my family.*" This assumes that respondents have families and ask for emotional support; for those who do not have a family or who do not seek help from their family, it is difficult to answer the question.
- *The question and answer options don't match.* It is important that the question match the options for the answer, a task that seems simple but is often done incorrectly. For example, the question, "*Have you had pain in the last week?*" is

sometimes matched with response options of "*never*," "*seldom*," "*often*," "*very often*," which is grammatically incorrect and can be confusing to respondents. (The question should be changed to "*How often have you had pain in the last week?*" or the answer should be changed to "*yes*" or "*no*.") Another common problem occurs when questions about intensity are given agree/disagree options. For example, a respondent may be given the statement "*I am sometimes depressed*" and then asked to respond with "*agree*" or "*disagree*." For those who are often depressed, it is unclear how to respond; disagreeing with this statement could mean that the person is often depressed or never depressed. In such a case, it is usually clearer to use a simple question about how often the person feels depressed matched with options about frequency (*never, sometimes, often*).

Scales and Scores to Measure Abstract Variables

It is difficult to quantitatively assess abstract concepts, such as quality of life, from single questions. Therefore abstract characteristics are commonly measured by generating scores from a series of questions that are organized into a scale.

Using multiple items to assess a concept may have other advantages over single questions or several questions asked in different ways that cannot be combined. Compared with the alternative approaches, multi-item scales can increase the range of possible responses (e.g., a multi-item quality-of-life scale might generate scores that range from 1 to 100 whereas a single question rating quality of life might produce four or five responses from "poor" to "excellent"). A disadvantage of multi-item scales is that they produce results (*quality of life = 46.2*) that can be difficult to understand intuitively.

Likert scales are commonly used to quantify attitudes, behaviors, and domains of health-related quality of life. These scales provide respondents with a list of statements or questions and asks them to select a response that best represents the rank or degree of their answer. Each response is assigned a number of points.

For each item, circle the one number that best represents your opinion:

	Strongly Agree	Agree	Neutral	Disagree	Strongly Disagree
a. Smoking in public places should be illegal.	1	2	3	4	5
b. Advertisements for cigarettes should be banned.	1	2	3	4	5
c. Public funds should be spent for antismoking campaigns.	1	2	3	4	5

An investigator can compute an overall score for a respondent's answers by simply summing the score for each item, or averaging the points for all nonmissing items. For example, a person who answered that he or she strongly agreed that smoking in public places should be illegal (one point) and advertisements for cigarettes be banned (one point) but disagreed that public funds should be spent for antismoking advertising (four points) would have a total score of 6. Simply adding up or averaging item scores assumes that all the items have the same weight and that each item is measuring the same general characteristic.

The **internal consistency** of a scale can be tested statistically using measures such as **Cronbach's alpha** (1) that assess the overall consistency of a scale. Cronbach's alpha is calculated from the correlations between scores on individual items. Values of this measure above 0.70 are usually acceptable, and 0.80 or more is excellent. Lower values for internal consistency indicate that some of the individual items may be measuring different characteristics.

Creating New Questionnaires and Scales

Sometimes an investigator needs to measure a characteristic for which there is no standard questionnaire or interview approach. When no adequate measure can be found of a concept that is important to the research, it is necessary to create new questions or develop a new scale. The task can range from the creation of a single new question about a minor variable in one study (*How frequently do you cut your toenails?*) to developing and testing a new multi-item scale for measuring the primary outcome (*sexual quality of life*) for a major study or line of investigation. At the simplest end of this spectrum, the investigator may use good judgment and basic principles of writing good questions to develop an item that should then be pretested to make sure it is clear and produces appropriate answers. At the other extreme, developing a new instrument to measure an important concept may need a systematic approach that can take years from initial draft to final product.

The latter process often begins by generating potential items for the instrument from interviews with individuals and **focus groups** (small groups of people who are relevant to the research question and who are invited to spend 1 or 2 hours discussing specific topics pertaining to the study with a group leader). Once the instrument has been drafted, the next step is to invite critical review by peers, mentors, and experts. The investigator then proceeds with the iterative sequence of pretesting, revising, shortening, and validating that is described in the next section. The development of the National Eye Institute Visual Function Questionnaire illustrates this process (Example 15.3).

Example 15.3 Development of a New Multi-Item Instrument

The National Eye Institute Visual Function Questionnaire exemplifies the painstaking development and testing of a multi-item instrument. Mangione and colleagues devoted several years to creating and testing the scale because it was intended to serve as a primary measurement of outcome of many studies of eye disease (2–4). They began by interviewing patients with eye diseases about the ways that the conditions affected their lives. Then they organized focus groups of patients with the diseases and analyzed transcripts of these sessions to choose relevant questions and response options. They produced and pretested a long questionnaire that was administered to hundreds of participants in several studies. They used data from these studies to identify items that made the largest contribution to variation in scores from person to person and to shorten the questionnaire from 51 to 25 items.

Because the creation and validation of new multi-item instruments is time consuming, it should generally only be undertaken for variables that are central to a study, and when existing measures are inadequate or inappropriate for the people who will be included in the study.

STEPS IN ASSEMBLING THE INSTRUMENTS FOR THE STUDY

There are a number of steps in developing a set of instruments for a particular study.

Make a List of Variables

Before designing an interview or questionnaire instrument, the researcher should write a detailed list of the information to be collected and concepts to be measured in the study. It can be helpful to list the role of each item (e.g., predictors, outcomes, and potential confounders) in answering the main research questions.

Collect Existing Measures

Assemble a file of questions or instruments that are available for measuring each variable. When there are several alternative methods, it is useful to create an electronic file for each variable to be measured and then to find and file copies of candidate questions or instruments for each item. It is important to use the best possible instruments to measure the main predictors and outcomes of a study, so most of the effort of collecting alternative instruments should focus on these **major variables**.

There are several sources for instruments. A good place to start is to collect instruments from other investigators who have conducted studies that included measurements of interest. Many standard instruments have been compiled and reviewed in books, review articles, and electronic sources accessed through NIH, CDC or other Web sites. There are collections of instruments on the Web that can be found by searching for key terms such as "health outcomes questionnaires." Instruments can also be found by examining published studies of similar topics and by calling or writing the authors.

Borrowing instruments from other studies has the advantage of saving development time and allowing results to be compared with those of other studies. On the other hand, existing instruments may not be entirely appropriate for the question or the population, or they may be too long. It is ideal to use existing instruments without modification. However, if some of the items are inappropriate (as may occur when a questionnaire developed for one cultural group is applied to a different setting), it may be necessary to delete, change, or add a few items.

If a good established instrument is too long, the investigator can contact those who developed the instrument to see if they have shorter versions. Deleting items from established scales risks changing the meaning of scores and endangering comparisons of the findings with results from studies that used the intact scale. Shortening a scale can also diminish its reproducibility or its sensitivity to detect changes. However, it is sometimes acceptable to delete sections or "subscales" that are not essential to the study while leaving other parts intact.

Compose a Draft

The first draft of the instrument should include more questions about the topic than will eventually be included in the instrument. The first draft should be formatted just as a final questionnaire would be.

Revise

The investigator should read the first draft carefully, attempting to answer each question as if he were a respondent and trying to imagine all possible ways to misinterpret questions. The goal is to identify words or phrases that might be confusing or misunderstood by even a few respondents and to find abstract words or jargon that could be translated into simpler, more concrete terms. Questions that are complex should be split into two or more questions. Colleagues and experts in questionnaire design should be asked to review the instrument, considering the content of the items as well as clarity.

Shorten the Set of Instruments for the Study

Studies usually collect more data than will be analyzed. Long interviews, questionnaires, and examinations may tire respondents and thereby decrease the accuracy and reproducibility of their responses. When the instrument is sent by mail, people are less likely to respond to long questionnaires than to short questionnaires. It is important to resist the temptation to include additional questions or measures "just in case" they might produce interesting data. Questions that are not essential to answering the main research question increase the amount of effort involved in obtaining, entering, cleaning, and analyzing data. Time devoted to unnecessary or marginally valuable data can detract from other efforts and decrease the overall quality and productivity of the study.

To decide if a concept is essential, it is useful to think ahead to analyzing and reporting the results of the study. Sketching out the final tables will help to ensure that all needed variables are included and to identify those that are less important. If there is any doubt about whether an item or measure will be used in later analyses, it is usually best to leave it out.

Pretest

Pretests should be done to clarify, refine, and time the instrument. For key measurements, large pilot studies may be valuable to find out whether each question produces an adequate range of responses and to test the validity and reproducibility of the instrument (Chapter 17).

Validate

Questionnaires and interviews can be assessed for validity (an aspect of accuracy) and for reproducibility (precision) in the same fashion as any other type of measurement (Chapter 4). The process begins with choosing questions that have **face validity**, a subjective but important judgment that the items assess the characteristics of interest, and continues with efforts to establish **content validity** and **construct validity**. Whenever feasible, new instruments can then be compared with established **gold standard** approaches to measuring the condition of interest. Ultimately, the **predictive validity** of an instrument can be assessed by correlating measurements with future outcomes.

If an instrument is intended to measure change, then its responsiveness can be tested by applying it to patients before and after receiving treatments considered effective by other measures. For example, a new instrument designed to measure quality of life in people with impaired visual acuity might include questions that have face validity (*"Are you able to read a newspaper without glasses or contact lenses?"*). Answers could be compared with the responses to an existing validated instrument (Example 15.3) among patients with severe cataracts and among those with normal eye examinations. The responsiveness of the instrument to change could be tested by comparing responses of patients with cataracts before and after curative surgery. The process of validating new instruments is time consuming and expensive, and worthwhile only if existing instruments are inadequate for the research question or population to be studied.

ADMINISTERING THE INSTRUMENTS

Questionnaires versus Interviews

There are two basic approaches to collecting data about attitudes, behaviors, knowledge, health, and personal history. Questionnaires are instruments that respondents administer to themselves, and interviews are those that are administered verbally by an interviewer. Each approach has advantages and disadvantages.

Questionnaires are generally a more efficient and uniform way to administer simple questions, such as those about age or habits of tobacco use. Questionnaires are less expensive than interviews because they do not require as much time from research staff, and they are more standardizable. **Interviews** are usually better for collecting answers to complicated questions that require explanation or guidance, and interviewers can make sure that responses are complete. Interviews may be necessary when participants will have variable ability to read and understand questions. However, interviews are more costly and time consuming, and they have the disadvantage that the responses may be influenced by the relationship between interviewer and respondent.

Both types of instruments can be standardized, but questionnaires have the advantage because interviews are inevitably administered at least a little differently each time. Both methods of collecting information are susceptible to errors caused by imperfect memory; both are also affected by the respondent's tendency to give socially acceptable answers, although not necessarily to the same degree.

Interviewing

The skill of the interviewer can have a substantial impact on the quality of the responses. **Standardizing** the interview procedure from one interview to the next is the key to maximizing reproducibility. The interview must be conducted with uniform wording of questions and uniform nonverbal signals during the interview. Interviewers must be careful to avoid introducing their own biases into the responses by changing the words or the tone of their voice. This requires training and practice.

For the interviewer to comfortably read the questions verbatim, the interview should be written in language that resembles common speech. Questions that sound unnatural or stilted when they are said aloud will encourage interviewers to improvise their own, more natural but less standardized way of asking the question.

Sometimes it is necessary to follow up on a respondent's answers to encourage him to give an appropriate answer or to clarify the meaning of a response. This "**probing**" can also be standardized by writing standard phrases in the margins or beneath the text of each question. To a question about how many cups of coffee respondents drink on a typical day, some respondents might respond "*I'm not sure; it's different from day to day.*" The instrument could include the follow-up probe: "*Do the best you can; tell me approximately how many you drink on a typical day.*"

Interviews can be conducted in person or over the telephone. **Computer-assisted telephone interviewing** (CATI) can reduce some of the costs associated with interviews while retaining most of their advantages (4) The interviewer reads questions to the respondent as they appear on the computer screen, and answers are entered directly into a database as they are keyed in. This enables immediate checking of out-of-range values. **Interactive voice response** (IVR) systems replace the interviewer with computer-generated questions that collect subject responses by telephone keypad or voice recognition(5).

In-person interviews, however, may be necessary if the study requires direct observation of participants or physical examinations, or if potential participants do not have telephones (e.g., the homeless). Some elderly and ill persons are best reached through in-person interviews where they are living.

Methods of Administering Questionnaires

There are several methods of administering questionnaires. They can be given to subjects in person or administered through the mail, by e-mail, or through a Web site. Distributing questionnaires in person allows the researcher to explain the instructions before the participant starts answering the questions. When the research requires the participant to visit the research site for examinations, questionnaires can also be sent in advance of an appointment and answers checked for completeness before the participant leaves.

E-mailed questionnaires have several advantages over those sent by US Mail, although they can only be sent to participants who have access to and familiarity with the Internet. Questionnaires sent by e-mail allow respondents an easy way to provide data without a clinic visit that can be directly entered into databases. Questionnaires on Web sites or handheld devices can produce very clean data because answers can be automatically checked for missing and out-of-range values, the errors pointed out to the respondent, and the responses accepted only after the errors are corrected.

■ SUMMARY

1. For many clinical studies, the quality of the results depends on the quality and appropriateness of the **questionnaires** and **interviews.** Investigators should take the time and care to make sure the **instruments** are as **valid** and **reproducible** as possible before the study begins.

2. **Open-ended questions** allow subjects to answer without limitations imposed by the investigator, and **closed-ended questions** are easier to answer and analyze. The response options to a closed-ended question should be **exhaustive** and **mutually exclusive.**

3. Questions should be **clear, simple, neutral,** and **appropriate** for the population that will be studied. Investigators should examine potential questions from the viewpoint of potential participants, looking for **ambiguous terms** and common pitfalls such as **double-barreled questions, hidden assumptions**, and **answer options that do not match the question.**

4. The instrument should be **easy to read,** and interview questions should be comfortable to read out loud. The **format** should fit the method for electronic data entry and be spacious and uncluttered, with instructions and arrows that direct the respondent or interviewer.

5. To measure abstract variables such as attitudes or health status, questions can be combined into **multi-item scales** to produce a total score. Such scores assume that the questions measure a single characteristic and that the responses are **internally consistent.**

6. An investigator should search out and use **existing instruments** that are known to produce valid and reliable results. When it is necessary to modify existing measures or devise a new one, the investigator should start by collecting existing measures to be used as potential models and sources of ideas.

7. The whole set of instruments to be used in a study should be **pretested** and timed before the study begins. For new instruments, small initial pretests can improve the clarity of questions and instructions; later, larger pilot studies can test and refine the new instrument's **range, reproducibility,** and **validity.**

8. **Self-administered questionnaires** are more economical than **interviews**, they are more readily standardized, and the added privacy can enhance the validity of the responses. Interviews, on the other hand, can ensure more complete responses and enhance validity through improved understanding. Administration of instruments by **computer-assisted telephone interviewing, e-mail**, and the **Internet** can enhance the efficiency of a study.

APPENDIX 15.1

An Example of a Questionnaire about Smoking

The following items are taken from a self-administered questionnaire used in our Study of Osteoporotic Fractures. Note that the branching questions are followed by arrows that direct the subject to the next appropriate question and that the format is uncluttered with the responses consistently lined up on the left of each next area.

1. Have you smoked at least 100 cigarettes in your entire life?

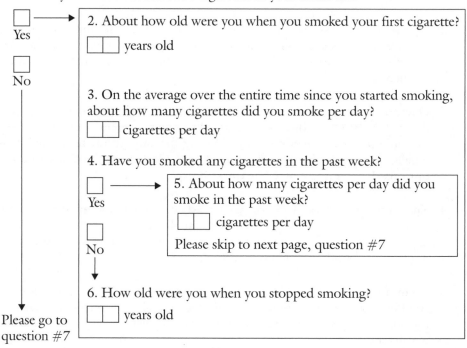

7. Have you ever lived for at least a year in the same household with someone who smoked cigarettes regularly?

☐ ⟶ 8. For about how many years, in total, have you lived with
Yes   someone who smoked cigarettes regularly at the time?

☐   ☐☐ years
No

            9. On the average over the entire time you lived with people who
               smoked, about how many cigarettes a day were smoked while
               you were at home?

               ☐☐ cigarettes per day

            10. Do you now live in the same household with someone who
                smokes cigarettes regularly?

                ☐
                Yes

                ☐
                No

11 etc.

REFERENCES

1. Bland JM, Altman DG. Cronbach's alpha. *BMJ* 1997;314:572.
2. Mangione CM, Berry S, Spritzer K, et al. Identifying the content area for the 51-item National Eye Institute Visual Function Questionnaire: results from focus groups with visually impaired persons. *Arch Ophthalmol* 1998;116:227–233.
3. Mangione CM, Lee PP, Pitts J, et al. Psychometric properties of the National Eye Institute Visual Function Questionnaire (NEI-VFQ). NEI-VFQ Field Test Investigators. *Arch Ophthalmol* 1998;116:1496–1504.
4. Anie KA, Jones PW, Hilton SR, et al. A computer-assisted telephone interview technique for assessment of asthma morbidity and drug use in adult asthma. *J Clin Epidemiol* 1996; 49:653–656.
5. Kobak KA, Greist JH, Jefferson JW, et al. Computer assessment of depression and anxiety over the phone using interactive voice response. *MD Comput* 1999;16:64–68.

16 Data Management

Michael A. Kohn

We have seen that undertaking a clinical research project requires choosing a study design, defining the population, and specifying the predictor and outcome variables. Ultimately, all information about the subjects and variables will reside in a computer **database** that will be used to store, update, and monitor the data, as well as format the data for statistical analysis. Simple study databases consisting of individual data tables can be maintained using **spreadsheet** or statistical software. More complex databases containing multiple interrelated data tables require **database management software.** Data management for a clinical research study involves defining the **data tables**, developing the **data entry** system, and **querying** the data for **monitoring** and **analysis.**

DATA TABLES

All computer databases consist of one or more data tables in which the **rows** correspond to records or **"entities"** and the **columns** correspond to fields or **"attributes".** For example, the simplest study databases consist of a single table in which each row corresponds to an individual study subject and each column corresponds to a subject-specific attribute such as name, birth date, sex, predictor or outcome status. Each row must have a column value or combination of column values that distinguishes it from the other rows. We recommend assigning a unique **identification number** ("subject ID") to each study participant. Using a unique subject identifier that has no meaning external to the study database simplifies the process of "de-linking" study data from personal identifiers for purposes of maintaining subject confidentiality.

Figure 16.1 shows a simplified data table for a cohort study of the association between neonatal jaundice and IQ score at age five (1). Each row in the table corresponds to a study subject, and each column corresponds to an attribute of that subject. The dichotomous predictor is "Jaundice," that is, whether the subject had

SubjectID	FName	DOB	Sex	Jaundice	ExDate	ExWght	ExHght	ExNPScor
2101	Robert	1/6/2005	M	☑	1/29/2010	23.9	118	104
2322	Helen	1/6/2005	F	☐	1/29/2010	18.3	109	94
2376	Amy	1/13/2005	F	☑	3/22/2010	18.5	117	85
2390	Alejandro	1/14/2005	M	☐				
2497	Isaiah	1/18/2005	M	☐	2/18/2010	20.5	121	74
2569	Joshua	1/23/2005	M	☑	2/13/2010	24.8	113	115
2819	Ryan	1/26/2005	M	☐				
3019	Morgan	1/29/2005	F	☐	2/9/2010	19.1	105	105
3031	Cody	2/15/2005	M	☐	4/16/2010	15.2	107	132
3290	Amy	2/16/2005	F	☑	4/12/2010	18.0	102	125
3374	Zachary	2/21/2005	M	☑				
3625	David	2/22/2005	M	☑	2/10/2010	19.2	114	134
3901	Jackson	2/28/2005	M	☐				

FIGURE 16.1. Simplified data table for a cohort study of the association between neonatal jaundice and IQ score at age 5. The dichotomous predictor is "Jaundice," that is whether the subject had neonatal jaundice, and the continuous outcome is "ExIQScor," which is the subject's IQ score at age 5.

neonatal jaundice, and the continuous outcome is "ExIQScor," which is the subject's IQ score at age 5.

If the study data are limited to a **single table** such as the table in Figure 16.1, they are easily accommodated in a spreadsheet or statistical package.[1] We often refer to a database consisting of a single, two-dimensional table as a **"flat-file"**.[2] Many statistical packages have added features to accommodate more than one table, but at their core, most remain single-table or flat-file databases.

The need to include more than one table in a study database (and move from spreadsheet or statistical software to data management software) often arises first when measurements are repeated on individual subjects. If the same study variable is measured on multiple occasions, then a separate table should be used to store the **repeated measurements.** The rows in this separate table correspond to individual examinations and include the examination date, the results of the exam, and most importantly, the subject identification number. In this **"relational database,"** the relationship between the table of subjects and the table of examinations is termed **one-to-many.**[3]

To improve precision and enable assessment of the interrater reliability in our infant jaundice study, the subjects receive the IQ exam multiple times from different examiners. This requires a second table of examinations in which each row corresponds to a discrete examination, and the columns represent examination date, examination results, and most importantly, the subject identification number (to link back to the subject table) (Fig. 16.2). In this two-table database structure, querying the examination table for all exams performed within a particular time period

[1] In the table shown in Fig. 16.1, the mean ($\pm$ standard deviation) IQ score for the 5 of 6 neonatal jaundice patients who had the outcome measured is 112.6 ($\pm$ 19.1). For the 4 of 7 controls with measurements, the mean is 101.3 ($\pm$ 24.2). t-test comparison of these means yields a P value of 0.46.

[2] The original meaning of the term "flat file" was a file consisting of a string of characters that could only be evaluated sequentially such as a tab-delimited text file.

[3] Strictly speaking, the term "relational" has little to do with the between-table relationships. In fact, "relation" is the formal term from mathematical set theory for a data table (2,3). However, the concept of a relational database as a collection of related tables is a useful heuristic.

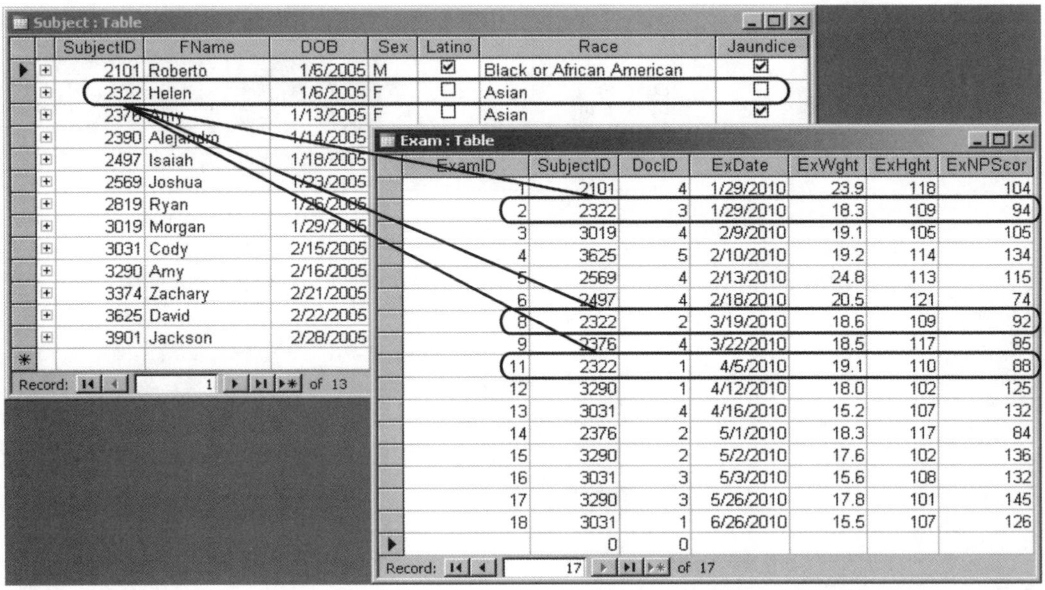

Subject : Table

	SubjectID	FName	DOB	Sex	Latino	Race	Jaundice
▶	2101	Roberto	1/6/2005	M	☑	Black or African American	☑
	2322	Helen	1/6/2005	F	☐	Asian	☐
	2376	Amy	1/13/2005	F	☐	Asian	☑
	2390	Alejandro	1/14/2005				
	2497	Isaiah	1/18/2005				
	2569	Joshua	1/23/2005				
	2819	Ryan	1/26/2005				
	3019	Morgan	1/29/2005				
	3031	Cody	2/15/2005				
	3290	Amy	2/16/2005				
	3374	Zachary	2/21/2005				
	3625	David	2/22/2005				
	3901	Jackson	2/28/2005				
*							

Record: 1 of 13

Exam : Table

	ExamID	SubjectID	DocID	ExDate	ExWght	ExHght	ExNPScor
	1	2101	4	1/29/2010	23.9	118	104
	2	2322	3	1/29/2010	18.3	109	94
	3	3019	4	2/9/2010	19.1	105	105
	4	3625	5	2/10/2010	19.2	114	134
	5	2569	4	2/13/2010	24.8	113	115
	6	2497	4	2/18/2010	20.5	121	74
	8	2322	2	3/19/2010	18.6	109	92
	9	2376	4	3/22/2010	18.5	117	85
	11	2322	1	4/5/2010	19.1	110	88
	12	3290	1	4/12/2010	18.0	102	125
	13	3031	4	4/16/2010	15.2	107	132
	14	2376	2	5/1/2010	18.3	117	84
	15	3290	2	5/2/2010	17.6	102	136
	16	3031	3	5/3/2010	15.6	108	132
	17	3290	3	5/26/2010	17.8	101	145
	18	3031	1	6/26/2010	15.5	107	126
▶		0	0				

Record: 17 of 17

FIGURE 16.2. The two-table infant jaundice study database has a table of study subjects in which each row corresponds to a single study subject and a table of examinations in which each row corresponds to a particular examination. Since a subject can have multiple examinations, the relationship between the two tables is one-to-many. The SubjectID field in the exam table links the exam-specific data to the subject-specific data.

requires searching a single exam date column. A change to a subject-specific field like birth date is made in one place, and consistency is preserved. Fields holding personal identifiers such as name and birth date appear only in the subject table with the other table(s) containing only the subject ID. The database can still accommodate subjects (such as Alejandro, Ryan, Zachary, and Jackson) who have no exams.

By structuring the database this way, instead of as a very wide and complex single table, we have eliminated redundant storage and the opportunity for inconsistencies. Relational database software will maintain **referential integrity,** meaning that it will not allow creation of an exam record for a subject who does not already exist in the subject table. Similarly, a subject may not be deleted unless and until all that subject's examinations have also been deleted.

Data Dictionaries, Data Types, and Domains

So far we have seen tables only in the spreadsheet view. Each column or field has a name and, implicitly, a data type and a definition. In the "Subject" table of Figure 16.2, "FName" is a text field that contains the subject's first name; "DOB" is a date field that contains the subject's birth date, and "Jaundice" is a yes/no field that indicates whether the study subject had neonatal jaundice. In the "Exam" table, "ExWght" is a real-number weight in kilograms and "ExIQScor" is an integer IQ score. The **data dictionary** makes these column definitions explicit. Figure 16.3 shows the subject and exam tables in table design (or "data dictionary") view. Note that the data dictionary is itself a table with rows representing fields and columns for field name, field type, and field description. Since the data

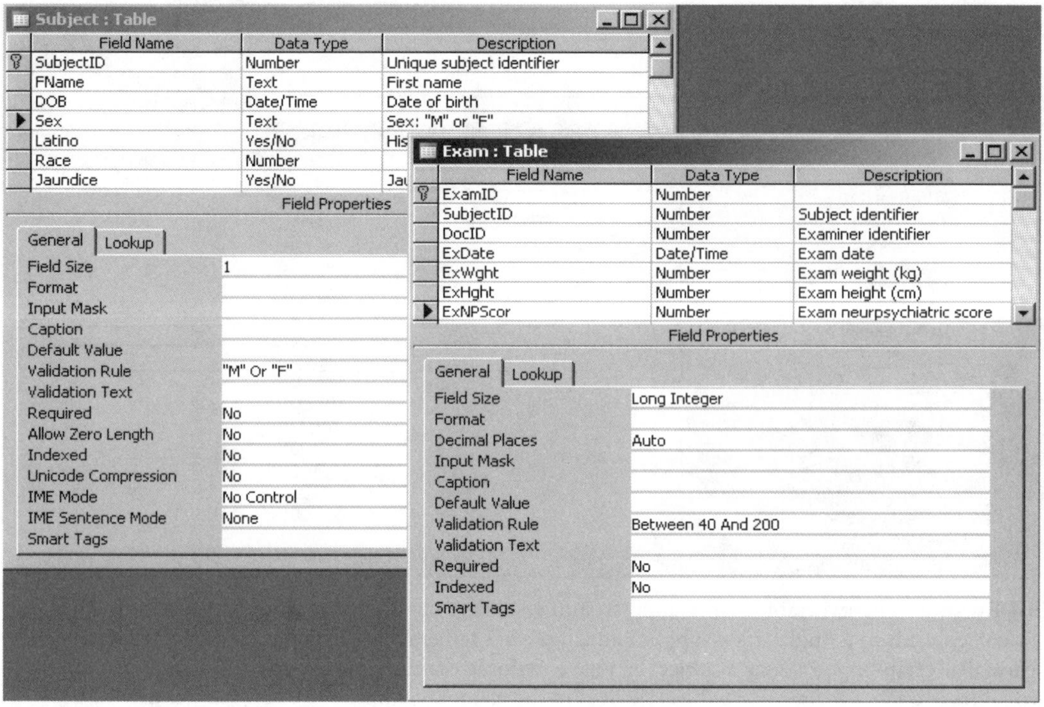

FIGURE 16.3. The table of study subjects ("Subject") and the table of measurements ("Exam") in "data dictionary" view. Each variable or field has a name, a data type, a description, and a domain or set of allowed values.

dictionary is a table of information about the database itself, it is referred to as "metadata".[4]

Each field also has a **domain** or range of allowed values. For example, the allowed values for the "Sex" field are "M" and "F".[5] The software will not allow entry of any other value in this field. Similarly, the "ExIQScor" field allows only integers between 40 and 200. Creating validation rules to define allowed values affords some protection against data entry errors. Some of the field types come with automatic validation rules. For example, the database management software will always reject a date of April 31.

Variable Names

Most spreadsheet, statistical, and database management programs allow long column headings or variable names. Philosophies and naming conventions abound. We recommend variable names that are short enough to type quickly, but long enough to be descriptive. Although they are often allowed by the software, we recommend avoiding spaces and special characters in variable names. It is generally better to use a variable name that describes the field rather than its location

---

[4] Although Figure 16.3 displays two data dictionaries, one for the "Subject" table and one for the "Exam" table, the entire database can be viewed as having a single data dictionary rather than one dictionary for each table. For each field in the database, the single data dictionary requires specification of the field's table name in addition to the field name, field type, field description, and range of allowed values.

[5] Another possibly preferable way to handle gender is to replace the "Sex" field with a "Male" field, and use 1 for yes (male sex) and 0 for no (female sex). This way the mean value for the field is the proportion of subjects who are male.

on the data collection form (e.g., "*EverSmokedCigarettes*" or "*eversmo*," instead of "*question1*.")

DATA ENTRY

Whether the study database consists of one or many tables and whether it uses spreadsheet, statistical, or database management software, a mechanism for populating the data tables is required.

Keyboard transcription. Historically, the common method for populating a study database has been to collect data on paper forms[6] and then transcribe the data by keyboard into the computer tables. The investigator or other members of the research team may fill out the paper form, or in some cases, the subject himself fills it out. Transcription can occur from the paper forms directly into the data tables (e.g, the response to question 3 on subject 10 goes into the cell at row 10, column 3) or through on-screen forms designed to make data entry easier and include automatic data validation checks. Transcription should occur as shortly as possible after the data collection, so that the subject and interviewer or data collector is still available if responses are found to be missing or out of range. Also, as discussed below, monitoring for data problems (e.g., outlier values) and preliminary analyses can only occur once the data are in the computer database.

If transcribing from paper forms, the investigator should consider **double data entry** to ensure the fidelity of the transcription. The database program compares the two values entered for each variable and presents a list of values that do not match. Discrepant entries are then checked on the original forms and corrected. Double data entry identifies data entry errors at the cost of doubling the time required for data entry. An alternative is to recheck or reenter a random proportion of the data. If the error rate is acceptably low, additional data editing is unlikely to be worth the effort and cost.

Machine-readable forms. Another alternative is to scan the data into the tables using **optical mark recognition (OMR)** and **optical character recognition (OCR)** software. Machine-readable forms can be created using this special software. When scanned or faxed, the handwritten information on these forms is read into the database. The obvious advantage is that keyboard data entry is not required. However, these systems are more difficult and costly to design and support. Because text is difficult to read accurately, machine-readable forms must be completed carefully, typically requiring that "bubbles" be filled in for categorical variables and that text be written clearly inside specific spaces. For this reason, machine-readable forms are often completed by trained study staff, rather than by study participants.

Most OMR/OCR programs provide a verification step. After the data forms are scanned or faxed, an image of the completed form and the data as they will appear in the database are presented on a computer screen. The person who is verifying the data must approve each coded value before it becomes part of the database. Systems for collecting data from machine-readable forms

[6]In clinical trials, the paper data collection form corresponding to a specific subject is commonly called a Case Report Form (CRF).

generally handle some types of data so well (bubbles, check boxes) that verification is not required, but accuracy should be tested before the study begins and retested during data collection. Machine-readable systems may be less accurate for other types of data, such as text, and it may be necessary to devote substantial time toward verification.

As with keyboard transcription, scanning of machine-readable forms should occur as shortly as possible after data collection.

Distributed data entry. If data collection occurs at multiple locations, the paper forms can be mailed or faxed to a central location for transcription or scanning into the computer database. Alternatively, the computer data entry can occur at each of the locations. In such distributed data entry, networked computers and the Internet allow direct entry into the central study database, often maintained on a server at the principle investigator's institution. Alternatively, data are stored on a local computer at the data collection site and batch transmitted by diskette, CD, tape, e-mail, or File Transfer Protocol (FTP). Government regulations require that electronic health information be either de-identified or transmitted securely (e.g., encrypted and password-protected).

Electronic data capture. Increasingly, research studies collect data using **on-screen forms**[7] or web pages, instead of paper data collection forms. This has many advantages:

- The data are keyed directly into the data tables without a second transcription step, which can be a source of error.
- The computer form can include validation checks and provide immediate feedback when an entered value is out of range.
- The computer form can also incorporate skip logic so that, for example, a question about packs per day appears only if the subject answered "yes" to a question about cigarette smoking.
- The form can still be filled out by a member of the study team or by the subject himself. When filling out a computer questionnaire, subjects may be more forthcoming about sensitive topics such as sexual behaviors and illicit drug use than during an in-person interview.
- The form may be viewed and data entered on portable, wireless devices such as handheld tablet computers and personal data assistants.

When using on-screen forms for electronic data capture, it sometimes makes sense to print out a paper record of the data immediately after collection. This is analogous to printing out a receipt after a transaction at the automated teller machine. The printout is a paper "snapshot" of the record immediately after data collection and may be used as the original or source document if a paper version is required.

Coded Responses versus Free Text

As mentioned above, defining a variable or field in a data table includes specifying its range of allowed values. For subsequent analysis, it is always preferable to limit responses to a range of coded values rather than allowing free-text responses. This is the same as the distinction made in Chapter 15 between "closed-ended" and "open-ended" questions. If the range of possible responses is unclear, initial data

---

[7]Since in clinical trials paper forms are called CRFs, electronic on-screen forms are called eCRFs.

collection during the pretesting of the study can allow free-text responses that will subsequently be used to develop coded response options.

A set of response options to a question should be **exhaustive** (all possible options are provided) and **mutually exclusive** (no two options can both be correct); response options can always be made collectively exhaustive by adding an "other" response. On-screen data collection forms and web pages provide three possible formats for displaying the mutually exclusive and collectively exhaustive response options: drop-down list, pick list (field list), or option group (Fig. 16.4.). These formats will be familiar to any research subject or data entry person who has worked with a computer form or web page. The drop-down list saves screen space but will not work if the screen form will be printed to paper for data collection. Both the pick list (which is just a drop-down list that is permanently dropped down) and the option group require more screen space, but provide a complete record when printed.

Questions with a set of mutually exclusive responses correspond to a single field in the data table. "All that apply" questions are not mutually exclusive, corresponding to as many yes/no fields as there are possible responses. By convention, response options for "all that apply" questions use square check boxes rather than the round radio buttons used for option groups with mutually exclusive responses (Fig. 16.5.). It is good practice to be consistent when coding yes/no (dichotomous) variables. In particular, 0 should always represent *no* or *absent*, and 1 should always represent *yes* or *present*. With this coding, the average value of the variable is interpretable as the proportion with the attribute.

Importing Measurements and Laboratory Results

Much study information, such as the baseline demographic information in the hospital registration system, the laboratory results in the laboratory's computer system, and the measurements made by dual energy x-ray absorptiometry scanners and Holter monitors, is already in digital electronic format. Where possible, these data should be incorporated directly in the study database to avoid the labor and potential transcription errors involved in reentering the data. For example, in the study of infant jaundice, the subject demographic data and contact information are obtained from the hospital database. Computer systems can often communicate with each other directly using a variety of protocols (web services, ODBC, XML, etc), and if this is not possible, they can produce text-delimited or fixed-column-width character files that the database software can import.

Back-end versus Front-end Software

Now that we have discussed data tables and data entry, we can make the distinction between the study database's back end and front end. The **back end** consists of the data tables themselves. The **front end** or "interface" consists of the on-screen forms or web pages used for entering, viewing, and editing the data. Table 16.1 lists some software programs used in data management for clinical research.

Simple study databases consisting of a single data table can use spreadsheet or statistical software for the back-end data table and the study personnel can enter data directly into the data table's cells, obviating the need for front-end data collection forms. More complex study databases consisting of multiple data tables require **relational database** software to maintain the back-end data tables. If the data are collected first on paper forms, entering the data will require scanning using OMR/OCR software or transcription through front-end forms or web pages. As discussed under "Electronic Data Capture" above, data may also be entered directly

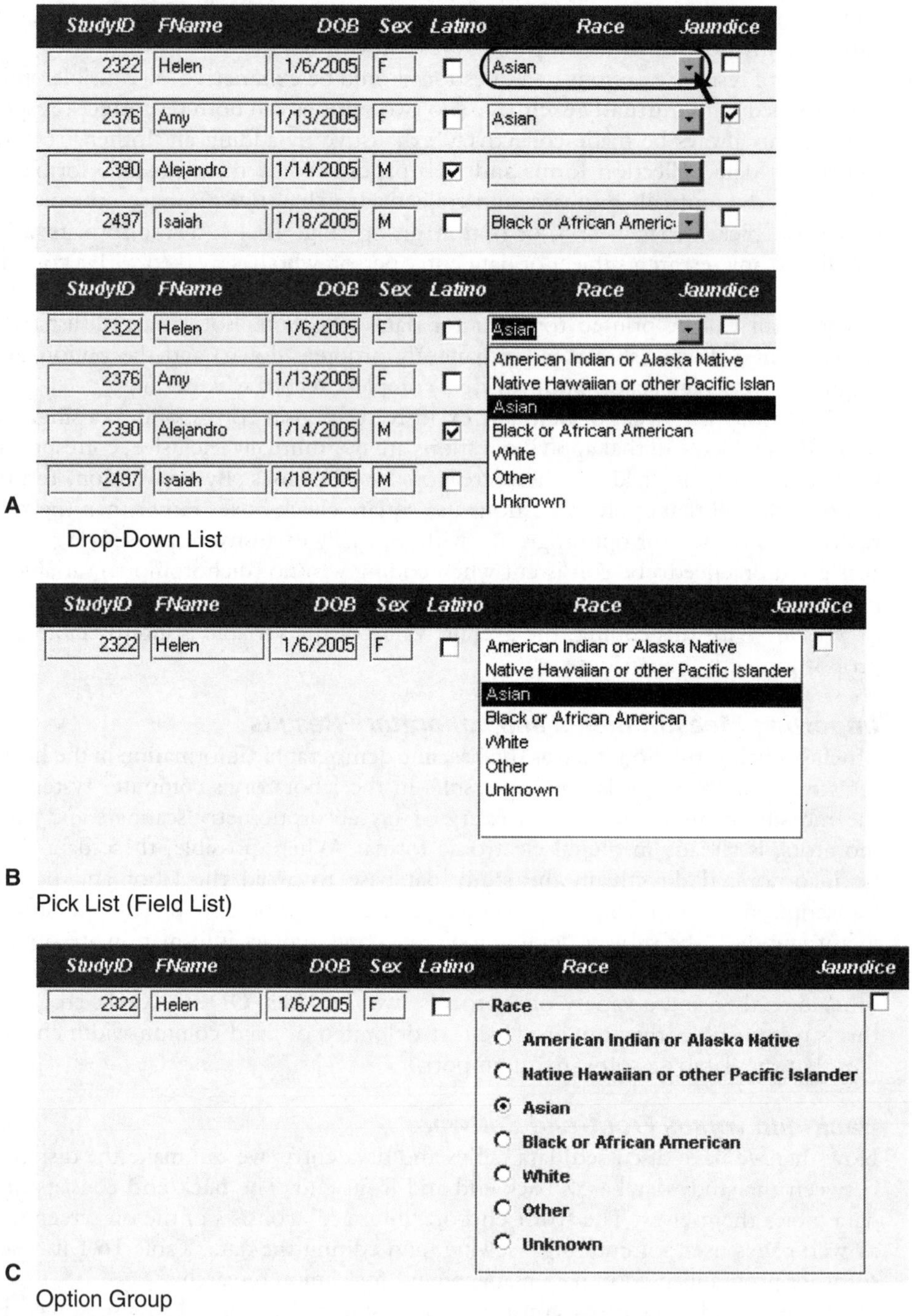

A   Drop-Down List

B   Pick List (Field List)

C   Option Group

FIGURE 16.4. Formats for entering from a mutually exclusive, collectively exhaustive list of responses. The drop-down list (**A**) saves screen space but will not work if the screen form will be printed to paper for data collection. Both the pick list (which is just a drop-down list that is permanently dropped down) (**B**) and the option group (**C**) require more screen space, but will work if printed.

TABLE 16.1	Some Software Programs Used in Research Data Management

Spreadsheet

  Excel

  Open Office Calc*

Statistical Analysis

  Statistical Analysis System (SAS)

  Statistical Package for the Social Sciences (SPSS)

  Stata

  R*

Form Scanning (Optical Mark Recognition) Software

  TeleForm

Integrated Desktop Database Systems (Back End and Front End)

  Access

  Filemaker Pro

  Open Office Base*

Enterprise Relational Database Systems (Back End)

  Oracle

  DB2

  SQL Server

  MySQL*

Interface Builders (Front End)

  Adobe Acrobat

  Front Page

  Dream Weaver

  Visual Studio

  JBuilder (Java)

  Eclipse (Java)

Integrated Web-Based Applications for Research Data Management

  Oracle Clinical

  Phase Forward Clintrial/InForm

  QuesGen

  Velos eResearch

  StudyTRAX

  Labmatrix

* Open source software.

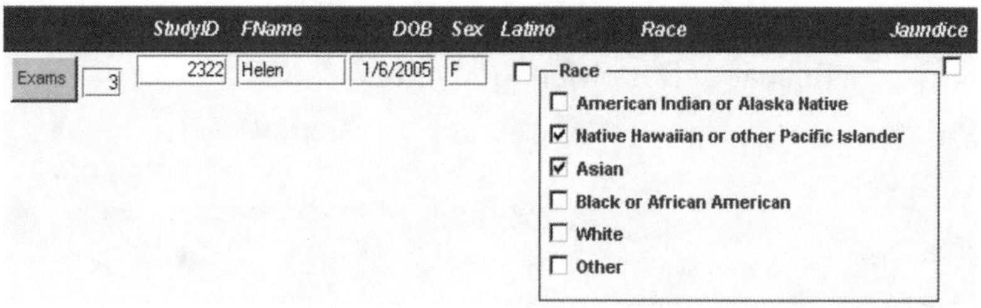

SubjectID	FName	DOB	Sex	Latino	AmerIndian	PacificIslander	Asian	AfricanAmerican	White	Other	Jaundice
2101	Robert	1/6/2005	M	☑	☐	☐	☑	☑	☐	☐	☑
2322	Helen	1/6/2005	F	☐	☐	☑	☑	☐	☐	☐	☐
2376	Amy	1/13/2005	F	☐	☐	☐	☑	☐	☐	☐	☑
2390	Alejandro	1/14/2005	M	☑	☐	☐	☐	☐	☐	☐	☐
2497	Isiah	1/18/2005	M	☐	☐	☐	☐	☑	☐	☐	☐
2569	Joshua	1/23/2005	M	☑	☐	☐	☐	☐	☐	☐	☑
2819	Ryan	1/26/2005	M	☐	☐	☐	☐	☐	☑	☐	☐

FIGURE 16.5. By convention, response options for "all that apply" questions use square check boxes. "All that apply" questions correspond to as many fields as there are possible responses.

into the front-end forms or web pages (with the option of printing out a paper "snapshot" of the record immediately after it is collected).

Some of the **statistical packages,** such as SAS, have developed data entry modules. **Integrated desktop database** programs, such as Access and Filemaker Pro, also provide extensive tools for the development of data forms. The so-called **"enterprise" database** programs, such as Oracle, SQL Server, and MySQL, are generally used for the back end, with the front end developed using separate software. Frequently, these enterprise databases are used in conjunction with a web browser–based front end.

Integrated applications, dedicated to research data management, with web-based front ends and enterprise back ends are beginning to appear (Table 16.1). At the time of publication, none of these was established in the research community, but this is a domain in which rapid progress is likely to take place.

EXTRACTING DATA (QUERIES)

Once the database has been created and data entered, the investigator will want to **organize, sort, filter**, and **view** ("query") the data. Queries are used for monitoring data entry, reporting study progress, and ultimately analyzing the results. The standard language for manipulating data in a relational database is called **Structured Query Language (SQL)** (pronounced "sequel").[8] All relational database software systems use one or another variant of SQL, but most provide a graphical interface for building queries that makes it unnecessary for the clinical researcher to learn SQL.

A query can **join** data from two or more tables, display only selected fields, and filter for records that meet certain criteria. Queries can also calculate values based on raw data fields from the tables. Figure 16.6 shows the results of a query on our infant jaundice database that filters for boys examined in January or February and

[8]SQL has 3 sublanguages: DDL—Data Definition Language, DML—Data Manipulation Language, and DCL—Data Control Language. Strictly speaking, DML is the SQL sublanguage used to view, organize, and extract data, as well as insert, update, and delete records.

SubjectID	Jaundice	Sex	ExDate	AgeInMonths	ExWght	ExHght	BMI
2101	☑	M	1/29/2010	60	23.9	118	17.2
3625	☑	M	2/10/2010	60	19.2	114	14.7
2569	☑	M	2/13/2010	61	24.8	113	19.4
2497	☐	M	2/18/2010	61	20.5	121	14.0

FIGURE 16.6. The results of a query on the infant jaundice database filtering for boys examined in January or February and calculating age in months (from birth date and date of exam) as well as body mass index (BMI—from weight and height).

calculates age in months (from birth date and date of exam) as well as body mass index (BMI—from weight and height). Note that the result of a query that joins two tables, displays only certain fields, selects rows based on special criteria, and calculates certain values, still looks like a table in spreadsheet view. One of the tenets of the relational database model is that operations on tables produce table-like results. The data in Figure 16.6 are easily exported to a statistical analysis package. (Note that no personal identifiers are included in the query.)

IDENTIFYING AND CORRECTING ERRORS IN THE DATA

The first step toward avoiding errors in the data is testing the data collection and management system as part of the overall pretesting for the study. The entire system (data tables, data entry forms, and queries) should be tested using dummy data.

We have discussed ways to enhance the fidelity of keyboard transcription, scanning of machine-readable forms, or electronic data capture once data collection begins. Values that are outside the permissible range should not get past the data entry process. However, the database should also be queried for missing values and outliers (extreme values that are nevertheless within the range of allowed values). For example, a weight of 30 kg might be within the range of allowed values for a 5-year old, but if it is 5 kg greater than any other weight in the dataset, it bears investigation. Many data entry systems are incapable of doing cross-field validation, which means that the data tables may contain field values that are within the allowed ranges but inconsistent with one another. For example, it would not make sense for a 30-kg 5-year-old to have a height of 100 cm. While the weight and height values are within range, the weight (extremely high for a 5-year old) is inconsistent with the height (extremely low for a 5-year old). A 5-year old simply cannot have a BMI of 30 kg/m^2. Such an inconsistency is easily identified using a query like the one depicted in Figure 16.6.

Missing values, outliers, inconsistencies, and other data problems are identified using queries and communicated to the study staff, who can respond to them by checking original source documents, interviewing the participant, or repeating the measurement. If the study relies on paper source documents, any resulting changes to the data should be highlighted (e.g., in red ink), dated, and signed. As discussed below, electronic databases should maintain an audit log of all data changes.

If data are collected by several investigators from different clinics or locations, means and medians should be compared across investigators and sites. Substantial differences by investigator or site can indicate systematic differences in measurement or data collection.

Data editing and cleaning should give higher priority to more important variables. For example, in a randomized trial, the most important variable is the outcome, and no errors should be tolerated. In contrast, errors in other variables, such as the date of a visit, may not substantially affect the results of analyses. Data editing is an iterative process. After errors are identified and corrected, editing procedures should be repeated until very few important errors are identified. At this point, the edited database is declared final or **"frozen,"** so that no further changes are permitted even if errors are discovered.

ANALYSIS OF THE DATA

Analyzing the data often requires creating new, derived variables based on the raw field values in the "frozen" dataset. For example, continuous variables may be dichotomized (*blood pressure above a cut point defined as hypertension*), new categories created (*specific drugs grouped as antibiotics*), and calculations made (*years of smoking x number of packs of cigarettes per day = pack years*). It is desirable to decide how missing data will be handled. "*Don't know*" is often recoded as a special category, combined with "*no*," or excluded as missing. If the study uses database software, queries can be used to derive the new variables prior to export to a statistical analysis package. Alternatively, derivation of the new fields can occur in the statistical package itself.

When multiple manuscripts are written based on the same database, it is desirable to use the same definitions of variables and handle missing data in the same way for each analysis. For example, it may be disconcerting for readers if the number of diabetic participants in the study varies. This could easily happen if diabetes is defined as self-reported diabetes in one analysis and reported use of hypoglycemic medications in another.

CONFIDENTIALITY AND SECURITY

As mentioned above, to protect research subject confidentiality, the database should assign a unique subject identifier (subject ID) that has no meaning external to the study database. In other words, the subject ID should not incorporate the subject's name, initials, birth date, or medical record number. Any database fields that contain personal identifiers should be deleted when the study is complete[9] and prior to sharing the data. If the database uses multiple tables, the personal identifiers can be kept in a separate table. Study databases that contain personal identifiers must be maintained on secure servers accessible only to authorized members of the research team, each of whom will have a user ID and password.

To be fully compliant with the Privacy Rule of the Health Insurance Portability and Accountability Act (HIPAA) (4), the database system should audit all viewing, entering, and changing of the data. Field level auditing allows determination of when a data element was changed, who made the change, and what change was made. This is necessary under the Code of Federal Regulations, Title 21, Part 11, (21 CFR 11) (5) if the electronic data will be used in an FDA New Drug Application without paper source documents.

The study database must be **backed up** regularly and **stored off-site.** Periodically, the back-up procedure should be tested by restoring a backed-up copy of the data. At the end of the study the original data, data dictionary, final database, and

---

[9]The table linking the subject ID to personal identifiers such as name, address, phone, and medical record number may be removed from the database but archived in a secure location should it ever be necessary to reidentify a subject.

the study analyses should be **archived** for future use. Such archives can be revisited in future years, allowing the investigator to respond to questions about the integrity of the data or analyses, perform further analyses to address new research questions and share data with other investigators.

SUMMARY

1. The study **database** consists of one or more data tables in which the rows correspond to **records** or "entities" (often participants) and the columns correspond to **fields** or "attributes" (often measurements).

2. The **data dictionary** specifies the **name, data type, description,** and **range of allowed values** for all the fields in the database.

3. The **data entry system** is the means by which the data tables are populated. Transcription from paper forms may require **double data entry** to ensure fidelity.

4. **Electronic data capture** through on-screen forms or web pages eliminates the transcription step. If required, a source document can be **printed** immediately after direct data entry.

5. A **spreadsheet** or statistical program is adequate for simple databases, but complex databases require the creation of a **relational database** using **database management software.**

6. Database **queries** sort and filter the data as well as calculate values based on the raw data fields. Queries are used to **monitor data entry, report on study progress,** and **format the results** for analysis.

7. To protect subject **confidentiality,** databases that contain **personal identifiers** must be stored on secure servers, with access restricted and audited.

8. Loss of the database must be prevented by regular **backups** and **off-site storage,** and by **archiving** copies of key versions of the database for future use.

REFERENCES

1. Newman TB, Liljestrand P, Jeremy RJ, et al. Five-year outcome of newborns with total serum bilirubin levels of 25 mg/dL or more. *N Engl J Med* 2006;354(18):1889–1900.
2. Codd EF. A relational model of data for large shared data banks. *Commun ACM* 1970;13(6): 377–387.
3. Date CJ. *An introduction to database systems*, 7th ed. Reading, MA: Addison Wesley, 2000.
4. NIH. *Protecting personal health information in research: understanding the HIPAA privacy rule*. NIH Publication #03-5388, September 25, 2003.
5. FDA. *Guidance for industry: computerized systems used in clinical trials (Draft guidance, Revision 1)*. September, 2004.

17 Implementing the Study and Quality Control

Deborah Grady and Stephen B. Hulley

Most of this book has dealt with the left-hand side of the clinical research model, addressing matters of design (Fig. 17.1). In this chapter we turn to the right hand, **implementation** side. Even the best of plans thoughtfully assembled in the armchair may work out differently in practice. Skilled research staff may be unavailable, study space less than optimal, participants less willing to enroll than anticipated, the intervention poorly tolerated, and the measurements challenging. The conclusions of a well-designed study can be marred by ignorance, carelessness, lack of training and standardization, and other errors in finalizing and implementing the protocol.

Successful study implementation begins with **assembling resources** including space, staff, and financial management for **study start-up.** The next task is to **finalize the protocol** through a process of **pretesting** and **pilot studies** of recruitment, measurement and intervention plans, in an effort to avoid the need for **protocol**

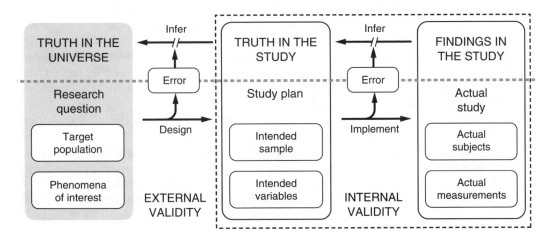

FIGURE 17.1. Implementing a research project.

revisions after data collection has begun. The study is then carried out with a systematic approach to **quality control** of **clinical** and **lab procedures** and of **data management** following the principles of **Good Clinical Practice** (GCP).

ASSEMBLING RESOURCES

Space

Conducting clinical research in which volunteer participants make study visits requires accessible, attractive, and sufficient space. Failing to successfully negotiate for space early in the study planning process can result in difficulty enrolling participants, poor adherence to study visits, incomplete data, and unhappy staff. Clinical research space must be easily accessible to participants and have adequate available parking. The space should be welcoming, comfortable, and spacious enough to accommodate staff, measurement equipment, and storage of study drug and study-related files. If there will be a physical examination, provision for privacy and hand-washing must be available. If the participants must go to other places for tests (such as the hospital laboratory or radiology department) these should be easily accessible. In some studies, such as those that enroll sick patients or deliver interventions that could be dangerous, access to cardiopulmonary resuscitation teams and equipment may be required.

Many university medical centers have clinical research centers that provide fully equipped research space that is staffed by experienced research staff. Clinical research centers often include the ability to make specialized measurements (such as caloric intake, bone density, and insulin clamp studies), and may provide access to other services (such as professional recruitment, database management, and statistical analysis). These centers provide an excellent option for carrying out clinical and translational research, but may require separate application and review procedures and reimbursement for services.

The Research Team

Research teams range in size from small—often just the investigator and a part-time research assistant—to multiple full-time staff for large studies. Regardless of size, all research teams must accomplish similar activities and fill similar roles, which are described in Table 17.1. Often, one person carries out several or many of these activities. However, some of these duties require special expertise, such as statistical programming and analyses. Some team members, such as the financial and human resources managers, are generally employed by the university or medical center, and provided by the investigator's department or unit. Regardless of the size of the study team, the principal investigator (PI) must make sure that each of the functions described in Table 17.1 is carried out.

After deciding on the number of team members and the distribution of duties, the next step is to work with a departmental administrator to find qualified and experienced job applicants. This can be difficult, because formal training for some research team members is variable, and job requirements vary from one study to the next. For example, the crucial position of project director may be filled by a person with a background in nursing, pharmacy, public health, laboratory services, or pharmaceutical research, and the duties of this position can vary widely.

TABLE 17.1	Functional Roles for Members of a Research Team*	
Role	**Function**	**Comment**
Principal investigator	Ultimately responsible for the design, conduct and quality of the study, and for reporting findings	
Project director/ clinic coordinator	Provides day-to-day management of all study activities	Experienced, responsible, meticulous, and with good interpersonal and organizational skills
Recruiter	Ensures that the desired number of eligible participants are enrolled	Knowledgeable and experienced with a range of recruitment techniques
Research assistant/clinic staff	Carries out study visit procedures and makes measurements	Physical examination or other specialized procedures may require special licenses or certification
Quality control coordinator	Ensures that all staff follow standard operating procedures (SOPs), and oversees quality control	Observes study procedures to ensure adherence to SOPs, may supervise audit by external groups such as U.S. Food and Drug Administration (FDA)
Data manager	Designs, tests, and implements the data entry, editing and storage system	
Programmer/analyst	Produces study reports that describe recruitment, adherence and data quality, conducts data analyses	Works under the supervision of the principle investigator (PI) and statistician
Statistician	Estimates sample size and power, designs analysis plan, interprets findings	Often plays a major role in overall study design and conduct
Administrative assistant	Provides clerical and administrative support, sets up meetings, etc.	Generally not eligible for federal direct cost support
Financial manager	Prepares budget and manages expenditures	Provides projections to help manage budget
Human resources manager	Assists in preparing job descriptions, hiring, evaluations	Helps manage personnel issues and problems

* In small studies, one person may take on several of these roles.

Most universities and medical centers have formal methods for posting job openings, but other avenues, such as newspaper and web-based advertisements, can be useful. The safest approach is to find staff of known competence, for example, someone working for a colleague whose project has ended.

Leadership and Team-Building

The quality of a study that involves more than one person on the research team begins with the integrity and leadership of the PI. The PI should ensure that all staff are properly trained and certified to carry out their duties. He should clearly convey the message that protection of human subjects, maintenance of privacy, completeness and accuracy of data, and fair presentation of research findings are paramount. He cannot watch every measurement made by colleagues and staff, but if he creates a sense that he is aware of all study activities and feels strongly about human subjects' protection and the quality of the data, most people will respond in kind. It is helpful to meet with each member of the team from time to time, expressing appreciation and discussing problems and solutions. A good leader is adept at delegating authority appropriately and at the same time setting up a hierarchical system of supervision that ensures sufficient oversight of all aspects of the study.

From the outset of the planning phase, the investigator should lead regular **staff meetings** with all members of the research team. Meetings should have the agenda distributed in advance, with progress reports from individuals who have been given responsibility for specific areas of the study. These meetings provide an opportunity to discover and solve problems, and to involve everyone in the process of developing the project and conducting the research. Staff meetings are enhanced by scientific discussions and updates related to the project. Regular staff meetings are a great source of morale and interest in the goals of the study and provide "on-the-job" education and training.

Most research-oriented universities and medical centers provide a wide range of **institutional resources** for conducting clinical research. These include human resources and financial management infrastructure, and centralized clinical research centers that provide space and experienced research staff. Many universities also have core laboratories where specialized measurements can be performed, centralized space and equipment for storage of biologic specimens or images, centralized database management services, professional recruitment centers, expertise regarding U.S. Food Drug Administration (FDA) and other regulatory issues, and libraries of study forms and documents. This infrastructure may not be readily apparent in a large sprawling institution, and investigators should seek to become familiar with their local resources before trying to do it themselves.

Study Start-up

At the beginning of the study, the PI must finalize the budget, develop and sign any contracts that are involved, define staff positions, hire and train staff, obtain institutional review board (IRB) approval, write the operations manual, develop and test forms, develop and test the database, and begin recruiting participants. This period of study activity is referred to as **study start-up**, and requires intensive effort before the first participant can be enrolled. Adequate time and planning for study start-up are important to the conduct of a high-quality study.

Adequate funding for conducting the study is crucial. The **budget** will have been prepared at the time the proposal is submitted for funding, well in advance of starting the study (Chapter 19). Most universities and medical centers employ staff with financial expertise to assist in the development of budgets (the **preaward manager**). It is a good idea to get to know this person well, and to thoroughly understand regulations related to various sources of funding.

In general, the rules for expending NIH and other public funding are considerably more restrictive than for industry or foundation funding. The total amount of the budget cannot be increased if the work turns out to be more costly than predicted, and shifting money across categories of expense (e.g., personnel, equipment, supplies, travel) usually requires approval by the sponsor. Universities and medical centers typically employ financial personnel whose main responsibility is to ensure that funds available to an investigator through grants and contracts are spent appropriately (the **postaward manager**). The postaward manager should prepare regular reports and projections that allow the investigator to make adjustments in the budget to make the best use of the available finances during the life of the study.

The budget for a study supported by a pharmaceutical company is part of a contract that incorporates the protocol and a clear delineation of the tasks to be carried out by the investigator and the sponsor. **Contracts** are legal documents that obligate the investigator to activities and describe the timing and amount of payment in return for specified "deliverables." University or medical center lawyers are needed to help develop such contracts and ensure that they protect the investigator's intellectual property rights, access to data, publication rights, and so forth. However, lawyers may not be familiar with the tasks required to complete a specific study, and input from the investigator is crucial, especially with regard to the scope of work.

Institutional Review Board Approval

The **IRB** must approve the study protocol, consent form and recruitment materials before recruitment can begin (Chapter 14). Investigators should be familiar with the requirements of their local IRB and the time required to obtain approval. IRB staff are generally very helpful in these matters, and should be contacted early on to discuss any procedural issues and design decisions that affect study participants.

Operations Manual and Forms Development

The study protocol is commonly expanded to create the **operations manual,** which includes the protocol, information on study organization and policies, and a detailed version of the methods section of the study protocol (Appendix 17.1). It specifies exactly how to recruit and enroll study participants, and describes all activities that occur at each visit—how randomization and blinding will be achieved, how each variable will be measured, quality control procedures, data management practices, and the statistical analysis plan. It should also include all of the questionnaires and forms that will be used in the study, with instructions on contacting the study participants; carrying out interviews, completing and coding study forms, entering and editing data, and collecting and processing specimens. An operations manual is essential for research carried out by several individuals, particularly when there is collaboration among investigators in more than one location. Even when a single investigator does all the work himself, operational definitions help reduce random variation and changes in measurement technique over time.

Design of the **data collection forms** will have an important influence on the quality of the data and the success of the study (Chapter 15). Before the first participant is recruited, the forms should be pretested. Any entry on a form that involves judgment requires explicit operational definitions that should be summarized briefly on the form itself and set out in more detail in the operations manual. The items should be coherent and their sequence clearly formatted, with arrows indicating when questions should be skipped (see Appendix 15.1). Pretesting will ensure clarity of meaning and ease of use. Labeling each page with the date, name, and ID number of the subject and staff safeguards the integrity of the data should pages become separated. Some studies use digital forms, handheld computers, personal digital assistants or other devices to collect data, bypassing the need to create paper forms. These devices must also be pretested during study start-up, and directions for their use included in the operations manual.

Database Design

Before the first participant is recruited, the database that will be used to enter, store, update, and monitor the data must be created and tested. Database design and management are discussed in Chapter 16. Depending on the type of database that will be used and the scope of the study, development and testing of the data entry and management system can require weeks to months after staff with the appropriate skills have been identified, hired, and trained. For very large studies, professional database design and management services are available, generally from organizations that provide professional research management (Clinical Research Organizations, or CROs).

Recruitment

Approaches to successfully recruiting the goal number of study participants are described in Chapter 3. We want to emphasize here that timely recruitment is the most difficult aspect of many studies. Adequate time, staff, resources, and expertise are essential, and should be planned well in advance of study start-up.

FINALIZING THE PROTOCOL

Pretests and Pilot Studies

Pretests and pilot studies are designed to evaluate the feasibility, efficiency and cost of study methods, the reproducibility and accuracy of measurements, and likely recruitment rates, outcome rates and effect sizes. The nature and scale of pretests and pilot studies depends on the study design and the needs of the study. For most studies, a series of pretests or a small pilot study serves very well, but for large, expensive studies a full-scale pilot study may be appropriate (1). It may be desirable to spend up to 10% of the eventual cost of the study to make sure that recruitment strategies will work, measurements are appropriate and sample size estimates are realistic.

Pretests are evaluations of specific questionnaires, measures, or procedures that can be carried out by study staff to assess their functionality, appropriateness and feasibility. For example, pretesting the data entry and database management system is generally done by having study staff complete forms with missing, out of range or illogical data, entering these data and testing to ensure that the data editing system identifies these errors.

Pilot studies enroll a small number of participants and require a protocol, approval by the IRB and informed consent. Important reasons for conducting a pilot study are to guide decisions about how to design recruitment approaches, measurements, and interventions. Evaluating the methods for **recruiting** study participants during a pilot study can provide rough estimates of the number who are available and willing to enroll, and test the efficiency of different recruitment approaches. Pilot studies can also give the investigator an idea of the nature of the populations he will be sampling—the distributions of age, sex, race, and other characteristics that may be important to the study. They can be designed to provide data on the feasibility of measurements, subjective reactions to each procedure and any discomfort it may have caused, whether there were questionnaire items that were not understood, and ways to improve the study.

Pilot studies may be particularly helpful for studies that involve a new **intervention,** where it is important to determine the dose or intensity, frequency, and duration of the intervention. For example, a pilot test of a new school-based AIDS education program designed to prevent HIV infection could help optimize effectiveness by determining the ideal duration of each training session and number of sessions per week.

Before the study begins, it is a good idea to test study procedures in a full-scale **dress rehearsal.** The purpose is to iron out problems with the final set of instruments and procedures. What appears to be a smooth, problem-free protocol on paper usually reveals logistic and substantive problems in practice, and the dress rehearsal will generate improvements in the approach. The investigator himself can serve as a **mock subject** to experience the study and the research team from that viewpoint.

Minor Protocol Revisions once Data Collection Has Begun

No matter how carefully the study is designed and the procedures pretested, problems inevitably appear once the study has begun. The general rule is to make as few changes as possible at this stage. Sometimes, however, protocol modifications can strengthen the study.

The decision as to whether a minor change will improve the integrity of the study is often a trade-off between the benefit that results from the improved methodology and the disadvantages of altering the uniformity of the study findings and spending time and money to change the system. Decisions that simply involve making an **operational definition** more specific are relatively easy. For example, in a study that excludes alcoholics, can a recovering alcoholic be included? This decision should be made in consultation with coinvestigators, but with adequate communication through memos and the operations manual to ensure that it is applied uniformly by all staff for the remainder of the study. Often minor adjustments of this sort do not require IRB approval, particularly if they do not involve changing the protocol that has been approved by the IRB, but the PI should ask an IRB staff member if there is any uncertainty.

Substantive Protocol Revisions once Data Collection Has Begun

Major changes in the study protocol, such as including different kinds of participants or changing the intervention or outcome, are a serious problem. Although there may be good reasons for making these changes, they must be undertaken with a view to analyzing and reporting the data separately if this will lead to a more appropriate interpretation of the findings. The judgments involved are illustrated by two examples from the Raloxifene Use for the Heart (RUTH) trial, a multicenter clinical trial of the effect of treatment with raloxifene on coronary events and breast cancer in 10,101 women at high risk for coronary heart disease (CHD) events. The initial definition of the primary outcome was the occurrence of nonfatal myocardial infarction (MI) or coronary death. Early in the trial, it was noted that the rate of this outcome was lower than expected, probably because new clinical cointerventions such as thrombolysis and percutaneous angioplasty lowered the risk. After careful consideration, the RUTH Executive Committee decided to change the primary outcome to include acute coronary syndromes other than MI. This change was made early in the trial; appropriate information had been collected on potential cardiac events to determine if these met the new criteria for acute coronary syndrome, allowing the study database to be searched for acute coronary syndrome events that had occurred before the change was made (1).

Also early in the RUTH trial, results from the Multiple Outcomes of Raloxifene Evaluation (MORE) trial showed that the relative risk of breast cancer was markedly reduced by treatment with raloxifene (2). These results were not conclusive, since the number of breast cancers was small, and there were concerns about generalizability since all women enrolled in MORE had osteoporosis. To determine if raloxifene would also reduce the risk of breast cancer in another population—older women without osteoporosis and at risk for CHD events—the RUTH Executive Committee decided to add breast cancer as a second primary outcome (1).

Each of these changes was major, requiring a protocol amendment, approval of the IRB at each clinical site, and approval of the FDA. These are examples of substantive revisions that enhanced feasibility or the information content of the study without compromising its overall integrity. Tinkering with the protocol is not always so successful. Substantive revisions should only be undertaken after weighing the pros and cons with members of the research team and appropriate advisors such as the DSMB and funding agency. The investigator must then deal with the potential impact of the change when he analyzes data and draws the study conclusions.

Closeout

At some point in all longitudinal studies and clinical trials, follow-up of participants stops. The period during which participants complete their last visit in the study is often called **"closeout."** Closeout of clinical studies presents several issues that deserve careful planning and implementation. At a minimum, at the closeout visit staff should thank participants for their time and effort and inform them that their participation was critical to the success of the study. In addition, closeout may include the following activities:

- participants (and their physicians) may be informed of the results of laboratory tests or other measurements that were performed during the study, either in person at the last visit or later by mail.
- in a blinded clinical trial, participants may be told their treatment status, either at the last visit, or by mail at the time all participants have completed the trial and the main data analyses are complete.
- a copy of the main manuscript based on the study results and a press release or other description of the findings written in lay language may be mailed to participants (and their physicians) at the time of presentation or publication.
- after all participants have completed the study, they may be invited to a reception during which the PI thanks them, discusses the results of the study, and answers questions.

QUALITY CONTROL DURING THE STUDY

Good Clinical Practice

A crucial aspect of clinical research is the approach to ensuring that all aspects of the study are of the highest quality. Guidelines for high-quality research, called **GCP**, were developed to apply specifically to clinical trials that test drugs requiring approval by the FDA or other regulatory agencies, and are defined as "a standard for the design, conduct, performance, monitoring, auditing, recording, analyses, and reporting of clinical trials that provides assurance that the data and reported results are credible and accurate, and that the rights, integrity, and confidentiality of trial subjects are protected."

Recently, these principles have been increasingly applied to clinical trials sponsored by federal and other public agencies, and to research designs other than trials (Table 17.2). GCP requirements are described in detail in the FDA Code of Federal Regulations Title 21 (3). The International Conference on Harmonization (4) provides quality control guidelines used by regulatory agencies in Europe, the United States and Japan.

GCP is best implemented by **standard operating procedures (SOPs)** for all study-related activities. The study protocol and operations manual can be considered SOPs, but often do not cover areas such as how staff are trained and certified, how the database is developed and tested, or how study files are maintained, kept confidential, and backed up. Many universities have staff who specialize in processes for meeting GCP guidelines and various templates and models for SOPs. GCP with respect to ethical conduct of research is addressed in Chapter 14, and in this chapter we focus on quality control of study procedures and data management.

Quality Control for Clinical Procedures

It is a good idea to assign one member of the research team to be the **quality control coordinator** who is responsible for implementing appropriate quality control techniques for all aspects of the study, supervising staff training and certification, and monitoring the use of quality control procedures during the study. The goal is to detect possible problems before they occur, and prevent them. The quality control coordinator may also be responsible for preparing for and acting as the contact person for audits by the IRB, FDA, study sponsor, or NIH. Quality control of clinical procedures begins during the planning phase and continues throughout the study (Table 17.3).

- *The operations manual.* The operations manual is a very important aspect of quality control that has been described earlier in this chapter. To illustrate, consider measuring blood pressure, a partially subjective outcome for which there is no

TABLE 17.2	Aspects of the Conduct of Clinical Research that are Covered by Good Clinical Practices

- The design is supported by preclinical, animal and other data as appropriate
- The study is conducted according to ethical research principles
- A written protocol is carefully followed
- Investigators and those providing clinical care are trained and qualified
- All clinical and laboratory procedures meet quality standards
- Data are reliable and accurate
- Complete and accurate records are maintained
- Statistical methods are prespecified and carefully followed
- The results are clearly and fairly reported

TABLE 17.3	Quality Control of Clinical Procedures*
Steps that precede the study	Develop a manual of operations

	Define recruitment strategies
	    Operational definitions of measurements
	    Standardized instruments and forms
	    Approach to managing and analyzing the data
	    Quality control systems
	    Systems for blinding participants and investigators

	Appoint quality control coordinator Train the research team and document this Certify the research team and document this
Steps during the study	Provide steady and caring leadership Hold regular staff meetings Special procedures for drug interventions Recertify the research team Periodic performance review Periodically compare measurements across technicians and over time

* Clinical procedures include blood pressure measurement, structured interview, chart review, etc.

feasible gold standard. The operations manual should give specific instructions for preparations before the clinic visit (including the timing of taking blood pressure medication); preparing the participant for the measurement (remove long-sleeved clothing, sit quietly for 5 minutes); choosing the proper size blood pressure cuff; locating the brachial artery and applying the cuff; inflating and deflating the cuff; and recognizing which sounds represent systolic and diastolic blood pressure.

- *Training and certification.* Standardized training of study staff is essential to high-quality research. All staff involved in the study should receive appropriate training before the study begins, and be certified as to competence with regard to key procedures and measurements. With regard to measurement of blood pressure, for example, members of the team can be trained in each aspect of the measurement, required to pass a written test on the relevant section of the operations manual and to obtain satisfactory readings on mock participants assessed simultaneously by the instructor using a double-headed stethoscope. The certification procedure should be supplemented during the study by scheduled recertifications and a log of training, certification and recertification should be maintained at the study site.

- *Performance review.* Supervisors should review the way clinical procedures are carried out by periodically sitting in on representative clinic visits or telephone calls. After obtaining the study participant's permission, the supervisor can be quietly present for at least one complete example of every kind of interview and technical procedure each member of his research team performs. This may seem awkward at first, but it soon becomes comfortable. It is helpful to use a standardized **checklist** (provided in advance and based on the protocol and operations manual) during these observations. Afterward, communication between the supervisor and the research team member can be facilitated by reviewing the checklist and resolving any quality control issues that were noted in a positive and nonpejorative fashion. The timing and results of performance reviews should be recorded in training logs.

Involving **peers** from the research team as reviewers is useful for building morale and teamwork, as well as for ensuring the consistent application of standardized approaches among members of the team who do the same thing. One advantage of using peers as observers in this system is that all members of the research team acquire a sense of ownership of the quality control process. Another advantage is that the observer often learns as much from observing someone else's performance as the person at the receiving end of the review procedure.

- *Periodic reports*. It is important to **tabulate data** on the technical quality of the clinical procedures and measurements at regular intervals. This can give clues to the presence of missing, inaccurate, or imprecise measurements. Differences among the members of a blood pressure screening team in the mean levels observed over the past 2 months, for example, can lead to the discovery of differences in their measurement techniques. Similarly, a gradual change over a period of months in the standard deviation of sets of readings can indicate a change in the technique for making the measurement. Periodic reports should also address the success of recruitment, the timeliness of data entry, the proportion of missing and out-of-range variables, the time to address data queries, and the success of follow-up and adherence to the intervention.

- *Special procedures for drug interventions*. Clinical trials that use drugs, particularly those that are blinded, require special attention to the quality control of labeling, drug delivery and storage, dispensing the medication and collecting unused medication. Providing the correct drug and dosage is ensured by carefully planning with the manufacturer and pharmacy the nature of the drug distribution approach, by overseeing its implementation, and occasionally by testing the composition of the blinded study medications to make sure they contain the correct constituents. Drug studies also require clear procedures and logs for tracking receipt of study medication, storage, distribution, and return by participants.

Quality Control for Laboratory Procedures

The quality of laboratory procedures can be controlled using many of the approaches described above for clinical procedures. In addition, the fact that specimens are being removed from the participants (creating the possibility of mislabeling) and the technical nature of laboratory tests, lead to special strategies summarized below (Table 17.4).

- *Attention to labeling*. When a participant's blood specimen or electrocardiogram is mistakenly labeled with another individual's name, it may be impossible to correct or even discover the error later. The only solution is prevention, **avoiding**

TABLE 17.4	Quality Control of Laboratory Procedures*
Steps that precede the study	Use strategies in Table 17.3
	Establish good labeling procedures
Steps during the study	Use strategies in Table 17.3
	Ensure/document proper function of equipment
	Use blinded duplicates or standard pools

* Laboratory procedures include blood tests, x-rays, electrocardiograms, radiology, pathology, etc.

transposition errors by carefully checking the participant's name and number when labeling each specimen. Computer printouts of labels for blood tubes and records speed the process of labeling and avoid the digit transpositions that can occur when numbers are handwritten. A good procedure when transferring serum from one tube to another is to label the new tube in advance and hold the two tubes next to each other, reading one out loud while checking the other; this can also be automated with scannable **bar codes.**

- *Blinding.* The task of blinding the observer is easy when it comes to measurements on specimens, and it is always a good idea to label specimens so that the technician has no knowledge of the study group or the value of other key variables. Even for apparently objective procedures, like an automated blood glucose determination, this precaution reduces opportunities for bias and provides a stronger methods section when reporting the results. However, blinding laboratory staff means that there must be clear procedures for reporting abnormal results to a member of the staff who is qualified to review the results and decide if the participant should be notified or other action should be taken. In clinical trials, there must also be strategies in place for (sometimes emergent) unblinding if laboratory measures indicate abnormalities that might be associated with the trial intervention and require immediate action.

- *Blinded duplicates and standard pools.* When specimens or images are sent to a central laboratory for chemical analysis or interpretation, it may be desirable to send blinded duplicates—a second specimen from a random subset of participants given a separate and fictitious ID number—through the same system. This strategy gives a measure of the precision of the laboratory technique. Another approach for serum specimens that can be stored frozen is to prepare a pool of serum at the outset and periodically send aliquots through the system that are blindly labeled with fictitious ID numbers. Measurements carried out on the serum pool at the outset, using the best available technique, establish its constituents; the pool is then used as a gold standard during the study, providing estimates of accuracy and precision. A third approach, for measurements that have inherent variability such as a Pap test or mammography readings, is to involve two independent, blinded readers. If both agree within predefined limits, the result is established. Discordant results may be resolved by discussion and consensus, or the opinion of a third reader.

- *Commercial laboratory contracts.* In some studies, biologic measures made on blood, sera, cells, or tissue are made under contract to commercial laboratories. The lab must be appropriately licensed and certified and a copy of these certifications should be on file in the study office. Commercial labs should guarantee timely service and provide standardized procedures for handling coded specimens, notifying investigators of abnormal results, and transferring data to the main database.

Quality Control for Data Management

The investigator should set up and pretest the data management system before the study begins (Chapter 16). This includes designing the forms for recording measurements, choosing computer hardware and software for data editing and management and designing the data editing parameters for missing, out-of-range and illogical entries, testing the data management system and planning dummy tabulations to ensure that the appropriate variables are collected (Table 17.5).

- *Missing data.* Missing data can be disastrous if they affect a large proportion of the measurements, and even a few missing values can sometimes bias the conclusions. A

TABLE 17.5	Quality Control of Data Management: Steps that Precede the Study

Be parsimonious: collect only needed variables
Select appropriate computer hardware and software for database management
Program the database to flag missing and out-of-range values
Test the database using missing and out-of-range values
Plan analyses and test with dummy tabulations
Design forms that are

>   Self-explanatory
>   Coherent (e.g., multiple-choice options are exhaustive and mutually exclusive)
>   Clearly formatted with boxes for data entry and arrows directing skip patterns
>   Printed in lower case using capitals, underlining, and bold font for emphasis
>   Esthetic and easy to read
>   Pretested and validated (see Chapter 15)
>   Labeled on every page with date, name, ID number, and/or bar code

study of the long-term sequelae of an operation that has a delayed mortality rate of 5%, for example, could seriously underestimate this complication if 10% of the participants were lost to follow-up and if death were a common reason for losing them. Erroneous conclusions due to missing data can sometimes be corrected after the fact—in this case by an intense effort to track down the missing participants—but often the measurement cannot be replaced. There are statistical techniques for **imputing missing values** based on other information (from baseline or from other follow-up visits) available for the participant. Although these techniques are useful, particularly for multivariate analysis in which the accumulation of missing data across a number of predictor variables could otherwise lead to large proportions of participants unavailable for analysis, they do not guarantee conclusions free of nonresponse bias if there are substantial numbers of missing observations.

The only good solution is to design and carry out the study in ways that avoid missing data, for example, by having a member of the research team check forms for completeness before the participant leaves the clinic, designing electronic data entry interfaces that do not allow skipped entries and designing the database so that missing data are immediately flagged for study staff (Table 17.6). Missing clinical

TABLE 17.6	Quality Control of Data Management: Steps during the Study

Flag or check for omissions and major errors while participant is still in the clinic
No errors or transpositions in ID number, name code, date on each page
All the correct forms for the specified visit have been filled out
No missing entries or faulty skip patterns
Entries are legible
Values of key variables are within permissible range
Values of key variables are consistent with each other (e.g., age and birth date)

Carry out periodic frequency distributions and variance measures to discover aberrant values
Create other periodic tabulations to discover errors (see Appendix 17.2)

measurements should be addressed while the participant is still in the clinic when it is relatively easy to correct errors that are discovered.

- *Inaccurate and imprecise data.* This is an insidious problem that often remains undiscovered, particularly when more than one person is involved in making the measurements. In the worst case, the investigator designs the study and leaves the collection of the data to his research assistants. When he returns to analyze the data, some of the measurements may be seriously biased by the consistent use of an inappropriate technique. This problem is particularly severe when the errors in the data cannot be detected after the fact. If interviews are carried out with leading questions or if blood pressure is measured differently in participants known to be receiving placebo, the database will include serious errors that are undetectable. The investigator will assume that the variables mean what he intended them to mean, and, ignorant of the problem, may draw conclusions from his study that are wrong.

  Staff training and certification, periodic performance reviews and regular evaluation of differences in mean or range of data generated by different staff members can help identify or prevent these problems. **Computerized editing** plays an important role, using data entry and management systems programmed to flag or not to allow submission of forms with missing, inconsistent, and out-of-range values. A standardized procedure should be in place for changing original data on any data form. Generally this should be done as soon after data collection as possible, and includes marking through the original entry (not erasing it), signing and dating the change. This provides an "**audit trail**" to justify changes in data and prevent fraud. On a computerized database, changing data generally requires generating a computer-based entry that is recorded with the date, staff ID, and reason for changing the data.

  Periodic tabulation and inspection of frequency distributions of important variables at regular intervals allows the investigator to assess the completeness and quality of the data at a time when correction of past errors may still be possible (e.g., by calling the participant or requesting that the participant return to the study offices), and when further errors in the remainder of the study can be prevented. A useful list of topics for quality control reports is provided in Appendix 17.2.

- *Fraudulent data.* Clinical investigators who lead research teams have to keep in mind the possibility of an unscrupulous colleague or employee who chooses fabrication of study information as the easiest way to get the job done. Approaches to guarding against such a disastrous event include taking great care in choosing colleagues and staff, developing a strong relationship with them so that ethical behavior is explicitly understood and rigorously followed by all, being alert to the possibility of fraud when data are examined, and making unscheduled checks of the primary source of the data to be sure that they are real.

Collaborative Multicenter Studies

Many research questions require larger numbers of participants than are available in a single center, and these are often addressed in collaborative studies carried out by research teams that work in several locations. Sometimes these are all in the same city or state, and a single investigator can oversee all the research teams. Often, however, collaborative studies are carried out by investigators in cities thousands of miles apart with separate funding, and administrative and regulatory structures.

Multicenter studies of this sort require special steps to ensure that all centers are using the same study procedures and producing comparable data that can be combined in the analysis of the results. A **coordinating center** establishes a communication network, coordinates the development of the operations manual, forms, and other standardized quality control aspects of the trial, trains staff at each center who will make the measurements, and oversees data management, analysis, and publication. Collaborative studies often have distributed data entry systems with computers or scanners connected through the Internet.

There is also a need for establishing a governance system with a **steering committee** made up of the PIs and representatives of the funding institution, and with various subcommittees. One **subcommittee** needs to be responsible for **quality control** issues, developing the standardization procedures and the systems for training, certification, and performance review of study staff. These tend to be complicated and expensive, providing **centralized training** for relevant staff from each center, **site visits** for performance review and data audits by coordinating center staff and peers (Appendix 17.2).

In a multicenter study, changes in operational definitions and other study methods often result from questions raised by a clinical center that are answered by the relevant study staff or committee and posted on the Internet in a running list to make sure that everyone involved in the study is aware of changes. If a significant number of changes accumulate, dated revised pages in the operations manual should be prepared that include these changes. Small single site studies can follow a simpler pattern, making notes about changes that are dated and retained in the operations manual.

A Final Thought

A common error in research is the tendency to collect **too much data.** The fact that the baseline period is the only chance to measure baseline variables leads to a desire to include everything that might conceivably be of interest, and there is a tendency to have more follow-up visits and collect more data at them than is useful. Investigators tend to collect far more data than they will ever analyze or publish.

One problem with this approach is the time consumed by measuring less important things; participants become tired and annoyed, and the quality of more important measurements deteriorates. Another problem is the added size and complexity of the database, which makes quality control and data analysis more difficult. It is wise to question the need for every variable that will be collected and to eliminate many that are optional. Including a few intentional redundancies can improve the validity of important variables, but parsimony is the general rule.

▪ SUMMARY

1. Successful study implementation begins with **assembling resources** including space, staff, and budget for **study start-up.**

2. The next task is to finalize the protocol through a process of **pretesting** and **pilot studies** of the appropriateness and feasibility of plans for **recruitment, measurements, interventions** and **outcome ascertainment** in an effort to minimize the need for subsequent protocol revisions once data collection has begun.

3. **Minor protocol revisions** after the study has begun, such as adding an item to a questionnaire or modifying an operational definition are relatively **easily accomplished,** though IRB approval may sometimes be required and data analysis may be affected.

4. **Major protocol revisions** after the study has begun, such as a change in the nature of the intervention or primary outcome, have **major implications** and should be undertaken reluctantly and with the approval of key bodies such as the DSMB, IRB, and funding institution.

5. The study is then carried out with a systematic approach under the supervision of a **quality control coordinator,** following the principles of **GCP,** and including:
    a. Quality control for **clinical procedures—operations manual, staff training** and **certification, performance review, periodic reports** (on recruitment, visit adherence, and so forth), and **team meetings.**
    b. Quality control for **laboratory procedures—blinding** and systematically **labeling** specimens taken from study participants, and using **standard pools** and **blinded duplicates.**
    c. Quality control of the **data management**—designing forms and electronic systems to enable oversight of the **completeness, accuracy,** and **integrity** of collecting, editing, entering, and analyzing the data.

6. **Collaborative multicenter studies** have special systems for managing the study and quality control.

APPENDIX 17.1

Example of an Operations Manual Table of Contents[1]

Chapter 1. Study protocol
Chapter 2. Organization and policies
    Participating units (clinical centers, laboratories, coordinating center, etc.)
    Administration and governance (committees, funding agency, safety and data monitoring, etc.)
    Policy concerns (publications and presentations, ancillary studies, conflict of interest, etc.)
Chapter 3. Recruitment
    Eligibility and exclusion criteria
    Sampling design
    Recruitment approaches (publicity, referral contacts, screening, etc.)
    Informed consent
Chapter 4. Clinic visits
    Content of the baseline visit
    Content and timing of follow-up visits
    Follow-up procedures for nonresponders
Chapter 5. Randomization and blinding procedures
Chapter 6. Predictor variables
    Measurement procedures
    Intervention, including drug labeling, delivery and handling procedures
    Assessment of compliance
Chapter 7. Outcome variables
    Assessment and adjudication of primary outcomes
    Assessment and management of other outcomes and adverse events
Chapter 8. Quality control
    Overview and responsibilities
    Training in procedures
    Certification of staff
    Equipment maintenance
    Peer review and site visits
    Periodic reports
Chapter 9. Data management
    Data collection and recording
    Data entry
    Editing, storage, and backup
    Confidentiality
    Analysis plans
Chapter 10. Data analysis
Appendices
    Letters to participants, primary providers, and so on
    Questionnaires, forms
    Details on procedures, criteria, and so on

[1] N.B. This is a model for a large multicenter trial. The manual of operations for a small study can be less elaborate.

APPENDIX 17.2

Quality Control Tables and Checklists

I. Tabulations for monitoring performance characteristics.[2]
  A. Clinic characteristics
    1. Recruitment
      a. Number of participants screened for enrollment; number rejected and tabulation of reasons for rejection
      b. Cumulative graph of number recruited compared with that required to achieve recruitment goal
    2. Follow-up
      a. Number of completed follow-up examinations for each expected visit; number seen within specified time frame
      b. Number of dropouts and participants who cannot be located for follow-up
    3. Data quantity and quality
      a. Number of forms completed, number that generated edit messages, and number of unanswered edit queries
      b. Number of forms missing
    4. Protocol adherence
      a. Number of ineligible participants enrolled
      b. Summary of data on pill counts and other adherence measures by treatment group
  B. Data center characteristics
    1. Number of forms received and number awaiting data entry
    2. Cumulative list of coding and protocol changes
    3. Timetable indicating completed and unfinished tasks
  C. Central laboratory characteristics
    1. Number of samples received and number analyzed
    2. Number of samples inadequately identified, lost, or destroyed
    3. Number of samples requiring reanalysis and tabulation of reasons
    4. Mean and variance of blind duplicate differences, and secular trend analyses based on repeat determinations of known standards
  D. Reading center characteristics
    1. Number of records received and read
    2. Number of records received that were improperly labeled or had other deficiencies (tabulate deficiencies)
    3. Analyses of repeat readings as a check on reproducibility of readings and as a means of monitoring for time shifts in the reading process

II. Site visit components:
  A. Site visit to clinical center
    1. Private meeting of the site visitors with the PI
    2. Meeting of the site visitors with members of the clinic staff
    3. Inspection of examining and record storage facilities

[2]Tables should contain results for the entire study period, and, when appropriate, for the time period covered since production of the last report. Rates and comparisons among staff and participating units should be provided when appropriate.

4. Comparison of data contained on randomly selected data forms with those contained in the computer data file
5. Review of file of data forms and related records to assess completeness and security against loss or misuse
6. Observation of clinic personnel carrying out specified procedures
7. Check of operations manuals, forms, and other documents on file at the clinic to assess whether they are up-to-date
8. Observation or verbal walk through of certain procedures (e.g., the series of examinations needed to determine participant eligibility)
9. Conversations with actual study participants during or after enrollment as a check on the informed consent process
10. Private conversations with key support personnel to assess their practices and philosophy with regard to data collection
11. Private meeting with the PI chief concerning identified problems

B. Site visit to data center
1. Review of methods for inventorying data received from clinics
2. Review of methods for data management and verification
3. Assessment of the adequacy of methods for filing and storing paper records received from clinics, including the security of the storage area and methods for protecting records against loss or unauthorized use
4. Review of available computing resources
5. Review of method of randomization and of safeguards to protect against breakdowns in the randomization process
6. Review of data editing procedures
7. Review of computer data file structure and methods for maintaining the analysis database
8. Review of programming methods both for data management and analysis, including an assessment of program documentation
9. Comparison of information contained on original study forms with that in the computer data file
10. Review of methods for generating analysis data files and related data reports
11. Review of analysis philosophy
12. Review of methods for backing up the main data file
13. Review of master file of key study documents, such as handbooks, manuals, data forms, minutes of study committees, and so on, for completeness

REFERENCES

1. Mosca L, Barrett-Connor E, Wenger NK, et al. Design and methods of the Raloxifene Use for The Heart (RUTH) Study. *Am J Cardiol* 2001;88: 392–395.
2. MORE Investigators. The effect of raloxifene on risk of breast cancer in postmenopausal women: results from the MORE randomized trial. Multiple outcomes of raloxifene evaluation. *JAMA*. 1999;281: 2189–2197.
3. Information about Good Clinical Practices in FDA Code of Federal Regulations Title 21. www.accessdata.fda.gov/scripts/cdrh/cfdocs/cfcfr/cfrsearch.cfm, October, 2006.
4. Information about Good Clinical Practices in the European Medicines Agency International Conference on Harmonization, at www.google.com/search?hl=en&q=ICH&btnG=Google+Search, or at www.ich.org/, October, 2006.

18 Community and International Studies

Norman Hearst and Thomas E. Novotny

Most clinical research takes place in university medical centers or other academic institutions. Such sites offer many advantages for conducting research, including the obvious one of having experienced researchers. An established culture, reputation, and infrastructure for research facilitate the work of everyone from novice investigator to tenured professor. Success breeds more success, thereby concentrating clinical research in centers of excellence. This chapter, in contrast, deals with research that takes place outside of such centers.

We define **community research** as research that takes place outside the usual university or medical center setting and that is designed to meet the needs of the communities where it is conducted. **International research,** particularly in poor countries, can involve many of the same challenges of establishing a research program where none existed before. Community and international research both often involve **collaboration between local investigators** and colleagues from an established research center. Such collaboration can be productive and critical in solving long-standing or emerging health problems, but it can be **challenging** because of **physical distance, cultural differences, and funding constraints.**

WHY COMMUNITY AND INTERNATIONAL RESEARCH?

Community research is often the only way to address research questions that have to do with specific settings or populations. Research in academic medical centers tends to focus on priorities that may be quite different from those in their surrounding communities, let alone those in distant places. The "10/90 gap" in health research in which 90% of the global burden of disease receives only 10% of global research investment (1) is ample justification for more collaborative research that addresses the enormous health problems of low- and middle-income countries. Furthermore, participation in the research process has benefits for a community that go beyond the value of the information collected in a particular study.

TABLE 18.1	Examples of Research Questions Requiring Local Research

What are the rates of child car seat and seat belt use in a low-income neighborhood of Chicago?

What are the patterns of antimicrobial resistance of tuberculosis isolates in Uganda?

What is the impact of a worksite-based AIDS prevention campaign for migrant farm workers in Texas?

What proportion of coronary heart disease among women in Brazil is associated with cigarette smoking?

Local Questions

Many research questions require answers available only through **local research.** National or state level data from central sources may not accurately reflect local disease burdens or the distribution of risk factors in the local community. Interventions, especially those designed to change behavior, may not have the same effect in different settings. For example, the public health effectiveness of condom promotion as an AIDS prevention strategy is quite different in the United States than in Africa (2). Finding approaches that fit local needs requires local research (Table 18.1).

Biologic data on the pathophysiology of disease and the effectiveness of treatments are usually generalizable to a wide variety of populations and cultures. But even here there can be racial or genetic differences or differences based on disease etiology. The efficacy of antihypertensive drugs is different in patients of African and European descent (3). The causative agents and patterns of antimicrobial sensitivity for pneumonia are different in Bolivia and Boston.

Greater Generalizability

Community research is sometimes useful for producing results that are more **generalizable.** For example, patients with back pain who are seen at referral hospitals are very different from patients who present with back pain to primary care providers. Studies of the natural history of back pain or response to treatment at a tertiary care center therefore may be of limited use for clinical practice in the community.

Partly in response to this problem, several **practice-based research networks** have been organized in which physicians from community settings work together to study research questions of mutual interest (4). An example is the response to treatment of patients with carpal tunnel syndrome in primary care practices (5). Most patients improved with conservative therapy; few required referral to specialists or sophisticated diagnostic tests. This contrasted with the previous literature on the disease from academic medical centers, which had indicated that the majority of patients with carpal tunnel syndrome require surgery.

Issues of generalizability are also important in **international research.** Research findings from one country will not always apply in another. Although results generalize best to where the research was done, they may also be relevant for migrant populations that originated in the country of the research. Such migrant and displaced populations are of ever increasing importance in a world that had 175 million international migrants as of the year 2000 (6).

Building Local Capacity

Clinical research should not be the exclusive property of academic medical centers. The priorities of researchers in these sites are bound to reflect the issues they encounter in their daily practice or that they believe are of general scientific or economic importance. Conducting research in the community setting ensures that questions of local importance will also be addressed.

The value of **community participation** in research goes beyond the specific information collected in each study. Conducting research has a substantial positive ripple effect by raising local scholarly standards and encouraging creativity and independent thinking. Each project builds skills and confidence that allow local researchers to see themselves as full participants in the scientific process, not just consumers of knowledge produced elsewhere. This in turn encourages more research. Furthermore, participating in research can bring intellectual and financial resources to a community and help encourage local empowerment and self-sufficiency.

■ COMMUNITY RESEARCH

In theory, community research is much like any other research. The general approach outlined in this book applies just as well in a small town in rural America or Kathmandu as it does in San Francisco or London. In practice, the greatest challenge is finding experienced colleagues or mentors with whom to interact and learn. Such help may not be available locally. This often leads to an important early decision for would-be local investigators: to work alone or in collaboration with more established investigators based elsewhere.

Starting on Your Own
Getting started in research without the help of a more experienced colleague is like teaching oneself how to swim: it is not impossible, but it is difficult. Sometimes, however, it is the only option. Following a few rules may make the process easier.

- *Start simple.* It is seldom a good idea to begin research in a community with a randomized controlled trial. Small descriptive studies producing useful local data may make more sense—better a small success than a large failure. More ambitious projects can be saved for later. For example, a descriptive study of condom use among young men in Uganda conducted by a novice local researcher served as a first step toward a larger intervention trial on AIDS prevention in that community (7,8).
- *Think of local comparative advantage.* What questions can an investigator answer in his local setting better than anyone else? This usually means leaving the development of new laboratory techniques and treatments to the academic medical centers and drug companies of the world. It is often best for a young investigator to focus on health problems or populations that are unusual elsewhere, but common in his community.
- *Network.* As discussed in Chapter 2, networking is important for any investigator. A new investigator should make whatever contact he can with scientists elsewhere who are addressing similar research questions. If formal collaborators are not available, it may at least be possible to find someone to give feedback on a draft of a research protocol, a questionnaire, or a manuscript. Attending a scientific conference in one's field of interest is a good way to make such contacts. Contacts can also be made at a distance through telephone, letters, and e-mail. Complimenting a person's work (if not overdone) can be a good way to initiate such a contact.

Collaborative Research

Because it is difficult to get started on one's own, a good way to begin research in a community is often in collaboration with more experienced researchers based elsewhere. There are two main models for such collaboration: top-down and bottom-up (9).

The **top-down** model refers to studies that originate in an academic center and involve community investigators in the recruitment of patients and the conduct of the study. This occurs, for example, in large multicenter trials that invite hospitals and clinics to enroll patients into an established research protocol. This approach has the great advantage that it comes with built-in senior collaborators who are usually responsible for obtaining the necessary resources and clearances to conduct the study.

Although one can gain valuable experience through this sort of collaboration, opportunities to develop as a researcher may be limited. Just as important, the potential benefit to one's community may be no greater than if the study had been done elsewhere. Once the study is over, the academic center or drug company may cut off involvement quickly with little or nothing left behind in the community.

In the **bottom-up** model, established investigators provide guidance and technical assistance to local investigators and communities developing their own research agendas. Some academic medical centers offer training programs for community investigators or international researchers. If one can gain access to such a program or establish an equivalent relationship, this can be ideal for building local research capacity, especially when such a partnership is sustained on a long-term basis. But establishing an institutional relationship of this type is not easy. Supporting bottom-up community research can be time consuming and therefore expensive. Most funding agencies are more interested in sponsoring specific research projects than in building local research capacity. Even when funding to cover expenses is available, experienced investigators may prefer to spend their time conducting their own research rather than helping others get started.

Community researchers need to take advantage of the potential incentives they can offer to more established investigators with whom they would like to work. In the top-down model, the most important thing they can offer is access to subjects. In the bottom-up model, the incentives can include the intrinsic scientific merit of a study in the community, coauthorship of resulting publications, and the satisfaction of helping a less experienced colleague in a worthwhile endeavor.

To start a new research program, the ideal option may be to form a long-term partnership with an established research institution. Collaboration under such a structure can include a combination of top-down and bottom-up projects. It must be remembered, however, that good research collaboration is fundamentally between individual investigators. An academic institution may provide the climate, structure, and resources that support individual collaboration, but the individuals themselves must provide the cultural sensitivity, mutual respect, hard work, and long-term commitment to make it work.

INTERNATIONAL RESEARCH

International research often involves collaboration between groups with different levels of experience and resources and therefore is subject to many of the same issues as community research. However, international research brings **additional challenges.** The issues described below are especially important.

Barriers of Distance, Language, and Culture

Because of the **distances** involved, opportunities for face-to-face **communication** between international colleagues are limited. If at all possible, colleagues on both sides should make at least one site visit to each other's institutions. International conferences may sometimes provide additional opportunities to meet, but such opportunities are likely to be rare. Fortunately, wireless communications, faxes, and e-mail (perhaps with voice-over capability and wide-band video capacity) have made international communication easier, faster, and less expensive. Good communication is possible at any distance, but it requires effort on both sides. The most modern methods of communication are of no help if they are not used regularly. Lack of frequent communication and prompt response to queries made on either side is a sign that a long-distance collaboration may be in trouble.

Language differences are often superimposed on the communication barriers caused by distance. If the first language spoken by investigators at all sites is not the same, it is important that there be a language that everyone can use. Expecting all interactions to be in English places investigators in poor countries at a disadvantage. Foreign investigators who do not speak the local language are unlikely to have more than a superficial understanding of the country's culture and cannot participate fully in many key aspects of a study, including questionnaire development and conversations with study subjects and research assistants. This is especially important in studies with behavioral components.

Even when linguistic barriers are overcome, **cultural** differences can cause serious misunderstandings between investigators and their subjects or between investigators. Literal word-by-word translations of questionnaires may have different meanings, be culturally inappropriate, or omit key local factors. Institutional norms may be different. For example, in some settings, a foreign collaborator's department chief who had little direct involvement in a study might expect to be first author of the resulting publication. Such issues should be anticipated and clearly laid out in advance as part of the important process of gaining high-level local institutional support for the project. Patience, good will, and flexibility on all sides can usually surmount problems of this type. For larger projects, it may be advisable to include an anthropologist, ethicist, or other expert on cultural issues as part of the research team.

Frequent, clear, and open communication and prompt clarification of any questions or confusion are essential. When dealing with cultural and language differences, it is better to be repetitive and risk stating the obvious than to make incorrect assumptions about what the other person thinks. Written affiliation agreements that spell out mutual responsibilities and obligations may help clarify issues such as data ownership, authorship order, publication rights, and decisions regarding the framing of research results. Development of such agreements requires the personal and careful attention of collaborators from both sides.

Issues of Funding

Because of economic inequities, collaboration between institutions in rich and poor countries is generally only possible with **funding** originating from the rich country or, less often, from other rich countries or international organizations. An increasing number of large donor organizations are active in global health research, but often their support is limited to a specific research agenda. Donor funding tends to flow through the institution in the rich country, reinforcing the subordinate position of institutions in poor countries. As in any situation with an **unequal balance of power**, this creates a potential for exploitation. When investigators from rich countries control the purse strings, it is not uncommon for them to treat their counterparts in poor countries more like employees than colleagues. International donors and funding agencies need to be especially careful to discourage this and instead to promote true joint governance of collaborative activities.

Different practices of **financial management** are another potential area for conflict between cultures. Institutions in rich countries may attempt to impose accounting standards that are difficult or impossible to meet locally. Institutions in poor countries may load budgets with computers and other equipment that they expect to keep after the study is over. Although this is understandable given their needs and lack of alternative funding sources, it is important that any subsidies beyond the actual cost of conducting the research be clearly negotiated and that the potential for diversion of funds by institutions or individuals be minimized. Conversely, institutional overheads and higher investigator salaries often create the inequitable situation of the majority of funding for collaborative research staying in the rich country even when most of the work is in the poor country.

Source country institutions and donors should pay particular attention to building the research **administration capacity** of local partners. This could mean providing administrative and budgetary training or using consultants in the field to help with local administrative tasks. Effort invested in developing administrative capacity may pay off in improved responsiveness to deadlines, more efficient reporting, avoiding unnecessary conflict, and building a solid infrastructure for future research.

Ethical Issues

International research raises **ethical issues** that must be faced squarely. All the general ethical issues for research apply (Chapter 14). Because international research presents an enhanced potential for exploitation, it also requires additional considerations and safeguards.

What, for example, is the appropriate comparison group when testing new treatments in a poor country where conventional treatment is unavailable? Placebo controls are unethical when other effective treatments are the standard of care in a community. But what is the "standard of care" in a community where most people are too poor to afford proven treatments? On the one hand, it may not be possible for investigators to provide state-of-the-art treatment to every participant in a study. On the other hand, allowing placebo controls simply because people are poor may encourage drug companies and others to test their new treatments in poor countries without proper protections and benefits for volunteers. Studies in poor countries of expensive antiretroviral drugs have drawn new attention to these concerns (10,11).

A related issue has to do with testing treatments that, even if proven effective, are unlikely to be economically accessible to the population of the host country. Are such studies ethical, even if they follow all the usual rules? If not, what proportion of study subjects should be able to afford the new treatment to make the study ethical? These questions do not have simple answers. Established international conventions governing ethical research, such as the Declaration of Helsinki, have been challenged and are subject to multiple interpretations (12,13).

A key test may be to consider why the study is being conducted in a poor country in the first place. If the true goal is to gather information to help the people of that country, this should weigh in favor of the study. Ideally, the goal of research should be sustainable change and added value for the host country (14). If, on the other hand, the goal is expediency or to avoid obstacles to doing the study in a rich country, the study should be subject to all ethical requirements that would apply in the sponsoring country.

For this and other reasons, studies in poor countries that are directed or funded from elsewhere should be approved by **ethical review boards in both countries.** Although such approval is necessary, it does not guarantee that a study is ethical. Systems for ethical review of research in many poor countries are weak or nonexistent and can sometimes be manipulated by local investigators or politicians who stand to benefit from a study. Conversely, review boards in rich countries are sometimes ignorant of or insensitive to the special issues involved in international research. Official approval does not remove the final responsibility for the ethical conduct of research from the investigators themselves.

Less talked about but also important are ethical issues in the **treatment of collaborators** from poor countries. Several issues must be agreed upon in advance. Who owns the data that will be generated? Who needs whose permission to conduct and publish analyses? Will local investigators get the support they need to prepare manuscripts for international publication without having to pay for this by giving up first authorship? How long a commitment is being made on both sides? A large recent trial in several poor countries of voluntary counseling and testing to prevent HIV infection abruptly dropped its collaborating site in Indonesia (15). According to the investigators, this was because the outcome variable of interest (HIV seroconversion) turned out to be less common at that site than projected in the study's power calculations. Although this decision made practical sense, it was perceived by the Indonesians as a breach of faith.

Other ethical issues may have to do with **local economic and political realities.** For example, a planned clinical trial of pre-exposure HIV prophylaxis with tenofovir for commercial sex workers recently was cancelled although it had been cleared by multinational ethical review boards (16). The intended study subjects were concerned that they might end up with no source of medical care for problems related to HIV infection or drug effects and were not willing to participate without guarantees of lifetime health insurance. The Prime Minister of the country intervened to stop the trial.

Finally, an explicit goal of all international collaboration should be to increase **local research capacity.** What skills and equipment will the project leave behind when completed? What training activities will take place for project staff? Will local researchers participate in international conferences? Will this be only for high-level local investigators who already have many such opportunities, or will junior colleagues have a chance as well? Will the local researchers be true collaborators and principal authors of publications, or are they simply being hired to collect data? Scientists in poor countries should ask and expect clear answers to these questions. As summarized in Table 18.2, good **communication** and long-term commitment are recurring themes in successful international collaborative research.

Risks and Frustrations

Researchers from rich countries who contemplate becoming involved in international research need to start with a realistic appreciation of the difficulties and risks involved. Launching such work is usually a long, slow process. **Bureaucratic obstacles** are common on both ends. In countries that lack infrastructure and political stability, years of work can be vulnerable to major disruption from natural or manmade **catastrophe.** In extreme cases, these can threaten the safety of project staff or investigators. For example, important collaborative AIDS research programs that had

TABLE 18.2	Strategies to Improve International Collaborative Research

Scientists in poor countries
  Choose collaborators carefully
  Learn English (or other language of collaborators)
  Become familiar with the international scientific literature in area of study
  Be sure that collaboration will build local research capacity
  Clarify administrative and scientific expectations in advance

Scientists in rich countries
  Choose collaborators carefully
  Learn the local language and culture
  Be sensitive to local ethical issues
  Encourage local collaboration in all aspects of the research process
  Clarify administrative and scientific expectations in advance

Funding agencies
  Set funding priorities based on public health need
  Encourage true collaboration rather than a purely "top-down" model
  Recognize the importance of building local research capacity
  Make subsidies for local equipment and infrastructure explicit
  Be sure that overhead and high salaries in the rich country do not take too much of the budget

been built over many years were completely destroyed by recent civil wars in Rwanda and the Congo.

Less catastrophic and more common are the daily hardships and **health risks** that expatriate researchers may face, ranging from unsafe water and malaria to smog, common crime, and traffic accidents. Key requirements to help insure safety of researchers working abroad include evacuation and repatriation insurance, good pre-travel health advice, registration with their Embassy or Consulate in the host country, and awareness of any special risks or instability in the host country. The US Centers for Disease Control and Prevention website provides excellent health information (http://www.cdc.gov/travel/), and the US Department of State website provides up-to-date information on registration, evacuation, and safety for international travelers (http://www.state.gov/travelandbusiness/).

Another frustration for researchers in poor countries is the difficulty in **applying their findings.** Even when new strategies for preventing or treating disease can be successfully developed and proven to be effective, lack of political will and resources often thwarts their widespread application. Researchers need to be realistic in their expectations, gear their work toward investigating strategies that would be feasible to implement if found effective, and be prepared to act as advocates for improving the health of the populations they study.

The Rewards

Despite the difficulties, the need for more health research in many parts of the world is overwhelming. Many investigators in major academic centers wonder how much difference their work really makes. It often seems that there are plenty of other qualified people who could do the job just about as well as they do. By participating in international research, an investigator in a rich country can sometimes have a far greater and more immediate **impact on people's lives** than would be possible by staying within the walls of his own university. This impact comes not only from the research itself but also from doing one's own small part to foster international collaboration.

Many of the potential problems with international research have their positive aspects. Although funding is harder to obtain, the same amount of money can go much further (17). Cross-cultural collaboration is as rewarding as it is difficult. The chance to have meaningful involvement and make a real contribution in a foreign land is a rare privilege. Furthermore, it can teach unexpected lessons that **enrich careers** and lives. All stand to gain through increased collaboration and expanding the traditional settings for research

SUMMARY

1. **Community and international research** is necessary to discover **regional differences** in such things as the epidemiology of a disease or the cultural factors that determine which interventions will be effective.

2. **Local participation** in clinical research can have secondary benefits to the region such as enhanced levels of **scholarship** and **self-sufficiency.**

3. Although the theoretical issues involved in research are broadly applicable, **practical issues** such as acquiring funding and mentoring are **more difficult** in a **community setting;** tips for success include **starting small,** thinking of **local advantages,** and **networking.**

4. **Collaboration** between academic medical centers and **community researchers** can follow a **top-down model** (community investigators conduct studies that originate from the academic center) or a **bottom-up model** (investigators from the academic center help community investigators conduct their own research).

5. **International research** involves many of the same issues as community research with additional challenges related to **communication** and **language, cultural differences, funding, unequal balance of power, financial** and **administrative practices,** and **ethics.**

6. Overcoming these challenges can bring the rewards of **helping people in need,** a large **public health impact,** and rich **cross-cultural experiences.**

REFERENCES

1. Stevens P. Diseases of poverty and the 10/90 gap. November 2004. Available at: http://www.fightingdiseases.org/pdf/Diseases_of_Poverty_FINAL.pdf.
2. Hearst N, Chen S. Condom promotion for AIDS prevention in the developing world: is it working? *Stud Fam Plann* 2004;35(1):39–47.
3. Drugs for hypertension. *Med Lett Drugs Ther* 1999;41:23–28.
4. Nutting PA, Beasley JW, Werner JJ. Practice-based research networks answer primary care questions. *JAMA* 1999;281:686–688.
5. Miller RS, Ivenson DC, Fried RA, et al. Carpal tunnel syndrome in primary care: a report from ASPN. *J Fam Pract* 1994;38:337–344.

6. United Nations Population Division. The international migrant stock: a global view. 2002. Available at: http://www.iom.int/documents/officialtxt/en/unpd%5Fhandout.pdf.

7. Kamya M, McFarland W, Hudes ES, et al. Condom use with casual partners by men in Kampala, Uganda. *AIDS* 1997;11(Suppl 1):S61–S66.

8. Kajubi P, Kamya MR, Kamya S, et al. Increasing condom use without reducing HIV risk: results of a controlled community trial in Uganda. *J Acquir Immune Defic Syndr* 2005;40(1):77–82.

9. Hearst N, Mandel J. A research agenda for AIDS prevention in the developing world. *AIDS* 1997;11(Suppl 1):S1–S4.

10. Lurie P, Wolfe SM. Unethical trials of interventions to reduce perinatal transmission of the human immunodeficiency virus in developing countries. *N Engl J Med* 1997;337:853–856.

11. Perinatal HIV Intervention Research in Developing Countries Workshop Participants. Science, ethics, and the future of research into maternal-infant transmission of HIV-1. *Lancet* 1999;353:832–835.

12. Brennan TA. Proposed revisions to the Declaration of Helsinki: will they weaken the ethical principles underlying human research? *N Engl J Med* 1999;341:527–531.

13. Levine RJ. The need to revise the Declaration of Helsinki. *N Engl J Med* 1999;341:531–534.

14. Taylor D, Taylor CE. *Just and lasting change: when communities own their futures.* Baltimore, MD: JHU Press, 2002.

15. Kamenga MC, Sweat MD, De Zoysa I, et al. The voluntary HIV-1 counseling and testing efficacy study: design and methods. *AIDS Behav* 2000;4:5–14.

16. Page-Shafer K, Saphonn V, Sun LP, et al. HIV prevention research in a resource-limited setting: the experience of planning a trial in cambodia. *Lancet* 2005;366(9495):1499–1503.

17. Chequer P, Marins JRP, Possas C, et al. AIDS research in Brazil. *AIDS* 2005;19(Suppl 4):S1–S3.

19 Writing and Funding a Research Proposal

Steven R. Cummings and Stephen B. Hulley

The **protocol** is the detailed written plan of the study. Writing the protocol forces the investigator to organize, clarify, and refine all the elements of the study, and this enhances the scientific rigor and the efficiency of the project. Even if the investigator does not require funding for a study, a protocol is necessary for guiding the work. A **proposal** is a document written for the purpose of obtaining funds from granting agencies. It contains the study protocol, the budget, and other administrative and supporting information that is required by the specific agency or board. This chapter will focus on the structure of a proposal and on how to write one that will be successful in getting funded.

WRITING PROPOSALS

The task of preparing a proposal generally requires several months of organizing, writing, and revising. The following steps can help the project to get off to a good start.

- *Decide where the proposal will be submitted.* Every **funding agency** has its own unique process and requirements for proposals. Therefore, the investigator should start by deciding where the proposal will be submitted, determining the limit on amounts of funding, and obtaining detailed guidelines about how to craft the proposal for that particular agency.
- *Organize a team and designate a leader.* Most proposals are written by a team of several people who will eventually carry out the study. This team may be small (just the investigator and his mentor) or large (including collaborators, a biostatistician, a fiscal administrator, and support staff). It is important that this team include or have access to the main expertise needed for designing and implementing the study.

  One member of the team must assume the responsibility for leading the effort. Generally this individual is the **principal investigator** (PI), who will have the ultimate authority and accountability for the study. The PI should generally be an experienced scientist whose knowledge and wisdom are useful for design decisions and whose track record with previous studies increases the likelihood of a successful study and, therefore, of funding (reviewers give considerable weight to the value of experience). Some studies also have a Co-PI, often a junior scientist who will serve as the day-to-day manager of the study and coordinate the proposal-writing effort. Either the PI or the Co-PI must exert steady leadership, delegating responsibilities for writing and other tasks, setting deadlines, conducting periodic meetings of the team, and ensuring that all the necessary tasks are completed on time.

- *Follow the guidelines of the funding agency.* All funding sources provide written **guidelines** that the investigator must carefully study before starting to write the proposal. This information includes instructions for organizing the proposal, page limits, information on the amount of money that can be requested, and elements that must be included in the proposal.

  However, these guidelines do not contain all the important information that the investigator needs to know about the operations and the preferences of the funding agencies. The NIH and private foundations have **scientific administrators** whose job is to help investigators design their proposals to be more responsive to the agency's funding policies. Early in the development of the proposal it is a good idea to **discuss the plan** with an individual at the agency who can clarify what the agency prefers (such as budgetary limits and the scope and detail required in the proposal) and confirm that the research plan is within the bounds of the agency's interests. The initial contact can be made by e-mail or letter, but a series of telephone calls or even a visit is a better way to establish a relationship and get information that will lead to a fundable proposal.

  It is useful to make a **checklist** of the details that are required, and to carefully review the checklist before sending the proposal. Rejection of an otherwise excellent proposal for lack of adherence to details is a frustrating and avoidable experience.

- *Establish a timetable and meet periodically.* A schedule for completing the writing tasks keeps gentle pressure on team members to meet their obligations on time. In addition to addressing the scientific components specified by the funding agency, the **timetable** should take into account the administrative requirements of the institution that will sponsor the research. Universities often require a time-consuming review of the budget and subcontracts before a proposal can be submitted to the funding agency. Leaving these details to the end can precipitate a last-minute crisis that damages an otherwise well-done proposal.

  A timetable generally works best if it specifies deadlines for written products and if each individual participates in setting his own assignments. The timetable should be reviewed at periodic meetings of the writing team to check that the tasks are on schedule and the deadlines still realistic.

- *Find a model proposal.* It is helpful to borrow from a colleague a successful recent proposal to the agency from which funding is being sought. Successful applications illustrate in a concrete way the format and content of a good proposal. The investigator can find inspiration for new ideas from the model and then design and write a proposal that is even clearer, more logical, and more persuasive. It is also a good idea to borrow examples of written criticisms that have been provided by the agency for previous successful or unsuccessful proposals. This will illustrate the key points that are important to the scientists who will be reviewing the proposal.

  NIH proposals of interest can be identified by using the Internet to search the NIH "CRISP" (Computer Retrieval of Information on Scientific Projects) database of funded grants. Copies of funded proposals can be obtained by writing to the PI or, as a last resort, through the Freedom of Information Act.

- *Work from an outline.* Begin by setting out the proposal in outline form (Table 19.1). This provides a starting point for writing and is useful for organizing the tasks that need to be done. If several people will be working on the grant, the outline helps in assigning responsibilities for writing parts of the proposal. One of the most common road blocks to creating an outline is the feeling that an entire plan must be worked out before starting to write the first sentence. The investigator should put this notion aside and let his thoughts flow onto paper, creating the raw material for editing, refining, and getting specific advice from colleagues.

- *Review, pretest, and revise repeatedly.* Writing a proposal is an iterative process; there are usually many versions, each reflecting new ideas, advice, and pretest experiences. Before the final draft is written, the proposal should be critically reviewed by colleagues who are familiar with the subject matter and funding agency. Particular attention should go to the quality of the research question, the validity of the design and methods, and the clarity of the writing. It is better to have sharp and detailed criticism before the proposal is submitted than to have the project rejected because of failure to anticipate and address potential problems. When the proposal is nearly ready for submission, the final step is to review it carefully for internal consistency, format, adherence to agency guidelines, and typographical errors.

ELEMENTS OF A PROPOSAL

The most important elements of a **proposal** are set out in Table 19.1 in the sequence required by the NIH. Some funding institutions may require less information or a different format, and the investigator should organize the proposal according to the guidelines of the agency that will receive the proposal (generally available on the Web).

The Beginning

The **title** should be descriptive and concise. It provides the first impression and a lasting reminder of the content and design of the study. A good title manages to summarize these elements, achieving brevity by avoiding unnecessary phrases like "A study to determine the...." In an NIH grant application, the choice of words in the title is important because it can influence the decision on which study section (review group) and institute will receive the protocol.

The **abstract** is a concise summary of the protocol that should begin with the research question and rationale, then set out the design and methods, and conclude with a statement of the importance of potential findings of the study. Most agencies require that the abstract be kept within a limited number of words, so it is best to use efficient and descriptive terms. The abstract will generally be written after the other protocol elements are settled, and it should go through enough revisions to ensure that it is first rate. This will be the only page read by some reviewers, and a convenient reminder of the specifics of the proposal for everyone else. It must therefore stand on its own, incorporating all the main features of the proposed study and persuasively revealing the strengths.

TABLE 19.1	Main Elements of a Proposal, Based on the **NIH** Model

Title

Abstract

Administrative parts

    Budget and budget justification

    Biosketches of investigators

    Resources, equipment, physical facilities

Specific aims

Background and significance

Preliminary studies and experience of the investigators

Methods

    Overview of design

    Study subjects

        Selection criteria

        Design for sampling

        Plans for recruitment

    Measurements

        Main predictor variables (intervention, if an experiment)

        Potential confounding variables

        Outcome variables

    Statistical issues

        Approach to statistical analyses

        Hypotheses, sample size, and power

    Quality control and data management

    Timetable and organizational chart

    Limitations and issues

Ethical considerations

References

Appendices and collaborative agreements

The Administrative Parts

Almost all agencies require an administrative section that includes a budget and a description of the qualifications of personnel and the institution and access to equipment, space, and expertise.

The **budget** section is generally organized according to guidelines from the funding institution. The NIH, for example, has a prescribed format that requires a detailed budget for the first 12-month period and a summary budget for the entire proposed project period (usually 3–5 years). The detailed 12-month budget includes the following categories of expenses: personnel (including names and positions of all persons involved in the project, the percent of time each will devote to the project, and the dollar amounts of salary and fringe benefits listed separately for each individual); consultant costs; equipment (itemized); supplies (itemized); travel (itemized); patient care costs; alterations and renovations; consortium/contractual costs; and other expenses (e.g., the costs of telephones, mail, copying, illustration, publication, books, and fee-for-service contracts).

The budget should not be left until the last minute. Many elements require time (to get good estimates of the cost of space, equipment, and personnel). The best approach is to notify a knowledgeable administrator as soon as possible about the plan to submit a proposal and schedule regular meetings with him to review progress and a written timeline for finishing the administrative section. An administrator can begin working as soon as the outline of the proposal is formulated, recommending the amounts for budget items. Institutions have regulations that must be followed and deadlines to meet, and an experienced administrator can help the investigator anticipate institutional rules, pitfalls, and potential delays. The administrator can also be very helpful in drafting the text of the sections on budget and resources, and in collecting the biosketches, appendices, and other supporting materials.

The need for the amounts requested for each item of the budget must be fully explained in a **budget justification.** Salaries will generally comprise most of the overall cost of a typical clinical research project, so it is important to show the need for each person and his effort. Carefully conceived job descriptions for the investigators and other members of the research team should leave no doubt in the reviewers' minds that the estimated effort of each individual is essential to the success of the project.

Reviewers often look at the percentages of time committed by key members of the project. Occasionally, proposals may be criticized because key members of the research team have only a very small (5%) commitment of time listed in the budget and a large number of other studies listed in their "other support" (implying that they have too many other commitments to be able to devote the necessary energy to the proposed study). On the other hand, the reviewers may also balk at percentages that are inflated beyond the requirements of the job description.

Even the best-planned **budgets** will **change** as the needs of the study change or there are unexpected expenses and savings. In general, once the grant is awarded the investigator is allowed to spend money in different ways from those specified in the budget, provided that the changes are modest and the expenditures are all appropriate to the study. When the investigator wants to move money across categories or to make a substantial change (up or down) in the effort of key investigators, he may need to get approval from the funding agency. Agencies generally approve reasonable requests for rebudgeting so long as the investigator is not asking for an increase in total funds.

The **biosketches** of investigators are four-page resumes that include academic degrees, current and previous employment, honors, recent and pertinent publications, and descriptions of recent research grants and contracts. The sections on **resources** available to the project, including computer and technical equipment and office and laboratory space, often draw on "boilerplate" in previous grants by colleagues in the investigator's institution.

Aims and Significance

The **specific aims** are statements of the research question and plan using a concise format that specifies in concrete terms the desired outcome. When appropriate, aims may be expressed as testable hypotheses. Most research proposals have several, and after an introductory paragraph these should be presented in a logical sequence. Sometimes this means putting them in order of importance, and sometimes in chronological order (objectives served by baseline data first, then those related to follow-up). Sometimes, as in the following example, a logical approach is to present the administrative aims first, then the scientific aims:

1. *To recruit 400 healthy men, 40–59 years old into a randomized blinded trial of the effects of a testosterone patch.*
2. *To test the hypothesis that compared with men assigned to receive a placebo patch, those assigned to receive the testosterone patch will have*
   a. *less bone loss*
   b. *an increase in quadriceps muscle strength*
   c. *a decreased risk of falling.*

The specific aims section can also serve as an outline for organizing later sections; the components of the significance and methods sections should usually follow a parallel sequence.

When a study has many facets, it is tempting to impress the reader with a long and detailed listing of specific aims. This strategy may backfire, creating a proposal that is overly ambitious or cluttered. When numerous specific aims are possible, it is best to propose only the most important and interesting ones. In general, this should not exceed one page.

The **background and significance** section sets the proposal in context, describing the background in the field under study. It should be written, as much as possible, in a way that is comprehensible to someone who is not an expert in that field. Enough information should be given to make clear what this particular study will accomplish and why it is important. How, specifically, will the study findings advance understanding, change clinical practice, or influence policy?

The purpose of this section is to demonstrate that the investigator understands what has been accomplished, what the problems are, and what needs to be done. The appropriate breadth or detail of the review depends on the scope of the specific aims, the complexity of the field, and the expectations of the review panel. Reviewers usually appreciate a thoughtful critical review of the most important previous studies rather than an exhaustive superficial catalogue of previous publications.

The **preliminary studies** and **experience** of the investigators section should concisely describe relevant previous research and skills of the investigator; a limited number of preprints can be included in appendices. Emphasis should be placed on the importance of the previous work and on the reasons it should be continued or extended. **Pilot studies** that support the research question and the feasibility of the study are important to many types of proposals, especially when the research team has little previous experience in the area to be studied, when the question is novel, and when there may be doubts about the feasibility of the proposed procedures or recruitment of subjects. Results of these studies should be highlighted here, with details provided in the appendices.

The Scientific Methods

The **methods** section generally receives close scrutiny from reviewers, and it will later serve as the basis for the operations manual for carrying out the study. Weakness in the technical methods is a common reason that proposals fail to be approved or funded by the NIH. For these reasons, this section deserves careful attention to detail.

The first concern is how to organize the section. Sometimes agencies provide guidelines about how to organize the methods. If not, we recommend the components and sequence listed in Table 19.1. A detailed table of the contents of the methods section can be very helpful at this point, and an overview of the **design,** sometimes accompanied by a schematic diagram or table, is essential for orienting the reader (Table 19.2).

The other specific components of the methods section have been discussed in other parts of this book. The **subjects** and **measurements** (Chapters 3 and 4), **pretest plans, data management,** and **quality control** (Chapters 16 and 17) are the centerpiece of the proposal, and require sufficient detail so that sophisticated reviewers will understand exactly how the study will be performed and the reasons for the design choices. Long descriptions of some techniques, such as the details of biochemical assays or of questionnaires, can be put into an appendix unless they are crucial to the evaluation of scientific merit.

The **statistical section** should usually begin with the plans for analysis. This can be set out in the logical sequence, first the descriptive tabulations and then the approach to analyzing associations among variables. This will lead to the topic

TABLE 19.2	Study Timeline for a Randomized Trial of the Effect of Testosterone Administration on Risk Factors for Heart Disease, Prostate Cancer, and Fractures				
	Screening Visit	**Randomization**	**3 Months**	**6 Months**	**12 Months**
Medical history	X	—	—	—	X
Blood pressure	X	X	X	X	X
Prostate examination	X	—	—	—	X
Prostate specific antigen	X	—	—	—	X
Blood lipid levels	—	X	X	X	X
Markers of inflammation	—	X	—	—	X
Bone density	—	X	—	—	X
Markers of bone turnover	—	X	X	—	X
Handgrip strength	—	X	X	X	X
Adverse events	—	—	X	X	X

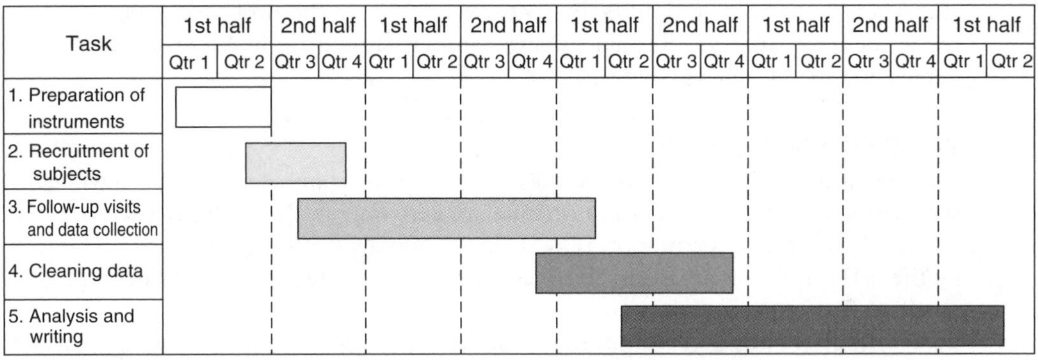

Task	1st half		2nd half		1st half		2nd half		1st half		2nd half		1st half		2nd half		1st half	
	Qtr 1	Qtr 2	Qtr 3	Qtr 4	Qtr 1	Qtr 2	Qtr 3	Qtr 4	Qtr 1	Qtr 2	Qtr 3	Qtr 4	Qtr 1	Qtr 2	Qtr 3	Qtr 4	Qtr 1	Qtr 2
1. Preparation of instruments																		
2. Recruitment of subjects																		
3. Follow-up visits and data collection																		
4. Cleaning data																		
5. Analysis and writing																		

FIGURE 19.1. A hypothetical timetable.

of **sample size** (Chapters 5 and 6), which should begin with a statement of the null hypotheses and the choice of statistical test before giving the sample size and power estimates at the specified alpha, and effect size. Most NIH review panels attach considerable importance to the statistical section, so it is a good idea to involve a statistician in writing, or at least in reviewing, this component of the proposal.

The proposal must provide a realistic work plan and **timetable,** including dates when each major phase of the study will be started and completed (Fig. 19.1). Similar timetables can be prepared for staffing patterns and other components of the project. For large studies, an organizational chart describing the research team should indicate levels of authority and accountability, and show how the team will function.

Final Pieces

The **human subjects** section is devoted to the ethical issues raised by the study, setting forth the issues of safety, privacy, and confidentiality. This section should indicate the specific plans to inform potential subjects of the risks and benefits, and to obtain their consent to participate (Chapter 14). It is an appropriate place to describe the inclusion of women, children and participants from minority groups, as required of NIH proposals, expanding on information provided in the methods section.

The **references** send a message about the investigator's familiarity with a field. They should be comprehensive but parsimonious, up to date and balanced—not an exhaustive and unselected list. Each reference should be cited accurately; errors in these citations or misinterpretation of the work will be viewed negatively by reviewers who are familiar with the field of research.

Information that is important for all reviewers to understand about the research plan should generally *not* be put in an **appendix**; in NIH study sections only the primary and secondary reviewers—usually about three—receive the appendices. However the appendices are useful for detailed technical and supporting material can be mentioned or described briefly in the main text. Examples are highly relevant preprints or in-progress reports by the investigators, questionnaires, and long descriptions of measurements that might be a useful reference for a reviewer.

The proposed use and value of each **consultant** should be described, accompanied by a signed letter of agreement from the individual and a copy of his biosketch. (Investigators with effort listed in the budget should not provide letters, because they are officially part of the proposal.) An explanation of the programmatic and administrative arrangements between the applicant organization and **collaborating institutions,**

labs, and so on should be included, accompanied by letters of commitment from responsible officials addressed to the investigator.

Writing Proposals for Career Development Awards

The research plan is only one element of proposals for **career development awards.** These proposals emphasize descriptions of the candidate and his strategy for developing a career in research, including plans for training in research. They generally require evidence of commitment from a mentor who has a strong track record in research and mentoring, and from the applicants institution (1). The requirements and criteria for review of applications for NIH career development awards are available on the NIH Web site.

CHARACTERISTICS OF GOOD PROPOSALS

A good proposal for a research project has several attributes. First is the **scientific quality of the research plan**: it must be based on a good research question, use a design and methods that are rigorous and feasible, and have a research team with sufficient experience, skill, and commitment to carry it out (2,3).

Clarity of presentation is one of the most important determinants of the fate of grant applications. Even if the research question is important and the study plan excellent, a poor presentation can leave the reviewer confused and uninterested. The proposal should be concise and engaging, and not lose the attention of the reviewer with writing that wanders vaguely through peripheral topics. A proposal that is well organized, thoughtfully written, attractively presented, and free of errors reassures the reader that the conduct of research is likely to be of similar quality.

Reviewers are often overwhelmed by a large stack of lengthy proposals, so the merits of the project must stand out in a way that will not be missed even with a quick and cursory reading. Clear **outlines,** short sections with meaningful **subheadings,** brief point-by-point **summaries,** concise **tables,** and simple **diagrams** can guide the reviewer's understanding of the most important features of the proposal. It is good to leave some **white space** on the pages.

Most reviewers are sophisticated, and are **put off by overstatement** and other heavy-handed forms of grantsmanship. Proposals that exaggerate the importance of the project or overestimate what it can accomplish will generate skepticism. Writing with enthusiasm is a good idea, but the investigator should be realistic about the limitations of the project. Most reviewers are adept at identifying potential problems in the design or feasibility of a research project.

Rather than ignore **potential flaws,** an investigator can address them explicitly, discussing the advantages and disadvantages of the various trade-offs in reaching the chosen plan. It is a mistake to overemphasize these problems, however, for this may lead a reviewer to focus disproportionately on the weaker aspects of the proposal and to overlook its strengths. The goal is to reassure the reviewer that the investigator has anticipated the potential problems and has a realistic and thoughtful approach to dealing with them. If the investigator thinks of issues that are not fully resolved in the main body of the proposal, it may be useful to pose these as questions with thoughtful and balanced answers in a **"Questions and Issues"** section at the end of the methods section.

A final round of **scientific review** by skilled scientists who have not been centrally involved, at a point in time when substantial changes are still possible, can be extraordinarily helpful to the proposal as well as a rewarding collegial experience. The investigator should leave time in the last week or two before the deadline to have someone with excellent **writing skills** read the proposal for clarity, grammatical errors, and spelling errors that are missed by word-processing spell- and grammar-check programs.

FINDING SUPPORT FOR RESEARCH

Investigators should be alert to opportunities to conduct good research without formal proposals for funding. For example, a beginning researcher may himself analyze data sets that have been collected by others, or receive small amounts of staff time from senior scientists or his department to conduct small studies. Conducting research without funding of formal proposals is generally quicker and simpler but has the disadvantage that the projects must be inexpensive and limited in scope. Furthermore, academic institutions often base decisions about advancement in part on a faculty member's track record of garnering external funding for research. There are four main sources of funds for medical research:

- **the government** (notably NIH, but also Centers for Disease Control and Prevention (CDC), and many other federal, state and county agencies);
- **private nonprofit institutions** (notably foundations and professional societies);
- **profit-making corporations** (notably pharmaceutical companies); and
- **intramural resources** (e.g., from the investigator's university).

Getting support from these sources is a complex and competitive process that favors investigators with **experience** and **tenacity,** and beginning investigators are well advised to find a mentor with these characteristics. In the sections below, we focus on several of the most important of these; for a complete listing, try the The American Association for the Advancement of Science (AAAS) Web site (4).

National Institutes of Health Grants and Contracts
It takes 8 to 10 months from the time a successful application is submitted to NIH until it receives funding. During this time the application goes through a process of initial administrative review by NIH staff, advisory **peer review,** final recommendation about funding by the Council of an institute, and decision about funding by the institute director (5). The peer review process, although laborious and somewhat capricious, is reasonably fair and tends to enhance the quality of medical research in the same way that journal reviewers enhance the quality of the medical literature.

The NIH offers many types of grants and contracts (6). The"**R**" **awards** (such as R01 and smaller R03 and R21 awards) support research projects conceived by the investigator on a topic of his choosing or written in response to a publicized request by one of the institutes at NIH. The "**K**" **awards** (such as K-08 or K-23 awards) support training and development of the careers of junior or midlevel investigators. An excellent way to begin a research career, K-awards generally provide substantial support for the young investigator's salary and modest support for research projects (1).

Institute-initiative proposals are designed to stimulate research in areas designated by NIH advisory committees, and take the form of either Requests for Proposals (**RFPs**) or Requests for Applications (**RFAs**). Under an RFP, the investigator contracts to perform certain research activities determined by the NIH. Under an RFA, the investigator conducts research in a topic area defined by the NIH, but the specific research question and study plan are proposed by the investigator. RFPs use the **contract** mechanism to reimburse the contractor for the costs involved in achieving the planned objectives, and RFAs use the **grant** mechanism to support activities that are more open-ended.

Grant applications are usually reviewed by one of many NIH **"study sections."** Each of these has a specific focus and is composed of experts in those areas drawn from institutions around the country. A list of the study sections and their current membership is available on the NIH Web site (5), and many investigators use this information to make sure their applications will be responsive to the particular individuals who may provide their peer review. Proposals for K-awards are usually reviewed by study sections comprised of experts in a general area of research sponsored by the particular NIH Institute. Proposals sent in response to an RFA or RFP are usually reviewed by *ad hoc* committees of peers that follow the same procedures as the study sections in passing on the merits of a proposal.

When an investigator submits a grant application to the NIH, it is assigned by the Center for Scientific Review (**CSR**) to a particular study section (Fig. 19.2). After review and discussion, each member of the study section assigns a priority score of 1 to 3 for each of the applications judged to be in the upper half. (A few applications are deferred to the next cycle 4 months later, pending clarification of points that were unclear, and the rest are not reviewed.) This is done by secret ballot, and the

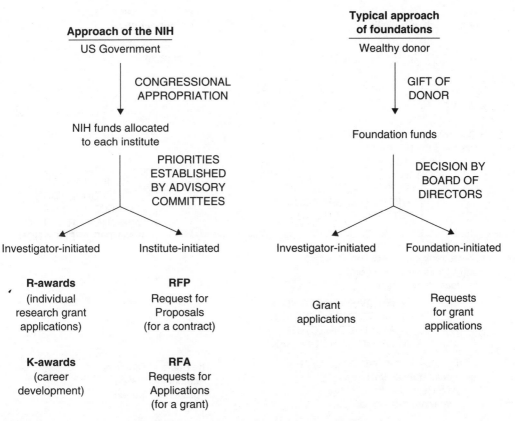

FIGURE 19.2. Overview of NIH and foundation funding sources and mechanisms.

average is computed and multiplied by 100 to yield a score from 100 (best) to 300 (worst). This score is compared with other scores from the study section to generate a percentile rank.

The CSR also assigns each grant application to a particular **institute** at NIH. Each institute then funds the grants assigned to it, in order of priority score (tempered by an advisory council review and sometimes over-ridden by the institute director), until the budget it has received from Congress is exhausted (Fig. 19.3). If an application is of interest to more than one institute, the PI should request dual assignment and the second institute may provide funds if the primary institute cannot, or the institutes may share funding.

The investigator should decide in advance, with advice from senior colleagues, on the outcome he prefers for the two key assignments that are made by the CSR—to a study section and to an institute. Study sections vary a great deal not only in topic area but also in the stringency and nature of their review, and there is a considerable difference among institutes in the extent and quality of the competition. Although the assignments are not fully controllable, the investigator can influence them by (a) choosing words in the title and abstract that make it obvious what the best assignment would be; (b) stating his preference in the cover letter for the application; (c) asking the NIH scientist in charge of the study section of choice (the "scientific review administrator") or the NIH scientist who will handle the grant at the institute of choice for advice on how to steer the application.

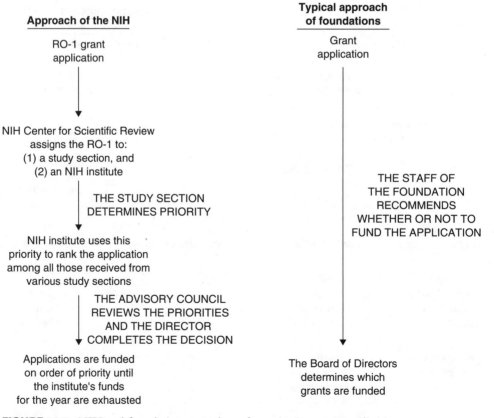

FIGURE 19.3. NIH and foundation procedures for reviewing grant applications.

After an application has been reviewed by the appropriate committee, the investigator receives written notification of the committee's action. This **summary statement** includes the score, percentile, and detailed comments and criticisms from the committee members who reviewed the application.

Applications that are not funded, as is often the case for the first submission, can be revised and submitted up to two more times. If the reviewers' criticisms suggest that the application can be made more acceptable to the committee, then a thoughtfully revised version may have an excellent chance of obtaining funding when it is resubmitted. An investigator need not automatically make all the changes suggested by reviewers, but he should adopt revisions that will satisfy the reviewer's criticisms wherever possible and justify any decision not to do so. A good format for the introduction of a resubmission is to quote each major criticism from the summary statement and then state the corresponding response and changes in the proposal, which should be earmarked in the text.

Grants from Foundations and Professional Societies

Private foundations (such as The Robert Wood Johnson Foundation) generally restrict their funding to specific areas of interest. Some disease-based foundations and **professional societies** (such as the American Heart Association and American Cancer Society) also sponsor small research programs, many of which are designed to support junior investigators. The total amount of research support is far smaller than that provided by NIH, and most foundations have the goal of using this money to fill the gaps, funding projects of merit that for one or another reason would not be funded by NIH. A few foundations offer career development awards that usually provide less financial support than NIH K-awards, and are focused on specific areas such as quality of health care. The Foundation Center (7) maintains a searchable directory of foundations, their Web sites, and contact information along with advice about how to write effective proposals to foundations. Decisions about funding follow procedures that vary from one institution to another but that usually respond rapidly to relatively short proposals (Fig. 19.3). The decisions are often made by an executive process rather than by peer review. Typically, the staff of the foundation makes a recommendation that is ratified by a board of directors.

To determine whether a foundation might be interested in a particular proposal, an investigator should consult with his senior mentors, and check foundation Web sites. The Website will generally describe the goals and purposes of the foundation and often list projects that have recently been funded. If it appears that the foundation might be an appropriate source of support, it is best to contact the appropriate staff member of the foundation to describe the project, determine the potential interest, and get guidance about how to submit a proposal. Many foundations ask that investigators send a short (three- to five-page) letter describing the background and principal goals of the project, the qualifications of the investigators, and the approximate duration and costs of the research. If the proposal is of sufficient interest, the foundation may request a more detailed proposal.

Research Support from Industry

Corporations that make drugs and devices (referred to as "industry") are a major source of funding, especially for randomized trials of new treatments. Large companies generally accept applications for investigator-initiated research that may include small pilot studies about the effects or mechanisms of action of a treatment, or epidemiologic studies about conditions of interest to the company. They will often supply the drug and a matching placebo for an investigator's research. Companies may provide small grants to support educational programs in areas of their interest. However, the most common form of industry support for clinical research is payment to enroll participants into large trials that are designed, conducted and analyzed by the company.

Requests for support for research or educational programs, or to participate as a site in a trial, generally begin by contacting the local or regional representative for the company. If the company is interested in the topic, the investigator may be asked to submit a relatively short application and complete forms about the request. Companies often give preference to requests from **"opinion leaders,"** clinicians or investigators who are well known and whose views may influence how other clinicians prescribe drugs or use devices. Therefore, a young investigator seeking industry support should generally get the help of a well-known mentor in contacting the company and submitting the application.

The **contracts** for support from profit-making companies can be a mixed experience. For participation in clinical trials, companies generally pay investigators a fixed fee for each participant included in the trial and the trial closes enrollment when the desired study-wide goal has been met. An investigator may enroll enough participants to receive funding that exceeds his costs, in which case he may retain the surplus as a long-term unrestricted account, but he will lose money if he recruits too few participants to achieve the needed economy of scale.

Funding from industry, particularly from marketing departments, is often channeled into topics and activities intended to increase the sales of the company's product (8). Investigators generally have more control over results of investigator-initiated work funded by industry than when they are one of many investigators in large industry-sponsored trials. Multicenter studies are generally analyzed by company statisticians and often written by industry-funded medical writers.

Industry conducts research primarily to make profit from the sale of drugs and devices. This motivation may influence employees of the company to put findings about their products in the most favorable light. All medical research (regardless of the source of support) is susceptible to various extrascientific influences. Because society places a premium on a favorable result, negative results are often dull and hard to publish even though we all recognize that a conclusive negative finding may be as important as a conclusive positive one. Investigators can create some **safeguards** against undue influence of financial and social pressures. It is important that contracts with companies include clear terms providing investigators with meaningful access to data. Investigators should seek involvement in publishing and presenting the results of the studies provided that they are able to design, request, and carefully review the analyses, write all, or key sections, of papers and produce their own slides for presentation of results at meetings. Manuscripts and presentations should be reviewed by publication committees, most of whose members are scientists involved in the trial but not affiliated with the company.

One **advantage** of corporate support is that it is the only practical way to address some research questions. There would be no other source of funds, for example, for testing a new antibiotic that is not yet on the market. Another advantage is the relative speed with which this source of funding can be acquired; decisions about small investigator-initiated proposals are made within a few months and drug companies are often eager to sign up qualified investigators to participate in their multicenter clinical trials. Additionally, most pharmaceutical companies place a high premium on maintaining a reputation for integrity (which enhances their dealings with the vigilant U.S. Food and Drug Administration (FDA) and their stature with the public), and the research expertise, measurement instruments, statistical support and financial resources they provide can improve the quality of the research.

Intramural Support

Universities often have local research funds for their own investigators that can be discovered through the **Dean's office.** Grants from these intramural funds are generally limited to relatively small amounts, but they are usually available much more quickly (weeks to months) and to a higher proportion of applicants than grants from the NIH or private foundations. Intramural funds may be restricted to special purposes, such as pilot studies that may lead to external funding, or the purchase of equipment that will permit a study to be done by scientists whose salary is supported by training funds. Such funds are often earmarked for **junior faculty** members or **fellows** and provide a unique opportunity for a beginning investigator to acquire the experience of leading a funded project.

■ SUMMARY

1. The **protocol** is the detailed written plan of the study. It is the scientific component of a **proposal** for funding, which also contains administrative and supporting information required by the funding agency.

2. An investigator who is working on a research protocol should begin by getting advice from senior colleagues about the choice of **funding agency.** The next steps are to study that agency's written **guidelines** and to contact the **scientific administrator** in the agency for advice.

3. The process of writing a proposal, which often takes much longer than expected, includes organizing a **team** with the necessary expertise, designating a **project leader,** establishing a **timetable** for written products, finding a **model proposal, outlining the proposal** along agency guidelines, and reviewing progress at regular **meetings.** The proposal should be **reviewed** by knowledgeable colleagues, revised often, and **polished** at the end with attention to detail.

4. A good proposal requires not only a good **research question, study plan,** and **research team,** but also a good **presentation:** the proposal must communicate clearly and concisely, following a logical outline and indicating the advantages and disadvantages of trade-offs in the study plan. The **merits** of the proposal should stand out so that they will not be missed by a busy reviewer.

5. There are four main sources of support for clinical research:
   a. The **NIH** and other governmental sources are the **largest** providers of support, using a complex system of peer and administrative review that moves slowly but encourages **good science.**
   b. **Foundations and societies** are often interested in promising research questions that escape NIH funding, and have review procedures that are quicker but more parochial than those of NIH.
   c. **Manufacturers of drugs and devices** are a very large source of support that is usually channeled to company-run studies of new drugs and medical devices,

but corporations value partnerships with leading scientists and support some investigator-initiated research.

d. **Intramural funds** tend to have favorable funding rates for getting small amounts of money quickly, and are suitable for pilot studies and beginning investigators.

REFERENCES

1. Gill TM, McDermott MM, Ibrahim SA, et al. Getting funded: career development awards for aspiring clinical investigators. *J Gen Intern Med* 2004;19:472–478.
2. Inouye SK, Fiellin DA. An evidence-based guide to writing grant proposals for clinical research. *Ann Intern Med* 2005;142:274–282.
3. Advice about how to write successful NIH applications: http://www.niaid.nih.gov/ncn/grants/default.htm and http://ora.stanford.edu/ora/ratd/nih_04.asp.
4. General advice from AAAS about how to obtain research funding. http://sciencecareers.sciencemag.org/funding.
5. Information about types of NIH funding: http://grants.nih.gov/grants/oer.htm.
6. Description of the NIH grant review and funding process: cms.csr.nih.gov.
7. Information from the Foundation Center about applying for funding from foundations: http://fdncenter.org/.
8. Davidoff F, DeAngelis CD, Drazen JM, et al. Sponsorship, authorship, and accountability. *JAMA* 2001;286:1232–1234.

Exercises

CHAPTER 1. GETTING STARTED: THE ANATOMY AND PHYSIOLOGY OF CLINICAL RESEARCH

For each of the following summaries of studies, write a single sentence that specifies the design and research question; the latter should include the main predictor and outcome variables, and the population sampled. Think about the main inference that can be drawn from the study: To what phenomena and which populations can the findings be generalized? What are the potential errors in drawing and applying these inferences?

1. Giving vitamin D to patients with vitamin D deficiency can improve strength, but little is known about any influence it may have on the ordinary weakness of aging. We selected 38 men 70 years of age and greater from a hypertension treatment clinic and randomly assigned them to receive either vitamin D_3 or identical placebo. Muscle strength of the quadriceps, measured with an isokinetic dynamometer after 6 months of treatment, was similar in the two groups. (Grady D et al., *JCEM* 1991;73:1111–7)

2. A random sample of high school students was surveyed in the fall about frequency of watching wrestling on television and fighting at school and on dates. The same subjects were surveyed again in the spring. The adjusted odds of reporting fighting with a date in the spring survey increased by 14% (OR = 1.14, 95% CI 1.06 − 1.22) for each episode of wrestling the students reported having watched in the 2-week period before the fall survey. (DuRant RH et al., *Pediatrics* 2006;118:e265–72)

3. To assess whether the sedative effects of psychotropic drugs might cause hip fractures, we studied 1,021 women with hip fractures and an equal number without hip fracture among elderly Medicaid enrollees. Women who had taken short-acting tranquilizers had no increased risk of hip fracture, but those who had taken tranquilizers with half-lives exceeding 24 hours did have an increased risk (odds ratio, 1.8; 95% CI 1.3 to 2.4). (Ray WA et al., *NEJM* 1987;316:363–9)

4. Knowledge about AIDS was studied among 1,526 teen-aged boys and girls in 12 secondary schools in Zimbabwe. Ninety-three percent of the children thought that it was an infection caused by having sexual relations, and 10% believed that it could be contracted from toilet seats.

CHAPTER 2. CONCEIVING THE RESEARCH QUESTION

Consider the following research questions. First, write each question in a single sentence that specifies a study design, predictor, outcome, and population. Then discuss whether this research question and the design you have chosen meet the FINER (Feasible, Interesting, Novel, Ethical, Relevant) criteria. Rewrite the question and design until you have overcome any problems in meeting these criteria.

1. What is the relationship between depression and health?
2. Does eating red meat cause cancer?
3. Can relaxation exercises decrease anxiety during a mammogram?
4. Are there proteomic markers for coronary atherosclerosis?

CHAPTER 3. CHOOSING THE STUDY SUBJECTS: SPECIFICATION, SAMPLING, AND RECRUITMENT

1. The research question is: "What are the factors that cause people to start smoking?" The investigator decides on a cross-sectional sample of high school students, invites eleventh graders in her suburban high school to participate, and studies those who volunteer. Discuss the suitability of this sample for the target population of interest.
2. Suppose that the investigator decides to avoid the bias associated with choosing volunteers by designing a 25% random sample of the entire eleventh grade, and that the actual sample turns out to be 70% female. If it is known that roughly equal numbers of boys and girls are enrolled in the school, then the disproportion in the sex distribution represents an error in drawing the sample. Could this have occurred through random error, systematic error, or both? Explain your answer.
3. The research question is, "What is the prevalence of alcohol and drug use among persons who attend rock concerts?" Classify the following sampling schemes for selecting individuals to fill out a brief questionnaire, commenting on feasibility and whether the results will be generalizable to all people who attend rock concerts.
   a. As each patron entered the theater, she is asked to throw a die. All patrons who throw a 6 are selected.
   b. As each patron entered the theater, she is asked to throw a die. Men who throw a 1 and women who throw an even number are selected.
   c. Tickets to the concert are known to be numbered serially. Each patron whose ticket number ends in 1 is selected.
   d. After all the patrons are seated, five rows are chosen at random by drawing from a shuffled set of cards that has one card for each theater row. All patrons in those five rows are selected.
   e. The first 27 patrons who enter the theater are selected.
   f. Some tickets were sold by mail and some were sold at the box office just before the performance. Whenever there were three or more people waiting in line to

buy tickets at the box office, the last person in line (who had the most time available) was selected.

  g. When patrons began to leave after the performance, those who seemed willing and able to answer questions were selected.

CHAPTER 4. PLANNING THE MEASUREMENTS: PRECISION AND ACCURACY

1. Classify the following variables as dichotomous, nominal, ordinal, continuous, or ordered discrete. Could any of them be modified to increase power, and how?
   a. Sex
   b. Age
   c. Education (high school degree/no degree)
   d. Education (highest year of schooling)
   e. History of heart attack (present/absent)
   f. Number of alcohol drinks per day
   g. Depression (none, mild, moderate, severe)
   h. Percent occlusion of coronary arteries
   i. Hair color
   j. Body weight (obese/not obese)
2. The research question is, "Does body weight at age 1 year predict the number of drop-in clinic visits during the following year?" The investigator plans a prospective cohort study, measuring body weight using an infant scale. Several problems are noted during pretesting. Are these problems due to lack of accuracy, lack of precision, or both? Is the problem mainly due to observer, subject, or instrument variability, and what could be done about it?
   a. During calibration of the scale, a 10-pound reference weight weighs 10.5 pounds.
   b. The scale seems to give variable results; weighing the 10-pound reference weight 20 times gives a mean of 10.01 ± 1.00 (standard deviation) pounds.
   c. Some babies are scared and when they try to climb off the scale the observer holds them on it to complete the measurement.
   d. Some babies are "squirmy," and the pointer on the scale swings up and down wildly.
   e. Some of the babies arrive for the examination immediately after being fed, whereas others are hungry; some of the babies have wet diapers.

CHAPTER 5. GETTING READY TO ESTIMATE SAMPLE SIZE: HYPOTHESES AND UNDERLYING PRINCIPLES

1. Define the concepts in **boldface.**
   An investigator is interested in designing a study with sufficient **sample size** to determine whether body mass index is associated with stomach cancer in women between 50 and 75 years of age. She is planning a case–control study with equal numbers of cases and controls. The **null hypothesis** is that there is no difference in mean body mass index between cases of stomach cancer and controls; she has chosen an **alternative hypothesis** with two sides. She would like to have a **power**

of 0.80, at a **level of statistical significance** (α) of 0.05, to be able to detect an **effect size** of a difference in body mass index of 1 kg/m^2 between cases and controls. Review of the literature indicates that the **variability** of body mass index among women is a standard deviation of 2.5 kg/m^2.

2. Which of the following is likely to be an example of a Type I error? A Type II error? Neither?

   a. A randomized trial finds that subjects treated with a new analgesic medication had greater mean declines in their pain scores during a study than did those treated with placebo ($P = 0.03$).

   b. A 10-year study reports that 110 subjects who smoke do not have a greater incidence of lung cancer than 294 non-smokers ($P = 0.31$).

   c. An investigator concludes that "Our study is the first to find that use of alcohol reduces the risk of diabetes in men less than 50 years of age ($P < 0.05$)."

CHAPTER 6. ESTIMATING SAMPLE SIZE AND POWER: APPLICATIONS AND EXAMPLES

1. Review exercise 1 of Chapter 5. Determine how many cases of stomach cancer would be required for the study. What if the investigator wanted a power of 0.90? Or a level of statistical significance of 0.01?

   Extra credit: Suppose the investigator only had access to 60 cases. What could she do?

2. Muscle strength declines with advancing age. Preliminary evidence suggests that part of this loss of muscle strength might be due to progressive deficiency of dehydroepiandrosterone (DHEA). Investigators plan a randomized trial to administer DHEA or identical placebo for 6 months to elderly subjects, and then measure muscle strength. Previous studies have reported a mean grip strength in elderly persons of 20 kg with a standard deviation of 8 kg. Assuming α(two-sided) = 0.05 and $\beta = 0.10$, how many subjects would be required to demonstrate a 10% or greater difference between strength in the treated and placebo groups? How many subjects would be needed if $\beta = 0.20$?

3. In exercise 2, sample size calculations indicated more subjects were needed than can be enrolled. A colleague points out that elderly people have great differences in grip strength. This accounts for much of the variability in the strength measured after treatment and might be obscuring the treatment effect. She suggests that you measure strength at baseline and again after treatment, using the change in strength as the outcome variable. A small pilot study shows that the standard deviation of the change in strength during a 6-month period is only 2 kg. How many subjects would be required per group using this design, assuming α(two-sided) = 0.05 and $\beta = 0.10$?

4. An investigator suspects that left-handedness is more common in dyslexic than in nondyslexic third graders. Previous studies indicated that about 10% of people are left-handed and that dyslexia is uncommon. A case–control study is planned that will select all the dyslexic students in a school district as cases, with an equal number of nondyslexic students randomly selected as controls. What sample size would be required to show that the odds ratio for dyslexia is 2.0 among left-handed students compared with right-handed students? Assume $\alpha = 0.05$ (two-sided) and $\beta = 0.20$.

5. An investigator seeks to determine the mean IQ of medical students in her institution, with a 99% CI of ± 3 points. A small pilot study suggests that IQ scores among medical students range from about 130 to 170. Approximately what sample size is needed?

CHAPTER 7. DESIGNING A COHORT STUDY

1. The research question is, "Does vitamin B_{12} deficiency cause hip fractures in the elderly?"
   a. Briefly outline a study plan to address this research question with a prospective cohort study.
   b. An alternative approach would be to compare evidence of vitamin B_{12} deficiency in women who have had previous hip fracture with that in women who have not. Compared with this "case–control" approach, list at least one advantage and one disadvantage of your prospective cohort study. (If you like, you can come back to this question after you have read Chapter 8.)
   c. Could the cohort study be designed as a retrospective study, and how would this affect these advantages or disadvantages?

CHAPTER 8. DESIGNING CROSS-SECTIONAL AND CASE–CONTROL STUDIES

1. The research question is, "How much does a family history of ovarian cancer increase the risk for ovarian cancer?" The investigator plans a case–control study to answer this question.
   a. How should she pick the cases?
   b. How should she pick the controls?
   c. Comment on potential sources of bias in the sampling of cases and controls.
   d. How would she measure "family history of ovarian cancer" as the predictor variable of interest? Comment on the sources of bias in this measurement.
   e. What measure of association would she use, and what test of statistical significance?
   f. Do you think the case–control method is an appropriate approach to this research question? Discuss the advantages and disadvantages of the case–control design relative to other possibilities for this research question.
2. The research question is, "Does maternal height or weight predict infant birth weight?" During a 12-month period an investigator assembles data on consecutive newborns in a large maternity hospital. The study is limited to term newborns as defined by delivery 38 to 42 weeks after the mother's last menstrual period. In the maternity ward, the investigator measures each infant's birth weight and the mother's height and weight. Based on the data obtained, the investigator concludes that birth weight is strongly dependent on both maternal height and weight.
   a. What kind of study is this?
   b. Explain why you agree or disagree with the investigator's conclusions?
3. The investigator wants to investigate the relationship between playing video games involving car racing and the risk of being involved in a real car crash (as the driver). She has two research questions, one that addresses the long-term effects of habitual

use of these games, and the other that tests whether use of such games in the hour immediately preceding driving increases short-term risk. What are some designs she might consider?

CHAPTER 9. ENHANCING CAUSAL INFERENCE IN OBSERVATIONAL STUDIES

(This is out favorite exercise)

1. The investigator undertakes a case–control study to address the research question, "Does eating more fruits and vegetables reduce the risk of coronary heart disease (CHD) in the elderly?" Suppose that her study shows that people in the control group report a higher intake of fruits and vegetables than people with CHD.

    What are the possible explanations for this inverse association between intake of fruits and vegetables and CHD? How could each of these possibilities be altered in the design phase of the study? How could they be addressed in the analysis phase?

    Give special attention to the possibility that the association between eating fruits and vegetables and CHD may be confounded by exercise (if people who eat more fruits and vegetables also exercise more, and this is the cause of their lower CHD rates). What approaches could you use to cope with exercise as a possible confounder, and what are the advantages and disadvantages of each plan?

CHAPTER 10. DESIGNING A RANDOMIZED BLINDED TRIAL

1. A herbal extract, huperzine, has been used in China as a remedy for dementia and preliminary studies in animals and humans have been promising. The investigator would like to test whether this new treatment might decrease the progression of Alzheimer's disease. Studies have found that plasma level of Abeta (1–40) is a biomarker for Alzheimer's disease: elevated levels are associated with a significantly increased risk of developing dementia and the levels of Abeta (1–40) increase with the progression of dementia. In planning a trial to test the efficacy of huperzine for prevention of dementia in elderly patients with mild cognitive impairment, the investigator considers two potential outcome measurements: change in Abeta (1–40) levels or incidence of a clinical diagnosis of dementia.
    a. List one advantage and one disadvantage of using Abeta (1–40) as the primary outcome for your trial.
    b. List one advantage and one disadvantage of using diagnosis of dementia as the primary outcome for the trial.
2. A large (>200 person per arm) trial of huperzine is being planned. The primary aim is to test whether this herbal extract decreases the incidence of a clinical diagnosis of dementia among elderly men and women who have mild cognitive impairment.
    a. Huperzine is expected to occasionally cause gastrointestinal symptoms, including diarrhea, nausea, and vomiting. Describe a plan for assessing adverse effects of this new treatment on symptoms or diseases besides cognitive impairment.
    b. Describe a general plan for baseline data collection: what types of information should be collected?

c. People who carry an Apoε4 allele have an increased risk of dementia. List one reason in favor and one against using stratified blocked randomization instead of simple randomization to assure a balance of people with the Apoε4 genotype in the treatment and control group.

CHAPTER 11. ALTERNATIVE TRIAL DESIGNS AND IMPLEMENTATION ISSUES

Topical finasteride is moderately effective in treating male pattern baldness and is approved by the U.S. Food and Drug Administration (FDA) for treating this condition. Statins have been found to increase hair growth in rodents and they act by a different pathway than does finasteride. Imagine that a start-up company wants to obtain FDA approval for marketing a new topical statin (HairStat) for the treatment of male pattern baldness.

1. Describe a phase I trial of HairStat for male pattern baldness. What would be the treatment group(s)? What type of outcomes?
2. The company wants to compare the efficacy of HairStat to finasteride. List at least one advantage and disadvantage the following approaches to testing the relative effectiveness of finasteride and the topical statin.
   a. Randomize bald men to either finasteride or topical statin.
   b. In a factorial design, randomly assign men to finasteride and statin, finasteride and statin-placebo, finasteride-placebo and statin, and double placebo.
3. Imagine that the company plans a 1-year placebo-controlled study of HairStat for treatment of baldness. The outcome is change in rating of the amount of hair in photographs of the bald region that is undergoing treatment. Follow-up visits (with photographs) are scheduled every 3 months. Outline a plan—with at least 2 elements—for encouraging compliance with the study and return for visits to assess the outcome.
4. Twenty percent of the men in the HairStat versus placebo trial did not return for the 3-month follow-up visit and 40% stopped by 1 year. Some stopped because a rash developed on their scalp. List one disadvantage and one advantage of analyzing the effect of treatment on hair growth by a strict intention-to-treat approach.
5. In the intention-to-treat analysis, HairStat increased hair growth (rated from comparison of photographs, masked to treatment) by about 20% ($P = 0.06$). Subsequent analyses showed that hair growth was 45% greater in men younger than age 40 than in older men ($P = 0.01$ in that subgroup). What are the problems with the company's conclusion that HairStat is effective for treating baldness in men younger than age 40?

CHAPTER 12. DESIGNING STUDIES OF MEDICAL TESTS

1. You are interested in studying the erythrocyte sedimentation rate (ESR) as a test for pelvic inflammatory disease (PID) in women with abdominal pain.
   a. To do this, you will need to assemble groups of women who do and do not have PID. What would be the best way to sample these women?

b. How might the results be biased if you used final diagnosis of PID as the gold standard and those assigning that diagnosis were aware of the ESR?

c. You find that the sensitivity of an ESR of at least 20 mm/hr is 90%, but the specificity is only 50%. On the other hand, the sensitivity of an ESR of at least 50 mm/hr is only 75%, but the specificity is 85%. How should you present these results?

2. You are interested in studying the diagnostic yield of computed tomography (CT) head scans in children presenting to the emergency department (ED) with head injuries. You use a database in the radiology department to find reports of all CT scans done on patients less than 18 years old and ordered from the ED for head trauma. You then review the ED records of all those who had an abnormal CT scan to determine whether the abnormality could have been predicted from the physical examination.

a. Out of 200 scans, 10 show intracranial injuries. However, you determine that in 8 of the 10, there had been either a focal neurological examination or altered mental status. Since only 2 patients had abnormal scans that could not have been predicted from the physical examination, you conclude that the yield of "unexpected" intracranial injuries is only 2 in 200 (1%) in this setting. What is wrong with that conclusion?

b. What is wrong with using intracranial injuries as the outcome variable for this diagnostic yield study?

c. What would be some advantages of studying the effects of the test on medical decision making, rather than just the diagnostic yield?

3. You now wish to study the sensitivity and specificity of focal neurological findings to predict intracranial injuries. (Because of the small sample size of intracranial injuries, you increase the sample size by extending the study to several other EDs.) One problem you have studying focal neurological findings is that children who have them are much more likely to get a CT scan than children who do not. Explain how and why this will affect the sensitivity and specificity of such findings if:

a. Only children who had a CT scan are included in the study.

b. Eligible children with head injuries who did not have a CT scan are included, and assumed not to have had an intracranial injury if they recovered without neurosurgical intervention.

CHAPTER 13. UTILIZING EXISTING DATABASES

1. The research question is: "Do Latinos in the United States have higher rates of gallbladder disease than whites, African Americans, or Asian Americans?" What existing databases might enable you to determine race-, age- and sex-specific rates of gallbladder disease at low cost in time and money?

2. A research fellow became interested in the question of whether mild or moderate renal dysfunction increases risk for CHD events and death. Because of the expense and difficulty of conducting a study to generate primary data, he searched for an existing database that contained the variables he needed to answer his research question. He found that the cardiovascular health study (CHS), a large, NIH-funded multicenter cohort study of predictors of cardiovascular disease in older

men and women provided all of the variables required for his planned analysis. His mentor was able to introduce him to one of the key investigators in CHS who helped him prepare and submit a proposal for analyses that was approved by the CHS Steering Committee.

    a. What are the advantages of this approach to study this question?

    b. What are the disadvantages?

3. An investigator is interested in whether the effects of treatment with post-menopausal estrogen or selective estrogen receptor modulators (SERMs) vary depending on endogenous estrogen levels. How might this investigator answer this question using an ancillary study?

CHAPTER 14. ADDRESSING ETHICAL ISSUES

1. The research question is to identify genes that are associated with an increased risk of developing type 2 diabetes mellitus. The investigator finds that frozen blood samples and clinical data are available from a large prospective cohort study on risk factors for coronary artery disease. That study collected baseline data on diet, exercise, clinical characteristics, and measurements of cholesterol and hemoglobin A1c. Follow-up data are available on coronary endpoints and the development of diabetes. The proposed study will carry out DNA sequencing on participants; no new blood samples are required.

    a. Can the proposed study be done under the original consent for the cohort study?

    b. If the original consent did not provide permission for such a study, how can the current investigators carry out their proposed study?

    c. When designing new studies that collect blood samples, how can investigators plan for future studies to use their data and samples?

2. The investigator plans a phase III randomized controlled trial of a new cancer drug that has shown promise in treating colon cancer. In order to reduce sample size, he would like to carry out a placebo-controlled trial rather than comparing it to current therapy.

    a. What are the ethical concerns about a placebo control in this situation?

    b. Is it possible to carry out a placebo-controlled study in an ethically acceptable manner?

3. The investigator plans a preparedness study for a future HIV vaccine trial. The goals are to determine (a) if it is possible to recruit a cohort of participants who have a high seroconversion rate despite state-of-the-art HIV prevention counseling and (b) if the follow-up rate in the cohort will be sufficiently high to carry out a vaccine trial. Participants will be persons at increased risk for HIV, including injection drug users, persons who trade sex for money, and other persons with multiple sexual partners. Most participants will have low literacy and poor health literacy. The study will be an observational cohort study, following participants for 2 years to determine sero-incidence rates.

    a. What do the federal regulations require be disclosed to participants as part of informed consent?

    b. What steps can be taken to ensure that consent is truly informed in this context?

c. What is the investigators' responsibility during this observational study to reduce the risk HIV in these high-risk participants?

CHAPTER 15. DESIGNING QUESTIONNAIRES AND INTERVIEWS

1. As part of a study of alcohol and muscle strength, an investigator plans to use the following item for a self-response questionnaire to determine current use of alcohol:

   "How many drinks of beer, wine, or liquor do you drink each day?"

   _____ 0
   _____ 1–2
   _____ 3–4
   _____ 5–6
   _____ 7–8

   Briefly describe at least two problems with this item.
2. Write a short series of questions for a self-response questionnaire that will better assess current alcohol use.
3. Comment on the advantages and disadvantages of a self-response questionnaire versus a structured interview to assess risky sexual behavior.

CHAPTER 16. DATA MANAGEMENT

1. Refer to the first six items on the sample questionnaire about smoking in Appendix 15.1. You have responses for three study subjects:

Subject ID	Description of Smoking History
1001	Started smoking at age 17 and has continued to smoke an average of 30 cigarettes/day ever since
1002	Started smoking at age 21 and smoked 20 cigarettes/day until quitting 3 years ago at age 45
1003	Smoked a few cigarettes (<100) in high school

   Create a data table containing the responses of these subjects to the first six questions in Appendix 15.1. The table should have three rows (one for each subject) and seven columns (one for Subject ID, and one each for the six questions).
2. The PHTSE (Pre-Hospital Treatment of Status Epilepticus) Study (1,2) was a randomized blinded trial of lorazepam, diazepam, or placebo in the treatment of prehospital status epilepticus. The primary endpoint was termination of convulsions by hospital arrival. To enroll patients, paramedics contacted base hospital physicians by radio. The following are base-hospital physician data collection forms for two enrolled patients:

PHTSE

Base Hospital Physician Data Collection Form

PHTSE Subject ID : *189*

Study Drug Administration

Study Drug Kit #: A322

Date and Time of Administration : 3/12/94 17:39

(Use 24 hour clock)

Transport Evaluation

| | Seizure Stopped

Time Seizure Stopped _____:_____

(Use 24 hour clock)

Final ("End-Of-Run") Assessment

Time of Arrival at Receiving Hospital ED: 17:48

(Use 24 hour clock)

On arrival at the receiving hospital:

[X] 1 Seizure activity (active tonic/clonic convulsions) continued

[ ] 0 Seizure activity (active tonic/clonic convulsions) stopped
    Verbal GCS
        [   ] 1 No Verbal Response
        [   ] 2 Incomprehensible Speech
        [   ] 3 Inappropriate Speech
        [   ] 4 Confused Speech
        [   ] 5 Oriented

   PAGE ON-CALL PHTSE STUDY PERSONNEL !!

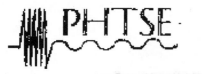

Base Hospital Physician Data Collection Form

PHTSE Subject ID : | **410** |

Study Drug Administration

Study Drug Kit #: | **B536** |

Date and Time of Administration : 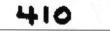 **12/01/98 01:35**

(Use 24 hour clock)

Transport Evaluation

☒ Seizure Stopped
Time Seizure Stopped **01:39**

(Use 24 hour clock)

Final ("End-Of-Run") Assessment

Time of Arrival at Receiving Hospital ED :   **01:53**

(Use 24 hour clock)

On arrival at the receiving hospital:

[ ]₁ Seizare activity (active tonic/clonic convulsions) continued

[☒]₀ Seizare activity (active tonic/clonic convulsions) stopped
Verbal GCS
   [   ]₁ No Verbal Response
   [   ]₂ Incomprehensible Speech
   [   ]₃ Inappropriate Speech
   [☒]₄ Confused Speech
   [   ]₅ Oriented

   PAGE ON-CALL PHTSE STUDY PERSONNEL !!

a. Display the data from these two data collection forms in a two-row data table.

b. Create a nine-field data dictionary for the data table in (a).

c. The paper data collection forms were completed by busy base hospital physicians who were called from the emergency department to a radio room. What are the advantages and disadvantages of using an on-screen computer form instead of a paper form? If you designed the study, which would you use?

3. The data collection forms in exercise 2 include a question about whether seizure activity continued on arrival at the receiving hospital (which was the primary outcome of the study). This data item was given the field name *HospArrSzAct* and was coded 1 for yes (seizure activity continued) and 0 for no (seizure activity stopped).

Interpret the average values for *HospArrSzAct* as displayed below:

	HospArrSzAct (1 = *Yes, seizure continued;* 0 = *No, seizure stopped*)	
	N	**Average**
Lorazepam	66	0.409
Diazepam	68	0.574
Placebo	71	0.789

REFERENCES

1. Lowenstein DH, Alldredge BK, Allen F, et al. The prehospital treatment of status epilepticus (PHTSE) study: design and methodology. *Control Clin Trials* 2001;22(3): 290–309.
2. Alldredge BK, Gelb AM, Isaacs SM, et al. A comparison of lorazepam, diazepam, and placebo for the treatment of out-of-hospital status epilepticus. *N Engl J Med* 2001;345(9): 631–637.

CHAPTER 17. IMPLEMENTING THE STUDY AND QUALITY CONTROL

1. An investigator studied the research question, "What are the predictors of death following hospitalization for myocardial infarction?" Research assistants collected detailed data from charts and conducted extensive interviews with 120 hospitalized patients followed over the course of 1 year. About 15% of the patients died during the follow-up period. When data collection was complete, one of the research assistants entered the data into a computer using a spreadsheet. When the data entry was complete, the investigator began to run analyses of the data. To his chagrin he discovered that about 10% to 20% of some predictor variables were missing, and others did not seem to make sense. Only 57% of the sample had been seen at the 1-year follow-up, now more than a year overdue for some subjects. You are called in to consult on the project.

a. What can the investigator do now to improve the quality of his data?

b. Briefly describe at least three ways that he could reduce missing values and errors in his next study.

CHAPTER 18. COMMUNITY AND INTERNATIONAL STUDIES

1. You wish to study the characteristics and clinical course of patients with abdominal pain of unclear etiology. You plan to enroll patients with abdominal pain in whom no specific cause can be identified after a standard battery of tests. There are two options for recruiting study subjects: (a) the G.I. clinic at your university medical center or (b) a local network of community clinics. What are the advantages and disadvantages of each approach?

2. You have been assigned to work with the Chinese Ministry of Health in a new program to prevent smoking-related diseases in China. Of the following research questions, to what degree does each require local research as opposed to research done elsewhere?
   a. What is the prevalence and distribution of cigarette smoking?
   b. What diseases are caused by smoking?
   c. What strategies are most effective for encouraging people to quit smoking?

CHAPTER 19. WRITING AND FUNDING A RESEARCH PROPOSAL

1. Search the NIH website (http://grants.nih.gov/grants/oer.htm) to find at least three types of investigator-initiated R-series grant awards.

2. Search the web for foundations that might be interested in the area of your research. List at least two.

3. A young investigator in physical therapy has interest and expertise in muscle physiology. A pharmaceutical company is testing a treatment that may increase the formation of skeletal muscle and invites him to recruit patients into a multicenter trial of the effect of the treatment on recovery from leg and hip fractures. The investigator would be paid a fee for each participant he enrolls in the trial. List at least two issues that the investigator should consider before contracting to participate in the trial.

Answers to Exercises

CHAPTER 1

1. This is a randomized blinded trial of whether treatment with vitamin D increases leg muscle strength in hypertensive men 70 years of age or greater.
2. This is a cohort study to examine whether watching wrestling on television predicts subsequent fighting on dates among high school students.
3. This is a case–control study of whether short- and long-acting psychotropic medications are associated with an increased risk for hip fracture among elderly women.
4. This is a cross-sectional descriptive study of the state of knowledge, among schoolchildren in Zimbabwe, about risk factors for AIDS.
   (We leave it to the reader to develop the inferences that can be drawn from these studies)

CHAPTER 2

1. One possible answer is "a cross-sectional study to determine whether depression is associated with health status among people in their early 20s." The possibility that "depression" and "health status" are related is Interesting and Relevant, and the question as stated is too vague to be able to judge whether it meets the other FINER criteria (Feasible, Novel and Ethical). How will depression and health status be measured, and in what population? Also it will be difficult to establish causality in a cross-sectional design—does depression lead to worse health or vice versa? A more specific design that could measure up to the FINER criteria (depending on how it is fleshed in) might be, "A cohort study to determine whether depression among college freshmen, assessed by the CES-D questionnaire predicts their health status as seniors, measured by the Rand General Health Questionnaire."
2. This is an Interesting research question that also needs to be made more specific. What is meant by red meat—does veal qualify? Any cancer, including skin cancer?

The research question and design could be rewritten: "A case–control study of whether the amount of beef consumed by elderly people is associated with occurrence of breast cancer over the next several decades?" This is less vague and certainly Ethical, but it may not be Feasible to produce a scientifically rigorous answer. The case–control design is suitable for cancer etiology, but subjects may have difficulty remembering how many servings of red meat they ate during different periods in their lifetime. The research question is not Novel—there have already been several studies of the association of eating meat and breast cancer, generally suggesting a small increase in risk among women who eat meat. Better data on meat consumption could be obtained with a prospective cohort study, but the low annual incidence of breast cancer would require a very large number of subjects followed for many years.

3. "A randomized clinical trial to test whether relaxation exercises decrease anxiety of middle-aged women during a mammogram" is a study that could be Feasible, Novel and Ethical, but this question may not be Interesting or Relevant enough to answer. Many women are anxious about having a mammogram and therefore delay or avoid the procedure. It is not the discomfort of the procedure itself, but the fear that a breast cancer will be diagnosed that creates anxiety. The relaxation exercise is unlikely to reduce this fear of finding cancer. In addition, such relaxation training will not be useful in getting more women to have a mammogram, because the intervention occurs only after the woman has already made the decision to have the test.

4. "A cross-sectional study to discover proteomic markers that help to distinguish coronary insufficiency from noncardiac causes in middle-aged men seen in the emergency room for chest pain." This study is Interesting, Novel and Ethical, and it is highly Relevant—better tests are needed to identify patients with substantial atherosclerotic plaque before undertaking expensive and invasive tests to explore their candidacy for coronary artery interventions. As to Feasibility, the study would not be a problem to carry out from a clinical standpoint, but the technical approaches to identifying individual proteomic markers among the thousands of proteins that circulate in the blood stream remain challenging.

CHAPTER 3

1. The target population (all eleventh graders, or more broadly, all high school students) may not be well suited to the research question if the antecedents of smoking take place at an earlier age—it might be better to study students in junior high. Also, the study sample (students at this one high school) may not adequately represent the target population—the causes of smoking differ in various cultural settings, and the investigator might do better to draw her sample from several high schools randomly selected from the whole region. Most important, the sampling design (calling for volunteers) is likely to attract students who are not representative of the accessible population in their smoking behavior.

2. The unrepresentative sample could have resulted from random error, but this would have been unlikely unless it was a very small sample. If the sample numbered ten, a 7 : 3 disproportion would occur fairly often as a result of chance; in fact, the probability of finding at least seven heads in ten tosses of a coin is 17% (plus another 17% chance of finding seven tails). But if the sample size were 100, the probability of finding at least 70 heads is less than 0.01%. This illustrates the fact

that the investigator can estimate the magnitude of the random component of sampling error once the sample has been acquired and that she can reduce it to any desired level by enlarging the sample size.

The unrepresentative sample could also have resulted from systematic error. The large proportion of females could have been due to different rates of participation among boys and girls. The strategies for preventing nonresponse bias include the spectrum of techniques for enhancing recruitment discussed in Chapter 3. The large proportion of females could also represent a technical mistake in enumerating or selecting the names to be sampled. The strategies for preventing mistakes include the appropriate use of pretesting and quality control procedures (Chapter 17).

3. a. Random sample (probability)
   b. Stratified random sample (probability), with a threefold over-sampling of women, perhaps because the investigator anticipated that few women would attend the concert
   c. Systematic sample (nonprobability)
   d. Cluster sample (probability)
   e. Consecutive sample (nonprobability)
   f. Convenience sample (nonprobability)
   g. Judgmental sample (nonprobability)

CHAPTER 4

1. a. Dichotomous
   b. Continuous
   c. Dichotomous
   d. Ordered discrete
   e. Dichotomous
   f. Ordered discrete
   g. Ordinal
   h. Continuous
   i. Nominal
   j. Dichotomous

   Power is increased by using an outcome variable that contains ordered information; that is, (d) has more power than (c). As to (j), use of body weight as a continuous outcome would offer far more power (carry more information) than presence or absence of obesity.

2. a. This is a problem with accuracy. It could be due to an observer not visualizing the reading correctly (a second observer could check the result), but more likely the scale needs to be adjusted.
   b. This is a problem with precision. The excessive variability could be an observer error, but more likely the scale needs refurbishing.
   c. This situation can reduce both accuracy and precision. Accuracy will suffer because the observer's hold on the baby will likely alter the observed weight; depending on technique, this might tend to consistently increase the observed weight or to consistently decrease it. This problem with the subjects might be solved by having the mother spend some time calming the baby; an alternative would be to weigh the parent with and without the baby, and take the difference.

d. This is primarily a problem with precision, because the pointer on the scale will vary around the true weight (if the scale is accurate). The problem is with the subjects and has the same solution as in (c).

e. This is mainly a problem with precision, since the babies' weights will vary, depending on whether or not they ate and wet their diapers before the examination. This problem of subject variability could be reduced by giving the mothers instructions not to feed the babies for 3 hours before the examination, and weighing all babies naked.

CHAPTER 5

1. Sample size = the projected number of subjects in a study that are required for the investigator to be able to detect a given effect size (at the specified levels of α and β)

   Null hypothesis = a statement of the research hypothesis that indicates that there is no difference between the groups being compared

   Alternative hypothesis = a statement of the research hypothesis that indicates that there is a difference between the groups being compared

   Power = the likelihood of detecting a statistically significant difference between the groups being compared (with a given sample size, at a given level of statistical significance) if the real difference in the population equals the effect size

   Level of statistical significance = the preset chance of falsely rejecting the null hypothesis

   Effect size = the minimum size of the difference in the two groups being compared that the investigator wishes to detect

2. a. Neither. This is a statistically significant result, and there is nothing to suggest that it represents a Type I error.

   b. The sample size was small and very few subjects would have developed lung cancer during the study. These negative results are almost certainly due to a Type II error, especially given extensive evidence from other studies that smoking causes lung cancer.

   c. There is no prior epidemiologic or pathophysiologic reason to believe that alcohol use reduces the risk of developing diabetes; this result is likely due to a Type I error.

CHAPTER 6

1. H_0: There is no difference in the body mass index of stomach cancer cases and controls.

   H_A (two-sided): There is a difference in the body mass index of stomach cancer cases and controls. Body mass index is a continuous variable and case–control is dichotomous, so a t-test should be used.

$$\text{Effect size} = 1 \text{ kg/m}^2$$
$$\text{Standard deviation} = 2.5 \text{ kg/m}^2$$
$$E/S = 0.4$$

From Appendix 6.A,

> If $\alpha = 0.05, \beta = 0.20,$ then 100 subjects are needed per group.
> If $\alpha = 0.05, \beta = 0.10,$ then 133 subjects are needed per group.
> If $\alpha = 0.01, \beta = 0.20,$ then 148 subjects are needed per group.

Extra credit: If the investigator only had access to 60 cases, only one of the following strategies for increasing power will help:

a. Use a continuous variable—body mass index is already being measured as a continuous variable.

b. Use a more precise variable—both weight and height are precise variables, and the standard deviation of body mass index is composed almost entirely of between-individual variation, which cannot be reduced.

c. Use paired measurements—not applicable; "change" in body mass index is not relevant in this situation

d. Use a more common outcome—not applicable.

e. Use unequal group sizes—the n of controls can be increased, as it is easy to find subjects without stomach cancer. For example, if the number of controls can be increased fourfold to 240, one can use the approximation formula on page 80:

$$n' = ([c + 1] \div 2c) \times n$$

where n' represents the "new" number of cases, c represents the control-to-case ratio (in this example, 4), and n represents the "old" number of cases (assuming a control per case). In this example,

$$n' = ([4 + 1] \div 8) \times 100 = (5/8) \times 100 = 63,$$

which is just about the number of cases that are available. Therefore, a study with 60 cases and 240 controls will have similar power as one with 100 cases and 100 controls.

2. H_0: There is no difference in mean strength between the DHEA-treated and placebo-treated groups.

 H_A: There is a difference in mean strength between the DHEA-treated and placebo-treated groups.

> $\alpha = 0.05$ (two-sided); $\beta = 0.10$
>
> Test $= t$ test
>
> Effect size $= 10\% \times 20$ kg $= 2$ kg
>
> Standard deviation $= 8$ kg

 The standardized effect size (E/S) is 0.25 (2 kg/8 kg). Looking at Appendix 6.A, go down the left column to 0.25, then across to the fifth column from the left, where α(two-sided) $= 0.05$ and $\beta = 0.10$. Approximately 338 subjects per group would be needed. If $\beta = 0.20$, then the sample size is 253 per group.

3. H_0: There is no difference in the mean change in strength between the DHEA-treated and placebo-treated groups.

H_A: There is a difference in mean change in strength between the DHEA-treated and placebo-treated groups.

$$\alpha = 0.05 \text{ (two-sided)}; \beta = 0.10$$
$$\text{Test} = t \text{ test}$$
$$\text{Effect size} = 10\% \times 20 \text{ kg} = 2 \text{ kg}$$
$$\text{Standard deviation} = 2 \text{ kg}$$

The standardized effect size (E/S) is 1.0 (2 kg/2 kg). Looking at Appendix 6.A, go down the left column to 1.0 then across to the fifth column from the left where α(two-sided) = 0.05 and β = 0.10. Approximately 23 subjects per group would be needed.

4. H_0: There is no difference in frequency of left-handedness in dyslexic and nondyslexic students.
   H_A: There is a difference in frequency of left-handedness in dyslexic and nondyslexic students.

$$\alpha = 0.05 \text{ (two-sided)}; \beta = 0.20$$
$$\text{Test} = \text{chi-squared test (both variables are dichotomous)}$$
$$\text{Effect size} = \text{odds ratio of 2.0}$$

Given that the proportion of nondyslexic students who are left-handed (P_2) is about 0.1, the investigator wants to be able to detect a proportion of dyslexic students who are left-handed (P_1) that will yield an odds ratio of 2.0. The sample size estimate will use a chi-squared test, and one needs to use Appendix 6.B. However, that appendix is set up for entering the two proportions, not the odds ratio, and all that is known is one of the proportions ($P_2 = 0.1$).

To calculate the value for P_1 that gives an odds ratio of 2, one can use the formula on page 69:

$$P_1 = \text{OR} \times P_2 \div ([1 - P_2] + [\text{OR} \times P_2]).$$

In this example:

$$P_1 = (2 \times 0.1) \div ([1 - 0.1] + [2 \times 0.1]) = 0.18$$

So P_1 is 0.18 and P_2 is 0.1. $P_1 - P_2$ is 0.08. The Table 6.B.2 in Appendix 6.B reveals a sample size of 318 per group.

Extra credit: Try this using the formula on page 87; just slog on through, carrying 6 places after the decimal. Then get an instant answer from the calculator on our website, www.epibiostat.ucsf.edu/dcr/

5. Standard deviation of IQ scores is about one-fourth of the "usual" range (which is $170 - 130 = 40$ points), or 10 points.

   Total width of the confidence interval = 6 (3 above and 3 below) Confidence level = 99%

   Standardized width of the confidence interval = total width/standard deviation $W/S = 0.6$

   Using Table 6.D, go down the W/S column to 0.60, then across to the 99% confidence level. About 74 medical students' IQ scores would need to be averaged to obtain a mean score with the specified confidence interval.

CHAPTER 7

1. a. Measure serum vitamin B_{12} levels in a cohort of white women more than 70 years of age and without a history of hip fractures and analyze the association with incident hip fractures observed over the next 5 years. (Choice of study subjects is based on the fact that hip fracture is most common in white women; the age cutoff is somewhat arbitrary, but based on the age at which hip fracture incidence rises rapidly and to substantial levels.) The use of reported dietary intake of foods rich in vitamin B_{12} instead of the serum level might be more expensive because dietary histories take a lot of time to collect and score and would certainly be a less precise and less accurate measurement.
   b. Advantages of the prospective cohort design for studying vitamin B_{12} sufficiency and hip fractures:
      • Temporal sequence (i.e., the hip fracture follows the vitamin B_{12} deficiency) helps establish a cause–effect relationship. Women who fracture their hips might become vitamin B_{12} deficient after the fracture because they have reduced food intake or received treatments to suppress acid (and vitamin B_{12}) production.
      • The prospective design allows you to design good methods for measuring the predictor variable (i.e., serum vitamin B_{12}).
      • The cohort design avoids the sampling bias that is always a possibility in case–control studies if the women with fractures come from a different accessible population than those without fractures.
      Disadvantage of the prospective cohort design:
      • A prospective cohort study will require many subjects followed for multiple years. The study will therefore be very expensive.
   c. A retrospective cohort study could be done if you could find a cohort with stored serum or records on dietary vitamin B_{12} intake and with reasonably complete follow-up to determine who developed hip fracture. The main advantage of this design is that it would be less time consuming and expensive. The major drawback is that measurements of vitamin B_{12} in the serum might be altered by the storage, and that measurements of potential confounders (such as age, race, physical activity, cigarette smoking, etc.) may not be available.

CHAPTER 8

1. a. The cases might consist of all women between 30 and 75 years of age with ovarian cancer reported to the Northern California Cancer Center Tumor Registry. This tumor registry has been shown to include nearly 100% of incident ovarian cancer cases in five San Francisco Bay Area counties.
   b. The controls might be a random sample of all women between 30 and 75 years of age from the same five counties in the San Francisco Bay Area. The random sample might be obtained by using random-digit dialing.
   c. The methods outlined for choosing cases and controls are aimed at obtaining all cancer cases and a random sample of those at risk in the target population (women 30 to 75 years old in five Bay Area counties). However, it is possible,

since ovarian cancer requires intensive therapy and is deadly, that some cases may be unwilling to enroll in the study or may die before they can be interviewed. If a family history of ovarian cancer is related to more aggressive forms of ovarian cancer, then the study might underestimate its relative risk, because those cases with a positive family history are less likely to survive long enough to be included in the sample of cases. If familial ovarian cancer is more benign than other ovarian cancers, the opposite could occur. Similarly, it is possible that healthy women who have a family member with ovarian cancer will be more interested in the study and more likely to enroll as a control than women who do not have a family member with ovarian cancer. In that case, the prevalence of family history of ovarian cancer in the control group will be artificially high, and the estimate of the risk for ovarian cancer due to family history will be falsely low. This problem might be minimized by not telling the potential control subjects exactly what the research question is or exactly which cancer is being are studied, if this can be done in a way that is acceptable to the IRB.

d. Family history of ovarian cancer is generally measured by asking subjects about how many female relatives they have, and how many of them have had ovarian cancer. Recall bias is a possible problem with this approach. Women with ovarian cancer, who may be concerned about the possibility of a genetic predisposition to their disease, may be more likely to remember or find out about relatives with ovarian cancer than healthy women who have not had reason to think about this possibility. In this case, the estimate of the association between family history and ovarian cancer may be falsely high.

In addition, women may confuse the gynecological cancers (cervical, uterine, and ovarian) and confuse benign gynecological tumors that require surgery with malignant tumors. This may cause misclassification (some women without a family history of ovarian cancer will report having the risk factor and be misclassified). If misclassification occurs equally in the cases and controls, the estimate of the association between family history and ovarian cancer will be falsely low. If this type of misclassification is more common in cases (who may be more likely to misinterpret the type of cancer or the reason for surgery in relatives), then the estimate of the association between family history and ovarian cancer will be falsely high. Misclassification could be decreased by checking pathological records of family members who are reported to have ovarian cancer to verify the diagnosis.

e. The simplest approach would be to dichotomize family history of ovarian cancer and use the odds ratio as the measure of association. The odds ratio approximates the relative risk because the outcome (ovarian cancer) is rare. A simple chi-square would then be the appropriate test of statistical significance. Alternatively, if family history were quantified (e.g., proportion of first- and second-degree female relatives affected), one could look for a dose–response, computing odds ratios at each level of exposure.

f. The case–control design is a reasonable way to answer this research question despite the problems of sampling bias, recall bias, and misclassification that are noted above. A nested case–control study is generally preferable if possible. The chief alternative would be a large cohort study, but because ovarian cancer is so rare, a cohort design is probably not feasible.

2. a. The study is cross-sectional because the potential predictors (maternal height and weight) are measured at essentially the same time as the outcome (infant birth weight).

b. Causal inference in cross-sectional observational studies depends on the time sequence of the predictor and outcome variables, and on the possible role of confounding variables. In this study, the mother's weight was measured just after delivery and reflects a combination of the mother's weight before she became pregnant and the amount of weight that she gained during pregnancy. Since the amount of weight gained during pregnancy may depend on the weight of the fetus, it is not clear which variable is the predictor. However, the mother's height measured just after delivery probably does not differ from her height if it had been measured before conception. It is reasonable therefore to conclude that maternal height is a predictor of birthweight. However, the phrase "dependent on" conveys a hint of causal inference that goes beyond the findings, since confounders like nutritional state of the mother may be operating.

3. Go for it–the sky's the limit.

CHAPTER 9

1. There are five possible explanations for the association between diet and CHD:
   a. Chance—the finding that people with CHD eat fewer fruits and vegetables was due to random error. As discussed in Chapter 5, the P value allows quantification of the magnitude of the observed difference compared with what might have been expected by chance alone. All else being equal, the smaller the P value, the less plausible chance is as an explanation.
   b. Bias—there was a systematic error (a difference between the research question and the way the study plan was carried out) with regard to the sample, predictor variable, or outcome variable. For example, the sample may be biased if the controls were patients at the same HMO, but were selected from those attending an annual health maintenance examination, as such patients may be more health conscious (and hence eat more fruits and vegetables) than the entire population at risk for CHD. The measurements of diet could be biased if people who have had a heart attack are more likely to recall poor dietary practices than controls (recall bias) or if unblinded interviewers asked the questions or recorded the answers differently in cases and controls. The likelihood of bias can be reduced by consulting with colleagues and carefully considering major design decisions such as selection of study subjects, and by blinding measurements wherever possible.
   c. Effect–cause—it is possible that having a heart attack reduced people's appetites, so that they ate less food in general (including less fruits and vegetables). The possibility of effect-cause can often be addressed by designing variables to examine the historical sequence—for example, by asking the cases if they changed their diet after their heart attack. In this instance, a strategy would be to express fruit and vegetable intake as percentage of total intake rather than as the absolute intake.
   d. Confounding—there may be other differences between those who eat more fruits and vegetables and those who eat fewer, and these other differences may be the actual cause of the lower rate of CHD. For example, people who eat more fruits and vegetables may exercise more. The strategies for addressing the latter possibility are as follows:

	Plan	Advantages	Disadvantages
Design Phase			
Specification	Enroll only people who report no regular exercise	Simple	Will limit the pool of eligible subjects, making recruitment more difficult. The study may not generalize to people that exercise.
Matching	Match each case to a control with similar exercise level	Eliminates the effect of exercise as a predictor of CHD, often with a slight increase in the precision (power) to observe diet as a predictor.	Requires extra effort to identify controls to match each case. Will waste cases if there is no control with a similar exercise level. Eliminates the opportunity to study the effect of exercise on CHD. Requires a matched statistical analysis model.
Analysis Phase			
Stratification	For the analysis, group the subjects into three or four exercise strata	Easy, comprehensible, and reversible	Can only reasonably evaluate a few strata and a few confounding variables before you find no cases (or controls) in a cell. Will lose some of the information contained in fitness measured as a continuous variable by switching to a categorical variable, and this may result in incomplete control of confounding.
Statistical adjustment (modeling)	Use logistic regression model to control for fitness as well as other potential confounders	Can reversibly control for all the information in fitness as a continuous predictor variable, while simultaneously controlling for other potential confounders such as age, race, and smoking	The statistical model might not fit the data, resulting in incomplete control of confounding and potentially misleading results. For example, the effect of diet or physical fitness may not be the same in smokers and nonsmokers. The important potential confounders must have been measured in advance. Sometimes it is difficult to understand and describe the results of the model, especially when variables are not dichotomous.

In addition to these four strategies for controlling confounding in observational studies, there is the ultimate solution: designing a randomized blinded trial.

e. Cause–effect—the fifth possible explanation is that eating fruits and vegetables really does reduce the rate of CHD events. This explanation is made likely partly by a process of exclusion, reaching the judgment that each of the other four explanations is unlikely and partly by seeking other evidence to support the causal hypothesis. An example of the latter is to consider the biologic evidence that there are components of fruits and vegetables (e.g., antioxidants) that are antiatherogenic.

CHAPTER 10

1. a. The advantage of using the biomarkers as the primary outcome of the trial is a smaller sample size and a shorter duration to determine whether the treatment reduces the level of the marker. The disadvantage is the uncertainty of whether change in the level of the marker induced by the treatment means that the treatment will reduce the progression of Alzheimer's disease.

   b. The clinical diagnosis of dementia is a more meaningful outcome of the trial that could improve clinical practice for prevention of dementia. On the other hand, such a trial would be large, long and expensive.

2. a. Participants should be asked at each follow-up visit whether they experience diarrhea, nausea, or vomiting. This could be done using a check box format that is easy to code and analyze. To find other unanticipated adverse effects, participants should also be asked to describe other symptoms, conditions or medical care (such as hospitalization or new prescription drugs) that have occurred since the previous visit. These would be asked in an open-ended way, but the responses can be coded for data entry.

   b. Baseline collection of data should include (a) measurement of the outcome (assessment of cognitive function), (b) risk factors for the outcome, such as hypertension or family history of dementia that might identify patients with the highest rate of the outcome and, perhaps, the greatest benefit from treatment; (c) information about how to contact the participant, family or doctor to allow more complete follow-up. Biological specimens should be stored to allow future measurement of factors, such as genotypes of enzymes that metabolize the drug, which could influence the effectiveness of the treatment.

   c. Stratified blocked randomization could guarantee that there would be a very similar number of participants with the Apoε4 genotype in the treatment and the placebo group. This could be especially important if the effect of the treatment is influenced by presence of the genotype. Stratified blocked randomization can avoid small random numerical imbalances of an important factor that could have relatively large impact on the outcome. On the other hand, this process makes the trial more complicated (assessing Apoε4 genotype before enrollment will delay randomization and raises issues that include how to counsel participants about the results.) The risk of a substantial imbalance in a relatively large trial (>200 per arm) is very low so that simple randomization would be good choice.

CHAPTER 11

1. The main goal of a phase I trial is to determine if the treatment is sufficiently safe and well tolerated to permit additional trials to find the best dose and test its clinical effectiveness. A phase I trial would use one or more potential human doses of the treatment with the main outcome of adverse events, such as the occurrence of rash. There would be no control group.

2. a. The comparison of two treatments without a placebo group has several disadvantages. This design cannot accurately determine the effectiveness of the new treatment: this requires comparison with a placebo. A large sample size may be needed to test whether the two treatments are equivalent or that the new treatment is not inferior. Equivalence or "noninferiority" trials have the advantage of assuring that all patients receive an active treatment and not a placebo, but this advantage is not important for a cosmetic problem.

   b. A factorial design that includes a placebo has the advantages of comparing each treatment to a placebo, and (if planned with adequate statistical power) testing whether the combination of treatments is better than either one alone. The obvious disadvantages are larger size, greater cost and complexity of the trial.

3. Adherence with the visits, protocol and study medication could be improved by:
   – employing friendly research staff who are enthusiastic about the study
   – reminders (by email, telephone or mail) of upcoming visits and the importance of adherence to treatment
   – reimbursement for travel, parking, and other expenses related to the study
   – consider a run-in period to exclude those more likely to miss follow-up visits or not adhere to treatment
   – other potential strategies listed in Table 11.2

4. The main disadvantage of intention-to-treat is that it includes participants who do not comply with the randomized treatment, and who therefore reduce the apparent magnitude of any effect that is observed for the whole randomized group. However, the disadvantages of using as-treated analyses in place of intention-to-treat are even greater—because participants who do not comply with the intervention usually differ from those who do comply in important ways, one no longer has a true randomized comparison and may incorrectly conclude that the HairStat is effective.

5. The conclusion that HairStat works better in younger men, based on a subgroup analysis, may be wrong and misleading because the result may be due to chance. The probability of finding a "significant" effect in a subgroup when there is no significant effect overall increases with the number of subgroups tested; it is not clear how many subgroups were tested to find this "significant" effect. The claim that the treatment is effective in men younger than age 40 implies that the treatment was ineffective—or even had the opposite effect—in older men. This result should also be reported and statistically tested for an interaction between age and the effect of treatment. The claim would be stronger if there were a biological basis for a greater effect in younger than older men and, for that reason, the subgroup analysis had been planned in advance.

CHAPTER 12

1. a. The best way to sample subjects for a diagnostic test is generally to sample patients at risk of a disease, before it is known who has the disease and who does

not. In this case, sampling women who present acutely to a clinic or emergency department with signs and symptoms consistent with pelvic inflammatory disease (PID) would probably be best. Comparing the erythrocyte sedimentation rates (ESRs) of women hospitalized with PID with those of a healthy control population (nurses, medical students) would be the worst approach, because both the spectrum of disease and especially the spectrum of nondisease are not representative of the groups in whom the test would be used clinically. (Those hospitalized for PID probably have more severe disease than average, and healthy volunteers are much less likely to have high ESRs than women with abdominal pain due to causes other than PID.)

b. If those assigning the final diagnosis used the ESR to help decide who had PID and who did not, both the sensitivity and specificity might be falsely high. The more those assigning the diagnosis relied on the ESR, the greater the bias in the study.

c. The best answer is that you should not use any particular cutoff for defining an abnormal result. Rather, you should graphically display the trade-off between sensitivity and specificity using a receiver operating characteristics (ROC) curve and present likelihood ratios for various ESR intervals (e.g., >20, 20 to 49, ≥50 mm/hr) rather than sensitivity and specificity at different cutoffs. This is illustrated by the table below, which can be created from the information in the question:

ESR	PID	No PID	Likelihood Ratio
≥ 50	75%	15%	5.00
20–49	15%	35%	0.43
< 20	10%	50%	0.20
	100%	**100%**	

The ROC curve could also be used to compare the ESR with one or more other tests such as a white blood cell count. This is illustrated in the hypothetical ROC curve below, which suggests that the ESR is superior to the WBC for predicting PID:

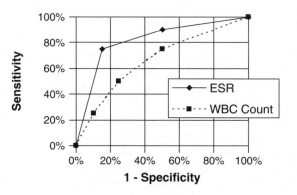

2. a. This problem illustrates the common error of excluding people from the numerator, without excluding them from the denominator. Although it is true that there were only two children with "unexpected" intracranial injuries,

the denominator for the yield must be the number of children with normal neurological examinations and mental status—probably a much smaller number than 200.

b. Unless the finding of an intracranial injury leads to changes in management and there is some way to estimate the effects of these management changes on outcome, it will be very hard to know what yield is sufficient to make the test worth doing. It would be better to use "intracranial injury requiring intervention" as the outcome in this study, although this will require some consensus on what injuries require intervention and some estimate of the effectiveness of these interventions for improving outcome.

c. The first advantage is the ability to examine possible benefits of normal results. For example, a normal CT scan might change the management plan from "admit for observation" to "send home." In diagnostic yield studies, normal results are generally assumed to be of little value. Second, as mentioned earlier, abnormal CT scan results might not lead to any changes in management (e.g., if no neurosurgery was required and the patient was going to be admitted anyway). Studying effects of tests on medical decision making helps to determine how much new information they provide, beyond what is already known at the time the test is ordered.

3. a. If only children who had a CT scan are included, the study will be susceptible to the first type of verification bias (Appendix 12B), in which sensitivity is falsely increased and specificity is falsely decreased, because children without focal neurologic abnormalities (who are either "false negatives" or "true negatives") will be underrepresented in the study.

b. If children with head injuries who did not have a CT scan are included, and assumed not to have an intracranial injury if they recover without neurosurgery, then the study will be susceptible to the second type of verification bias, "double gold standard bias" (Appendix 12C), which will tend to increase both sensitivity and specificity, if some intracranial injuries resolve without neurosurgery.

CHAPTER 13

1. Three possibilities:
   a. Analyze data from the National Health and Nutrition Examination Survey (NHANES). These national studies are conducted periodically and their results are available to any investigator at a nominal cost. They contain data from population-based samples that include variables on self-reported clinical history of gallbladder disease and the results of abdominal sonography.
   b. Analyze Medicare data on frequency of gallbladder surgery in patients more than 65 years of age in the United States or National Hospital Discharge Survey data on the frequency of such surgery for all ages. Both data sets contain a variable for race. Denominators could come from census data. Like the NHANES, these are very good population-based samples but have the problem of answering a somewhat different research question (i.e., what are the rates of surgical treatment for gallbladder disease). This may be different from the actual incidence of gallbladder disease due to factors such as access to care.
   c. Check local coroner records on the relation between gallbladder disease (as an incidental finding on autopsy) and race. Such a sample, however, may have biases as to who gets autopsied.

2. a. The main advantages are that using CHS data in a secondary data analysis was quick, easy, and inexpensive—especially compared to the time and expense of planning and conducting a large cohort study. In addition, the research fellow has since developed an on-going collaboration with the investigators in CHS and has been able to add more sophisticated measures of kidney function to CHS in an ancillary study.

   b. In some cases, the secondary dataset does not provide optimal measures of the predictor, outcome or potential confounding variables. It is important to be sure that the dataset will provide reasonable answers to the research question before investing the time and effort required to obtain access to the data.

3. There have been several large randomized controlled trials of the effect of estrogen and SERMs on various disease outcomes, including cardiovascular events, cancer and thromboembolic events. These trials include the Heart and Estrogen/Progestin Replacement Study, the Women's Health Initiative randomized trials, the Breast Cancer Prevention Trial, the Multiple Outcomes of Raloxifene Evaluation trial, and the Raloxifene Use for The Heart trial. The best place for this investigator to begin would be to determine if estrogen can be measured from stored frozen sera, and if so, determine if any of these large trials have stored sera that could be used for this measurement. The best design for this question is a nested case–control or case–cohort study. The investigator will likely need to write a proposal for this ancillary study, obtain approval from the trial Steering Committee and sponsor, and obtain funding to make the measurements (a relatively inexpensive prospect, since most of the costs of the study have already been covered by the main trial).

CHAPTER 14

1. a. It depends on whether the participants in the original study gave consent for their samples to be used in future studies and what kinds of studies were specified. The samples may have been collected to be used only to repeat the tests specified in the protocol, in case of lost samples or laboratory accidents. Or, the participants might have specified that the samples could be used in other studies of coronary artery disease. In these two situations, the original consent would not cover the proposed project.

   b. Under the Common Rule, a project can be carried out on existing specimens and data if the new investigator cannot identify the participants, either directly or with the assistance of someone else. Thus, if the new researcher receives samples and data labeled 0001, 0002, 0003, etc., and the code that links the samples and the identities of the participants is destroyed or not accessible to the new researcher, additional consent need not be obtained for the secondary study. The ethical justification is that such anonymization of materials protects participants from breaches of confidentiality, which is the major risk in research with existing materials and data. The presumption is that no one would object to their materials and data being used if there was no risk of breaches of confidentiality. Note, however, that some participants might find it objectionable for someone to sequence their DNA, even if confidentiality is maintained, since the DNA contains information that could lead ultimately to a loss of confidentiality. In other words, for some types of sensitive research, there may be ethical concerns about studies that are permitted under the federal regulations.

One way to resolve this dilemma is to have the IRB for the proposed study have strong input from lay and community members. In addition, the IRB might add ad hoc reviewers who represent groups who might have specific concerns about the proposed study, such as ethnic minority communities who have suffered discrimination from genetic research in the past. Another approach if the prospective study is still ongoing is that the investigators can to ask participants to give specific consent for the new study. If feasible, this approach best respects the wishes of participants.

c. When researchers collect new samples in a research project, it is prudent to ask permission to collect and store additional blood, to be used in future research studies. Storing samples allows future research to be carried out more efficiently than assembling a new cohort. Tiered consent is recommended: the participant is asked to consent (i) to the specific study (for example the original cohort study), (ii) to other research projects on the same general topic (such as risk of coronary artery disease), or (iii) to all other future research that is approved by an IRB and by a scientific review panel. To address the issues raised in (b), the participant might also be asked to consent specifically to research in which their DNA would be sequenced. The participant may agree to one, a few, or all options. Of course, it is impossible to describe future research. Hence consent for future studies is not really informed in the sense that the participant will not know the nature, risks, and benefits of future studies. The participant is being asked to trust that IRBs and scientific review panels will only permit future studies that are scientifically and ethically sound.

2. a. Withholding from the control group drugs that are known to be effective would subject them to harm and would therefore be unethical. Even if participants would give informed consent for participate in such a placebo-controlled trial, an IRB may not approve such a study, which violates the regulatory requirements that the risk/benefit balance be acceptable and that the risks be minimized.

b. The investigators should try to identify a subgroup of patients for whom no therapy has been shown to prolong survival (the most clinically significant end-point in most cancer treatments). For example, patients whose disease has progressed despite chemotherapy and have no options that are proven effective could be asked to participate in a placebo-controlled trial of the experimental intervention. An acceptable control arm could be placebo or best current treatment. This approach assumes that if the drug is active in previously untreated patients it will also be active after other treatments have failed. It is, of course, possible, that a drug that does not work in refractory disease may be effective as first-line treatment.

3. a. During informed consent, the investigators must discuss: (i) the nature of the study; (ii) the study intervention and the number and length of visits; (iii) the potential benefits and risks of participation (in this case primarily stigma and discrimination if confidentiality is breached); (iv) alternatives to participation in the trial, including HIV prevention measures that are available outside the trial; (v) the voluntary nature of participation and the right to withdraw at any time; (vi) protection of confidentiality consistent with state public health reporting requirements; and (vii) a commitment to answer questions about the study.

b. Investigators need to present information in a manner that participants can understand. Participants with low health literacy will not be able to comprehend a detailed written consent form. It would be useful for the researchers to consult with community and advocacy groups on how to present the information. Suggestions might include community meetings, videotapes, DVDs, and comic books. Extensive pretesting should be carried out. Furthermore, researchers should determine what misunderstandings about the study are common and revise the consent process to address them.

c. Even though the study is an observational study, researchers have an ethical obligation to provide information to participants about how to reduce their risk for HIV. There are both ethical and scientific reasons for doing so. Researchers have an ethical obligation to prevent harm to participants in their study. They may not withhold feasible public health measures that are known to prevent the fatal illness that is the end-point of the study. Such measures would include counseling, condoms, and referral to substance abuse treatment and needle exchange programs. The preparedness study offers an opportunity to develop and field-test these prevention interventions. Researchers must also invoke these co-interventions to prevent harm to participants in the subsequent vaccine trial, even though the power of the trial will be reduced.

CHAPTER 15

1. a. There is no definition of how big a "drink" is.
   b. There is no way to respond if the subject is drinking more than eight drinks per day.
   c. The question does not specify time—weekdays versus weekend, everyday versus less than daily.
   d. It may be better to specify a particular time frame (e.g., in the past 7 days).
2. a. Which of the following statements best describes how <u>often</u> you drank alcoholic beverage during the past year? An alcoholic beverage includes wine, liquor or mixed drinks. Select one of the 8 categories.

   ☐ Every day   ☐ 2–3 Times per month
   ☐ 5–6 Days per week   ☐ About once a month
   ☐ 3–4 Days per week   ☐ Less than 12 times a year
   ☐ 1–2 Days per week   ☐ Rarely or not at all

   b. During the past year, <u>how many</u> drinks did you <u>usually</u> have on a <u>typical day</u> <u>when you drank alcohol?</u> A drink is about 12 oz. of beer, 5 oz. of wine, or $1\frac{1}{2}$ oz. of hard liquor. 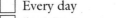 drinks
   c. During the past year, what is the <u>largest number</u> of alcoholic drinks you can recall drinking <u>during one day?</u> 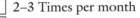 drinks
   d. About how old were you when you first started drinking alcoholic beverages?

      _____ years old. (if you have never consumed alcoholic beverages, write in "never" and go to question #7)

e. Was there ever a period when you drank quite a bit more than you do now?

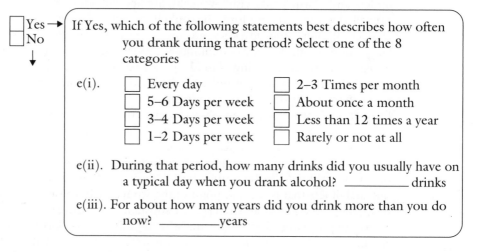

e(i).
- [ ] Every day
- [ ] 5–6 Days per week
- [ ] 3–4 Days per week
- [ ] 1–2 Days per week
- [ ] 2–3 Times per month
- [ ] About once a month
- [ ] Less than 12 times a year
- [ ] Rarely or not at all

e(ii). During that period, how many drinks did you usually have on a typical day when you drank alcohol? _____ drinks

e(iii). For about how many years did you drink more than you do now? _____ years

f. Have you ever had what might be considered a drinking problem?

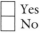
- [ ] Yes
- [ ] No

3. a. Obtaining data through interviews requires more staff training and time than a self-administered questionnaire and is therefore much more expensive.
   b. Some subjects do not like to tell another person the answer to sensitive questions in the area of sexual behavior.
   c. Unless the interviewers are well trained and the interviews are standardized, the information obtained may vary.
   d. However, interviewers can repeat and probe in a way that improves comprehension and produces more accurate and complete responses in some situations than a self-administered questionnaire.

CHAPTER 16

1.

SubjectID	EverSmoked100Cigs	AgeFirstCig	AvgCigsPerDay	PastWeekCigsAny	PastWeekCigsPerDay	AgeStoppedSmoking
1001	TRUE	17	30	TRUE	30	
1002	TRUE	21	20	FALSE		45
1003	FALSE			FALSE		

This is how the data might look in a spreadsheet program such as Excel. There are many acceptable possibilities for the field names (column headings). These field names use IntraCaps (capitals in the middle of the word to separate its parts). Database designers are about equally divided between those who like IntraCaps and those who hate them.

2. a.

SubjectID	KitNumber	AdminDate	AdminTime	SzStopPreHosp	SzStopPreHospTime	HospArrTime	HospArrSzAct	HospArrGCSV
189	A322	3/12/1994	17:39	FALSE		17:48	TRUE	
410	B536	12/1/1998	01:35	TRUE	01:39	01:53	FALSE	4

b.

Field Name	Data Type	Description	Validation Rule
SubjectID	Integer	Unique subject identifier	
KitNumber	Text(5)	5-character Investigational Pharmacy Code	
AdminDate	Date	Date study drug administered	
AdminTime	Time	Time study drug administered	
SzStopPreHosp	Yes/no	Did seizure stop during prehospital course?	
SzStopPreHospTime	Time	Time seizures stopped during prehospital course (blank if seizure did not stop)	
HospArrTime	Time	Hospital arrival time	
HospArrSzAct	Yes/no	Was there continued seizure activity on hospital arrival?	Check against SzStopPreHosp
HospArrGCSV	Integer	Verbal GCS on hospital arrival (blank if seizure continued)	Between 1 and 5

c. **Advantages of an on-screen form:**
   - No need for transcription from paper forms into the computer data tables
   - Immediate feedback on invalid entries
   - Programmed skip logic (if seizure stopped during prehospital course, computer form prompts for time seizure stopped, otherwise this field is disabled and skipped)
   - Can be made available via a web-browser at multiple sites simultaneously

   Disadvantages of an on-screen form:
   - Hardware requirement—a computer workstation
   - Some user training required

   Advantages of a paper form:
   - Ease and speed of use
   - Portability
   - Ability to enter unanticipated information or unstructured data (notes in the margin, responses that were not otherwise considered, etc.)

- Hardware requirement—a pen
- User training received by all data entry personnel in elementary school

Disadvantages of a paper form:

- Requires subsequent transcription into the computer database
- No interactive feedback or automated skip logic
- Data viewing and entry limited to one person in one place

Although data entry via on-screen data collection forms has many advantages and we recommend it for most research studies, in this study it is impractical. The simplest, fastest, and most user-friendly way to capture data on a nonvolatile medium is still to use a pen and paper.

d. When coded with 0 for *no* or *absent* and 1 for *yes* or *present*, the average value of a dichotomous (yes/no) variable is interpretable as the proportion with the attribute. Of those randomized to lorazepam, 40.9% (27 of 66) were still seizing on hospital arrival; of those randomized to diazepam, 57.4% (39 of 68) were still seizing; and of those randomized to placebo, 78.9% (56 of 71) were still seizing.

CHAPTER 17

1. a. Not enough! But here are some steps he can take:
   - Identify all missing and outlying values and recheck the paper forms to make sure that the data were entered correctly.
   - Retrieve missing data from charts.
   - Collect missing interview data from surviving patients (but this will not help for those who died or for those whose responses might have changed over time).
   - Make a special effort to find subjects who had been lost to follow-up, and at least get a telephone interview with them.
   - Obtain vital status, using the National Death Index or a firm that finds people.
   b. • Collect less data.
   - Check forms on site immediately after collecting the data to be certain that all items are complete and accurate.
     — Use interactive data entry with built-in checks for missing and out-of-range values.
     — Review this shortly after data collection so that missing data can be collected before the patient leaves the hospital (or dies).
   - Periodically tabulate the distributions of values for all items during the course of the study to identify missing values and potential errors.
   - Hold periodic team meetings to review progress.

CHAPTER 18

1. a. The G.I. clinic
   - *Advantages:* This is likely to be a convenient and accessible source of patients. The clinic staff probably has experience participating in research. Implementing a standard battery of diagnostic tests for patients with abdominal pain should not be difficult.

- *Disadvantages:* Patients in this clinic might be a highly selected subset of all patients presenting with abdominal pain. Your results may therefore have limited generalizability.
  b. Community clinics
    - *Advantages:* Here you can identify patients at first presentation without the selection and delay caused by the referral process. Community physicians may benefit from the opportunity to participate in research.
    - *Disadvantages:* These are mainly logistic. Identifying participating physicians and patients and implementing a standard research protocol will be a major organizational task, and quality control will be a challenge.

2. a. This can only be answered with local data. Research elsewhere will not help you.
   b. This is well known from the international literature. Repeating such research in China is unlikely to be an efficient use of resources.
   c. For this question, the generalizability of research from elsewhere is likely to be intermediate. Strategies for smoking cessation proven successful in other countries may serve as a basis for strategies to be tried in China, but you cannot be sure they will have the same success in China without local research. Previous studies in populations elsewhere with cultural ties to China, such as recent Chinese immigrants to the United States, may be helpful.

CHAPTER 19

3. The investigator may lose money if the study-wide enrollment of participants is finished before he can enroll enough participants to cover his costs. More importantly, he might have a very limited role in the analysis and reporting of the results by the company, which might be influenced by their incentive to market a successful product. The investigator should insure that he has the right to obtain and analyze the data from the trial. The potential for bias would be reduced if a steering committee of academic scientists oversees the analysis and publications, and the investigator should aspire to be a part of such a group.

SUBJECT INDEX

Note: Page numbers followed by *f* indicate figures; those followed by *t* indicate tables.